European Observatory on Health Systems and Policies Series

The European Observatory on Health Systems and Policies is an international project that builds on the commitment of all its partners to improving health care systems:

- World Health Organization Regional Office for Europe
- Government of Belgium
- Government of Finland
- Government of Greece
- Government of Norway
- Government of Spain
- Government of Sweden
- European Investment Bank
- Open Society Institute
- World Bank
- London School of Economics and Political Science
- London School of Hygiene & Tropical Medicine

Series Editors

Josep Figueras is Head of the Secretariat and Research Director of the European Observatory on Health Systems and Policies and Head of the European Centre for Health Policy, World Health Organization Regional Office for Europe.

Martin McKee is Research Director of the European Observatory on Health Systems and Policies and Professor of European Public Health at the London School of Hygiene & Tropical Medicine as well as a co-director of the School's European Centre on Health of Societies in Transition.

Elias Mossialos is Research Director of the European Observatory on Health Systems and Policies, Brian Abel-Smith Professor of Health Policy, Department of Social Policy, London School of Economics and Political Science and Co-Director of LSE Health and Social Care.

Richard B. Saltman is Research Director of the European Observatory on Health Systems and Policies and Professor of Health Policy and Management at the Rollins School of Public Health, Emory University in Atlanta, Georgia.

The series

The volumes in this series focus on key issues for health policy making in Europe. Each study explores the conceptual background, outcomes and lessons learned about the development of more equitable, more efficient and more effective health systems in Europe. With this focus, the series seeks to contribute to the evolution of a more evidence-based approach to policy formulation in the health sector.

These studies will be important to all those involved in formulating or evaluating national health care policies and, in particular, will be of use to health policy makers and advisers, who are under increasing pressure to rationalize the structure and funding of their health systems. Academics and students in the field of health policy will also find this series valuable in seeking to understand better the complex choices that confront the health systems of Europe.

The Observatory supports and promotes evidence-based health policy-making through comprehensive and rigorous analysis of the dynamics of health care systems in Europe.

European Observatory on Health Systems and Policies Series

Series Editors: Josep Figueras, Martin McKee, Elias Mossialos and Richard B. Saltman

Published titles

Funding health care: options for Europe
Elias Mossialos, Anna Dixon, Josep Figueras, Joe Kutzin (eds)

Health care in central Asia
Martin McKee, Judith Healy and Jane Falkingham (eds)

Health policy and European Union enlargement
Martin McKee, Laura MacLehose and Ellen Nolte (eds)

Hospitals in a changing Europe
Martin McKee and Judith Healy (eds)

Regulating entrepreneurial behaviour in European health care systems
Richard B. Saltman, Reinhard Busse and Elias Mossialos (eds)

Regulating pharmaceuticals in Europe: striving for efficiency, equity and quality
Elias Mossialos, Monique Mrazek and Tom Walley (eds)

Forthcoming titles

Effective purchasing for health gain
Josep Figueras, Ray Robinson and Elke Jakubowski (eds)

Mental Health Policy and Practice across Europe
Martin Knapp, David McDaid, Elias Mossialos and Graham Thornicroft (eds)

Social health insurance systems in western Europe
Richard B. Saltman, Reinhard Busse and Josep Figueras (eds)

European Observatory on Health Systems and Policies Series

Edited by Josep Figueras, Martin McKee, Elias Mossialos and Richard B. Saltman

Regulating pharmaceuticals in Europe: striving for efficiency, equity and quality

Edited by

Elias Mossialos

Monique Mrazek

Tom Walley

Open University Press

Open University Press
McGraw-Hill Education
McGraw-Hill House
Shoppenhangers Road
Maidenhead
Berkshire
England
SL6 2QL

email: enquiries@openup.co.uk
world wide web: www.openup.co.uk

and Two Penn Plaza, New York, NY101-2-2289
USA

First published 2004
Reprinted 2004

A catalogue record of this book is available from the British Library

ISBN 0 335 21465 7(pb)   0 335 21466 5 (hb)

Library of Congress Cataloging-in-Publication Data
CIP data applied for

Typeset by RefineCatch Limited, Bungay, Suffolk
Printed in Great Britain by MPG Books Ltd, Bodmin, Cornwall

Contents

List of boxes, figures and tables

List of contributors

Julia Abelson is Assistant Professor in the Department of Clinical Epidemiology and Biostatistics at McMaster University, Hamilton, Ontario.

Christa Altenstetter is Professor of Political Science at the Graduate School of the City University of New York (CUNY), and Queens College of CUNY.

Vittorio Bertele' is Head of the Regulatory Policies Laboratory at the 'Mario Negri' Institute for Pharmacological Research, Milan.

Christine Bond is Professor of Primary Care (Pharmacy) at the Department of General Practice and Primary Care, University of Aberdeen, and Consultant in Pharmaceutical Public Health, NHS Grampian.

Marcel L. Bouvy is a Community Pharmacist at the Academic Pharmacy Stevenshof and a researcher at both the SIR Institute for Pharmacy Practice Research, Leiden and the Department of Pharmacoepidemiology and Pharmaco-therapy, Utrecht University.

Colin Bradley is Professor of General Practice at University College Cork, and is Chief Editor of the *European Journal of General Practice*.

Steve Chapman is Professor of Prescribing Studies and Head of Department at the Department of Medicines Management, Keele University.

Anna Dixon is Lecturer in European Health Policy at the Department of Social Policy, The London School of Economics and Political Science.

Michael Drummond is Professor of Health Economics and Director of the Centre for Health Economics at the University of York.

Pierre Durieux is Associate Professor of Public Health at University Paris V and Hôpital Européen Georges Pompidou, Paris.

Edzard Ernst is Professor of Complementary Medicine at the Peninsula Medical School, Universities of Exeter and Plymouth.

Armin Fidler is the Health Sector Manager for Europe and Central Asia at the World Bank, and adjunct faculty at the George Washington University School of Public Health, Washington, DC.

Eric Fortess is Associate Professor of Health Administration at the Department of Public Management, Sawyer School of Management, Suffolk University.

Richard Frank is Margaret T. Morris Professor of Health Economics at Harvard Medical School, Boston, MA, and a Research Associate with the National Bureau of Economic Research, Cambridge, MA.

Silvio Garattini is Director of the 'Mario Negri' Institute for Pharmacological Research, Milan.

Leigh Hancher is Professor of European Law at the University of Tilburg, and Of Counsel at Allen & Overy, Amsterdam.

Ebba Holme Hansen is Professor of Social Pharmacy at the Danish University of Pharmaceutical Sciences and Director of the Research Centre for Quality in Medicine Use.

Steve Hudson is Boots Professor of Pharmaceutical Care, Department of Pharmaceutical Sciences at the Strathclyde Institute for Biomedical Sciences, University of Strathclyde.

Kees de Jonchere is Regional Adviser for Health Technology and Pharmaceuticals at the WHO Regional Office for Europe, Copenhagen.

Panos Kanavos is Lecturer in International Health Policy at the Department of Social Policy, The London School of Economics and Political Science.

Sjoerd Kooiker is Senior Researcher at the Social and Cultural Planning Office, The Hague.

Jean-Marc Leder is a Community Pharmacist in Paris and an expert in tobacco cessation.

Graham Lewis is Research Fellow at the Science and Technology Studies Unit (SATSU), Department of Sociology, University of York.

Donald W. Light is Professor of Comparative Health Care Systems at the University of Medicine and Dentistry of New Jersey, and a Senior Fellow at the Center for Bioethics at the University of Pennsylvania.

Alistair McGuire is Professor of Health Economics at LSE Health and Social Care, The London School of Economics and Political Science.

Elias Mossialos is Brian Abel-Smith Professor of Health Policy at the Department of Social Policy, The London School of Economics and Political Science, and a Research Director of the European Observatory on Health Systems and Policies.

Monique Mrazek is a Health Economist at the World Bank (Europe and Central Asia region). She was Research Officer in Health Economics at the European Observatory on Health Systems and Policies during the writing of this book.

Maria Pia Orru' is a Community Pharmacist in Cagliari, Italy.

Govin Permanand is Research Officer in Health and Pharmaceutical Policy at LSE Health and Social Care, The London School of Economics and Political Science.

Guenka Petrova is Associate Professor of Social Pharmacy and Pharmacoeconomics at the Faculty of Pharmacy, Medical University in Sofia.

Munir Pirmohamed is Professor of Clinical Pharmacology at the University of Liverpool, and a Consultant Physician at the Royal Liverpool and Broadgreen University Hospital, Liverpool.

Dennis Ross-Degnan is Associate Professor and Director of Research at the Department of Ambulatory Care and Prevention, Harvard Medical School and Harvard Pilgrim Health Care, Boston, MA.

Frans Rutten is Professor of Health Economics and Chair of the Institute for Health Policy and Management at Erasmus University Medical Centre, Rotterdam.

Steven Soumerai is Professor of Ambulatory Care and Prevention, and Director of Drug Policy Research at Harvard Medical School and Harvard Pilgrim Health Care, Boston, MA.

David Taylor is Professor of Pharmaceutical and Public Health Policy at the School of Pharmacy, University of London, and Chairman of the Camden and Islington NHS Mental Health and Social Care Trust.

Sarah Thomson is Research Officer in Health Policy at LSE Health and Social Care, The London School of Economics and Political Science, and Research Officer at the European Observatory on Health Systems and Policies.

Tom Walley is Professor of Clinical Pharmacology at the University of Liverpool, and Director of the UK National Health Technology Assessment Programme.

Series editors' introduction

European national policy makers broadly agree on the core objectives that their health care systems should pursue. The list is strikingly straightforward: universal access for all citizens, effective care for better health outcomes, efficient use of resources, high-quality services and responsiveness to patient concerns. It is a formula that resonates across the political spectrum and which, in various, sometimes inventive configurations, has played a role in most recent European national election campaigns.

Yet this clear consensus can only be observed at the abstract policy level. Once decision makers seek to translate their objectives into the nuts and bolts of health system organization, common principles rapidly devolve into divergent, occasionally contradictory, approaches. This is, of course, not a new phenomenon in the health sector. Different nations, with different histories, cultures and political experiences, have long since constructed quite different institutional arrangements for funding and delivering health care services.

The diversity of health system configurations that has developed in response to broadly common objectives leads quite naturally to questions about the advantages and disadvantages inherent in different arrangements, and which approach is 'better' or even 'best' given a particular context and set of policy priorities. These concerns have intensified over the last decade as policy makers have sought to improve health system performance through what has become a European-wide wave of health system reforms. The search for comparative advantage has triggered – in health policy as in clinical medicine – increased attention to its knowledge base, and to the possibility of overcoming at least part of existing institutional divergence through more evidence-based health policy making.

The volumes published in the European Observatory series are intended to provide precisely this kind of cross-national health policy analysis. Drawing on an extensive network of experts and policy makers working in a variety of academic and administrative capacities, these studies seek to synthesize the available evidence on key health sector topics using a systematic methodology. Each volume explores the conceptual background, outcomes and lessons learned about the development of more equitable, more efficient and more effective health care systems in Europe. With this focus, the series seeks to contribute to the evolution of a more evidence-based approach to policy formulation in the health sector. While remaining sensitive to cultural, social and normative differences among countries, the studies explore a range of policy alternatives available for future decision making. By examining closely both the advantages and disadvantages of different policy approaches, these volumes fulfil a central mandates of the Observatory: to serve as a bridge between pure academic research and the needs of policy makers, and to stimulate the development of strategic responses suited to the real political world in which health sector reform must be implemented.

The European Observatory on Health Systems and Policies is a partnership that brings together three international agencies, six national governments, two research institutions and an international non-governmental organization. The partners are as follows: the World Health Organization Regional Office for Europe, which provides the Observatory secretariat; the governments of Belgium, Finland, Greece, Norway, Spain and Sweden; the European Investment Bank; the Open Society Institute; the World Bank; the London School of Hygiene & Tropical Medicine and the London School of Economics and Political Science.

In addition to the analytical and cross-national comparative studies published in this Open University Press series, the Observatory produces Health Care Systems in Transition (HiTs) profiles for the countries of Europe, the journal *Eurohealth* and the newsletter *Euro Observer*. Further information about Observatory publications and activities can be found on its website *www.observatory.dk*.

Josep Figueras, Martin McKee, Elias Mossialos and Richard B. Saltman

Foreword

Pharmaceuticals are a crucial component of delivering health care. Regulating pharmaceutical markets is a complex issue that involves the dynamic interplay of multiple actors and not just the physician who prescribes: pharmacists have an active role not only in dispensing but also in the selection of multi-sourced products and in product procurement. Moreover, today, patients are more informed about their own health and in some cases have been given financial incentives to make them more aware of their pharmaceutical consumption. The media as information providers on health and health care play an increasingly important role in shaping patients' expectations. Wholesalers can have an impact on the final retail price, while the pharmaceutical industry itself has an important role not only in terms of product development and pricing, but can also influence levels of drug utilization as a result of marketing and information dissemination. Certainly, the role and objectives of governments and insurance funds in setting regulation are complex and diverse. Internationalization and global trends have a growing influence on the provision of pharmaceuticals as well.

This volume sets out the approaches used by governments and regulators to manage pharmaceutical policy and spending across Europe, with the aim of highlighting how various policies impact on strategic objectives such as efficiency, quality, equity and cost control.

The book is a welcome addition to the body of literature already published on pharmaceutical policy and regulation. It attempts to consider the perspectives and regulatory influences on all the actors involved in the market for pharmaceuticals. Its specific contribution is that it offers a comprehensive analysis of all aspects of pharmaceutical regulation within the European context, and combines theoretical outlooks with the most current empirical evidence available.

Regulating Pharmaceuticals in Europe will provide policy makers and industry practitioners with a critical analysis of the broad range of issues impacting on the regulation of the pharmaceutical sector in Europe from a number of stakeholder perspectives. The evidence presented here will undoubtedly contribute to a greater transparency and understanding of the processes involved in regulating a complex sector, whose impact on the health of populations and on health care systems cannot be underestimated.

Marc Danzon
WHO Regional Director for Europe

Preface

All governments face pharmaceutical expenditures, which, in many countries, are rising at rates greater than gross domestic product and usually greater than other health care budgets. Many countries consider this to be a problem and make attempts to contain these expenditures. But governments have other responsibilities – to improve the quality of care their health service offers by meeting patient need, and to ensure equity in the services provided. They try to stretch limited budgets as far as possible by increasing the efficiency of their services. Some of these policies may be conflicting – for instance, increasing universal access to services and improving the quality of those services will increase costs but may increase efficiency.

The primary objective of this book is to examine comprehensively the approaches used to manage pharmaceutical expenditure through various actors across Europe and what impact these strategies have had on the efficiency, quality, equity and cost of pharmaceutical care. By efficiency, here we refer to technical efficiency defined by the best use of resources within a budget-constrained service. Allocative efficiency, which encompasses both health policy and industrial policy objectives, is broader and considers the overall costs and benefits arising from a pharmaceutical industry providing employment and export earnings as well as providing essential tools for prescribers. We do not address this wider meaning here, but acknowledge it as important. Claims by the pharmaceutical industry that attempts to constrain their profits will stifle expenditure and risk losing all of the wider social benefits should be treated with some caution. Within this context, it is part of the role of government to balance industrial and health policy.

Current market interventions affect pharmaceutical expenditure by targeting price, volume or both. These interventions affect either – or both – supply and demand. Supply-side measures either act directly on price or act indirectly to regulate pharmaceutical prices. These measures also indirectly affect volume. Demand-side measures include financial incentives or non-financial incentives targeting physicians, pharmacists and/or patients to control volumes directly and indirectly. However, this framework does not describe how these attempts to regulate actually affect efficiency, quality, equity and cost. The pursuit of efficiency requires not only the economic evaluation of competing pharmaceuticals to determine cost-effectiveness, but also the creation of incentives to ensure that doctors and pharmacists, in particular, translate clinical evidence into practice. Policy makers have to rank policy goals and recognize the trade-offs involved and the importance of context in translating evidence to practice.

This book addresses broad perspectives, encompassing the institutional, political and supranational; it describes, analyses and compares the successes and failures of specific initiatives to regulate the pharmaceutical market in Europe. Chapters 2–4 tackle specific topics related to political, legal and public health aspects of pharmaceutical regulation at national and European Union level. Ways to measure and monitor policy outcomes in the pharmaceutical sector are examined in Chapter 5. Chapters 6–13 tackle specific topics relating to supply- and demand-side measures (i.e. regulating pharmaceutical prices, reimbursement of pharmaceuticals, good prescribing practice, patients and their medicines, financial incentives for prescribing, regulating distribution and retail pharmacy, the role of hospital pharmacies, and the impact of cost sharing). Chapters 14–18 explore how regulations may vary in different segments of the pharmaceutical market for off-patent and over-the-counter drugs and the current and future implications of lifestyle drugs, biotechnology and alternative medicines.

Although the focus of this book is predominantly on policies in Western Europe, in Chapters 19 and 20 we examine the regulation of pharmaceutical markets in other countries with a very different historical and cultural background, specifically the Central and Eastern European countries and the Commonwealth of Independent States. These markets are not described well elsewhere in the literature, and we hope this adds an extra perspective for the reader. Finally, Chapter 21 examines important ethical issues related to approaches to managing pharmaceutical markets.

Regulating the pharmaceutical sector involves complex decision-making frameworks and policies. We hope this book has comprehensively outlined the important issues and that it will contribute to policy debates about improving efficiency, quality and equity in pharmaceutical care.

Elias Mossialos, Monique Mrazek and Tom Walley

Acknowledgements

This volume is part of a series of books undertaken by the European Observatory on Health Systems and Policies. We are very grateful to our authors, who responded promptly both in producing and later amending their chapters in light of several ongoing discussions.

We particularly appreciate the detailed and very constructive comments of our reviewers, Professor Jerry Avorn (Harvard Medical School), the late Professor Bernie O'Brien (McMaster University) and Dr Peter Clappison (Department of Health for England). We should also like to thank Dr Juan Rovira and Jai Shah for comments on particular chapters as well as Reinhard Busse and Alistair McGuire for their review of Chapter 1. Renee Hsia and Sherry Merkur provided much valued research assistance. We would also like to thank Anna Maresso, who edited successive versions of chapters and finalized the manuscript, and Jeffrey V. Lazarus, who was responsible for the book's delivery process and production.

Monique Mrazek would like to thank the Canadian Health Services Research Foundation for the research sponsorship that contributed to her work on Chapters 6, 11 and 14. Moreover, the Observatory is especially grateful to the Health Technology and Pharmaceuticals Unit, World Health Organization Regional Office for Europe, which provided the financial support for the authors' workshop that took place in London on 14–15 February 2003 to discuss earlier drafts of chapters. In addition to all the authors who provided detailed feedback on each other's chapters, special thanks are extended to all the other workshop participants, especially Jan Bultman, René Christensen, Elin Michelsen and Richard B. Saltman for useful comments.

Finally, while this book has benefited enormously from the contributions of numerous collaborators, responsibility for any errors remains with the editors.

chapter one

Regulating pharmaceuticals in Europe: an overview

Elias Mossialos, Tom Walley and Monique Mrazek

Introduction

Governments try to regulate few markets as much as they do the pharmaceutical market. They have to balance contrasting objectives. First, governments must secure health policy objectives: protecting public health; guaranteeing patient access to safe and effective medicines; improving the quality of care; and ensuring that pharmaceutical expenditure does not become excessive so as to undermine these and other government objectives. Equity and efficiency (i.e. making best use of limited resources to increase population health) and meeting patient need are, therefore, perhaps the prime objectives. Health economists might equate efficiency with quality: doctors and patients would define quality as treating the patient appropriately – that is, what the patient needs for their condition and with only limited, if any, consideration of cost or cost-effectiveness. One of the roles of government in pharmaceutical policy is to provide the funding and framework that allows that quality of care.

Cost containment is thus not a main health policy objective in itself but is one of the few tools that governments employ in their attempts to manage pharmaceuticals and to achieve a balance between conflicting demands. Governments, therefore, have often seemed to concentrate on this as a regulatory measure, especially targeting the supply side of the market, namely the pharmaceutical industry; demand-side instruments are now also increasingly used. The success of these policies is varied and in many countries pharmaceutical expenditure nevertheless continues to rise. The impact of these cost-containment policies on efficiency and quality of care and prescribing is also often unclear. Governments may seek ideas for solutions from the experience of other countries, bearing in mind the different contexts in which they work.

There are also concerns about future developments, for example the impact of new technologies (such as the developments in pharmacogenetics) and, of course, the impact of demographic shifts in ageing populations.

Governments must also balance health policy objectives against those of industrial policy – that is, encouraging drug research and development, continued employment in the pharmaceutical sector, and a positive balance of trade with regard to drug exports. Governments must not, however, accept uncritically the claims from the industry that any constraint on profits will threaten truly valuable innovation. However, new drug developments that lead to improvements in health outcomes are valuable to society and truly innovative drugs should be appropriately rewarded.

In Europe, a variety of controls and incentives is used in different countries to try to balance effective and efficient spending on drugs against the need to promote a major industry. Regulating pharmaceutical markets is complex and involves a dynamic interplay between government and multiple actors, and not just the prescribing physician. Pharmacists have an active role not only in dispensing but also in selecting multi-sourced products and in product procurement. Wholesalers can affect the final retail price. The pharmaceutical industry itself has an extremely important influence not only on product development and pricing, but also on levels of drug utilization as a result of marketing and information dissemination. Finally, patients today are more informed about their own health and treatments and, in some countries, have been given financial incentives to make them more aware of their pharmaceutical consumption. All of these factors must be taken into account when trying to regulate pharmaceutical expenditures.

Many of these trade-offs, market structures and regulations do not exist for any other industrial sector. The pharmaceutical market is unique with regard to the extent and depth of its failure to meet the criteria for a perfect market (Abel-Smith and Grandjeat 1978; Jacobzone 2000; Dukes *et al.* 2003). There are market imperfections in both supply (generally related to patent protection, the process and length of regulatory approval and brand loyalty) and demand sides (there is a four-tiered structure of demand where the physician prescribes, the pharmacist dispenses, the patient consumes and a third party pays). Other fundamental characteristics of pharmaceutical and health care markets that make them less ideal for allocation solely by market mechanisms include the existence of indivisibilities and externalities.

These issues are discussed in individual chapters throughout this book. In this chapter, we provide an overview of the policies and the systems by which countries try to address efficiency, equity and quality. It is difficult to assess which of the different approaches has been the most effective: they are rarely applied singly, and it is often impossible to disentangle the influence of each in an overall effect. Many of the effects observed may be context specific, and may not indicate a universal truth as to which policies are the most likely to bring about a change. Even where interventions have been studied individually, the quality of the evidence may be weak: this will be considered for each approach in turn.

Trends in pharmaceutical expenditure in the EU member states

Although most health care in European Union (EU) member states is publicly funded, this is not universally the case in the pharmaceutical sector, where levels of private expenditure are often high (see Table 1.1). Pharmaceutical expenditure is predominantly private in Belgium, Denmark and, until recently, Italy (OECD 2002). Between 1980 and 2000, the public share of total expenditure on pharmaceuticals declined in nine of 14 EU member states for which data exist, largely because of attempts to contain health care costs (Mossialos and Le Grand 1999). The decline was small in Sweden, the Netherlands, Portugal and the UK, but substantial in Italy and Belgium. Conversely, some countries saw an increase in the share of public expenditure on pharmaceuticals – significant in Ireland, more modest in France and Spain. Countries with low total pharmaceutical expenditure as a percentage of gross domestic product (GDP) include Ireland, Luxembourg and Denmark, while those with high pharmaceutical expenditures in terms of GDP as well as percentage of total health expenditures include Italy, Portugal, France, Spain and Greece.[1]

Between 1995 and 2000, most countries increased their total pharmaceutical spending as a percentage of total health expenditure; the exceptions were Belgium, Ireland and Luxembourg (Table 1.1). Between 1990 and 2000 the unweighted average of per capita pharmaceutical expenditure (in US$ PPPs) in the EU member states (excluding Austria) increased by 79.9 per cent, prompting much greater attention to drug expenditures during the 1990s.

Most data on pharmaceutical spending, however, do not distinguish between different types of private expenditure. As a result, it is difficult to determine how much private expenditure arises from direct payments, such as spending on over-the-counter (OTC) products or prescribed products that are not reimbursed by the statutory health care system, and how much arises from user charges (i.e. co-payments for reimbursed products). Although OTC drugs are usually relatively inexpensive and are consumed by a large proportion of the population, the distributional impact of OTC drug expenditure on different population groups/patients is not easy to measure.

Additional methodological problems exist when performing cross-country comparisons of pharmaceutical expenditure and prices; biases include exchange rate fluctuations, differences in pharmaceutical prices between countries, and variations in private (out-of-pocket) and public coverage. To eliminate price level differences in inter-country comparisons, conversions using purchasing power parities (PPPs) equalize currencies to allow the purchase of the same basket of goods and services in different countries. Still, difficulties remain not only because pharmaceutical prices have weakly comparable volume indices, but also because figures for PPPs may be outdated. In addition, there are challenges in separating out factors that influence drug prices caused by the structure of the market in each country: different health system structures and financing, divergent regulatory and pricing policies, drug subsidies, production costs and product mix variations. Furthermore, consideration must be given to where price information is taken from within the distribution chain, as wholesale and retail prices are marked-up from the manufacturer's price – ideally, it should

Table 1.1 Pharmaceutical expenditure in EU member states (1980–2000*)

	Total expenditure on pharmaceuticals (% GDP)					Total expenditure on pharmaceuticals (% of total health expenditure)					Public expenditure on pharmaceuticals (% of total pharmaceutical expenditure)					Total per capita expenditure on pharmaceuticals (US$ PPPs)				
	1980	1985	1990	1995	2000*	1980	1985	1990	1995	2000*	1980	1985	1990	1995	2000*	1980	1985	1990	1995	2000*
Austria[e]	—	—	—	1.4	1.1[a]	—	—	13.2	10.4	14.1[a]	—	—	—	—	65.4[a]	—	—	—	—	270[a]
Belgium	1.1	1.1	1.1	1.4	1.4[c]	17.4	15.7	15.5	16.3	16.3[c]	57.3	51.0	46.8	43.0	44.7[c]	100	139	193	309	328[c]
Denmark	0.6	0.6	0.6	0.7	0.8	6.0	6.6	7.5	9.1	9.2	49.9	45.5	34.2	48.6	46.1	50	77	109	171	223
Finland	0.7	0.7	0.7	1.1	1.0	10.7	9.7	9.4	14.0	15.5	46.7	44.5	47.4	45.3	50.1	54	82	122	199	259
France	—	—	1.4	1.7	1.9	—	—	16.8	17.5	20.1	—	—	61.9	61.4	65.1	—	—	254	346	473
Germany	1.2	1.3	1.2	1.3	1.3[b]	13.4	13.8	14.3	12.3	12.7[b]	73.7	71.9	73.1	72.3	69.2[b]	110	172	228	269	312[b]
Greece	1.2	1.1	1.1	1.5	1.5	18.8	—	14.5	17.3	18.4	60.0	—	70.3	70.0	61.6	65	83	104	195	258
Ireland	0.9	0.8	0.7	0.7	0.6	10.9	9.9	11.3	9.7	9.6	52.7	60.7	65.0	78.3	83.9	50	58	88	126	187
Italy	—	—	1.7	1.5	1.9[d]	—	—	21.2	20.9	23.7[d]	—	—	62.8	38.3	53.3[d]	—	—	280	311	459[d]
Luxembourg	0.9	0.9	0.8	0.8	0.7[a]	14.5	14.7	14.9	12.0	11.7[a]	86.4	86.0	84.6	81.7	80.8[a]	88	132	223	255	307[a]
Netherlands	0.6	0.7	0.8	0.9	1.0	8.0	9.3	9.6	11.0	11.8	66.7	63.3	66.6	88.8	63.7	53	83	128	196	264
Portugal	1.1	1.5	1.5	1.9	2.0[b]	19.9	25.4	24.9	23.2	23.5[b]	68.6	64.7	62.3	63.3	66.1[c]	53	97	152	266	316[b]
Spain	1.1	1.1	1.2	1.4	1.4[c]	21.0	20.3	17.8	17.7	19.0[c]	64.0	62.5	71.7	75.8	78.1[c]	69	93	145	210	246[c]
Sweden	0.6	0.6	0.7	1.0	1.0[c]	6.5	7.0	8.0	12.5	12.8[c]	71.8	70.1	71.7	71.4	71.2[c]	55	82	120	202	227[c]
United Kingdom	0.7	0.8	0.8	1.1	1.1[c]	12.8	14.1	13.5	15.3	15.9[c]	67.6	64.1	66.6	63.5	64.2[c]	57	94	131	201	236[c]

Notes: *Or latest available year. Data from [a]1999, [b]1998, [c]1997, [d]2001. [e]Data for Austria from ÖBIG (Rosian *et al.* 2001).
Source: OECD (2002).

always be taken from the same point in each country, but this is not always possible.

Pharmaceutical regulation, legislation and market authorization

The relationship between the pharmaceutical industry and government is an important determinant of the government approach to managing pharmaceuticals at the national and EU level. Some issues such as aspects of market authorization have been harmonized and are uniform across EU member states. However, other aspects of regulating the pharmaceutical industry vary across Europe according to the balance between pursuing health policy versus industrial policy objectives at national levels. The pricing and reimbursement of pharmaceuticals differs from country to country across the EU: some countries negotiate pharmaceutical prices directly with industry, while others regulate company profits or set maximum reimbursement prices. Other countries have price–volume agreements with companies. Generally, objectives are similar but some countries are more willing to trade-off slightly higher pharmaceutical prices if they see a return from pharmaceutical companies in terms of research and development (R&D), employment and a positive balance of trade. These issues concerning the relationship between government and industry are important as company strategy and market structure are constantly changing.

Pharmaceutical policy making is highly politicized and involves a multiplicity of actors, including doctors, wholesalers, pharmacists, patients and patient advocacy groups, importers and the research-based and generics industries. Because these stakeholders often have competing interests, governments find it difficult to achieve their many objectives in managing pharmaceuticals (Davis 1996, 1997).

Although pharmaceutical policy is primarily determined at the national level by individual EU member states, there is nevertheless a considerable amount of relevant legislation at the EU level. The European Commission (EC) has an expanding role in this area, with the legal duty to advocate and reinforce the principles of European law, including the free movement of goods and undistorted competition. Hence, the EC's executive competence to launch policy initiatives and ultimately propose binding rules has encompassed three areas: (i) national prices, profit, and reimbursement, rational use and advertising; (ii) free movement and competition issues; and (iii) market access through harmonization and eventual centralized authorization procedures through the European Agency for the Evaluation of Medicinal Products (EMEA) (see Chapter 3). Yet interventions in profit and price controls have implications for many national processes and entire distribution chains, which blur the lines between industrial, health and health insurance policies (see Chapter 3). Despite the pharmaceutical industry's recurrent requests for the EC to remove certain forms of national pharmaceutical price regulation, the industry cannot be wholly protected from inter-brand competition from generics following patent expiration and intra-brand competition created by parallel importing from lower priced EU countries.

Inevitable in these attempts to harmonize market authorization and facilitating free movement is the need to address overcapacity in production facilities (Mossialos *et al.* 1994). Because merging fragmented markets will necessarily entail 'winners' and 'losers' (e.g. manufacturing will probably be moved to wherever production is cheapest), many countries have been reluctant to accept or even resistant to price deregulation because of the uncertainty of who will gain and who will lose. This shift may be less relevant for R&D units, but may eventually change these also. Both industrial policy and regulation of the EC's pharmaceutical sector remain shared competencies between the Community and the EU member states. The reasons are well documented in the literature (see Chapters 2 and 3). Briefly, the level at which regulation is attempted depends on whether one adopts an industrial or health policy perspective. Industrial policy is underpinned by wider harmonization powers than health policy, but they both exist concurrently. What should be noted, however, is that despite this potential conflict, the continuing development of European competencies in both fields means that policy is increasingly being decided at the supranational level. The Commission has no power to specify levels of national price controls or profit caps, but rather ensures that national procedures are efficient, transparent and fair. It is also important to note that the Commission is not the sole institution that can enforce the EU Treaty provisions, since parties claiming injuries in member states can insist on adherence to these provisions as well (see Chapter 3).

Parallel importing has been encouraged through European Court of Justice (ECJ) rulings removing divergent national intellectual property rights regarding copyrights, trademarks and patents. Furthermore, unnecessary national licensing regimes that prevent competition from generic products have been confronted through EU Treaty Articles 28EC and 30EC that endorse the free movement of goods. Claims by pharmaceutical companies against other companies based on intellectual property rights have not been well received, and the Court has repeatedly ruled that pharmaceutical companies must respect the rights of free movement (see Chapter 3).

Pricing and reimbursement, as well as incentives for R&D, are generally under national jurisdiction, reflecting the historical framework, the presence of the research-based industry and various other objectives pursued by different countries. National competencies also include, to some extent, market authorization. The challenge of constructing lucid and shared policy objectives becomes complicated, since several national ministries (health, finance and trade) are often involved in the setting of pharmaceutical policy (see Chapter 2).

Market authorization for pharmaceutical products, previously a wholly national procedure, is increasingly the responsibility of the EMEA.[2] The EMEA central approval process operates currently alongside a decentralized process run by the regulatory agencies of member states. EMEA centralized approval for new pharmaceutical products requires acceptance in all EU member states, and is mandatory for all new biotechnology products and orphan drugs (medicines for rare diseases). The centralized process has been reasonably successful and will broaden its scope to include generics. Companies can ask for market authorization of other new products either through the EMEA or through the decentralized or mutual recognition system (MRS). In this, a company can apply in one member state for approval and, when it receives such approval and if there are no specific objections from other countries, may then apply to market the drug in other member states with the expectation of speedy authorization. If a conflict arises between two member states, the EMEA resolves the dispute.

The EMEA is governed by a management board and has technical groups with advisory capacity for the scientific evaluation of medicinal, veterinary and orphan drug products. These groups consist of representatives from each member state and EMEA staff providing technical services. The Committee for Proprietary Medicinal Products (CPMP) provides scientific advice to help industry meet the guidelines for specific therapeutic areas, evaluates the dossiers to reach an opinion, handles appeals by pharmaceutical companies, and monitors a new medicine for safety.

There have been concerns, however, that the review process is inadequate. One weakness is the lack of evaluation of the comparative therapeutic value of new medicines, which instead is still often based on efficacy compared only to a placebo rather than on head-to-head trials against the existing practice or best current treatment. As a result, many drugs are approved that may not have much added clinical benefit, despite their often higher prices. Because of this lack of adequate comparative data, reliable comparative cost-effectiveness data cannot be generated, and medicines coming to the European market often cannot be adequately reviewed on economic grounds (although this is not a role of the EMEA). A review of 12 anticancer drugs approved by EMEA between 1995 and 2000 showed that these drugs were evaluated in small phase II trials only to demonstrate equivalence or non-inferiority to reference drugs (Garattini and Bertele' 2002). Endpoints in these evaluations were also short-term and subjective. As a result of the weak criteria needed for authorization, some of these approved drugs are not likely to meet the expectations of patients who believe that these new drugs signify substantial improvements in treatments (Garattini and Bertele' 2002).

There are a number of concerns regarding the operation of the EMEA (see Chapter 4). First, the EMEA is regulated by the EC Directorate-General of Enterprise; were it under the jurisdiction of the Directorate-General for Health and Consumer Protection, its objectives would perhaps be more aligned with the interests of patients and less with the interests of the pharmaceutical industry. Second, the financing of the EMEA is primarily through fees from the industry for market authorization. Yet because companies can also go through the decentralized (national) procedure, competition for funds exists between the EMEA, which operates the centralized procedure, and national licensing agencies, which operate the decentralized procedure. Ideally, the decentralized process should become obsolete. Any direct financial dependency of the EMEA on the industry should be avoided and the EU should fund the agency directly, with the industry paying fees to the EU. In addition to these uncomfortably intimate links between the EMEA and industry, the European Commission has recently suggested that the management board of EMEA should include representatives from the pharmaceutical industry. This would produce an inevitable conflict of interest. Similarly, some members of the CPMP also have mixed relationships: some members advise industry about medicines, but also have responsibilities for securing approval or dealing with appeals.

It has been argued that the EMEA should be able to perform (or contract out) independent research to verify the findings reported by the industry. Currently, unlike the Food and Drugs Administration (FDA) in the USA, the EMEA does not have internal staff capable of performing evaluations of submitted products. Instead, the EMEA asks national agencies to act as rapporteurs, to evaluate the medicine and report back to the EMEA. It is argued that companies also can nominate a national agency as a rapporteur to the CPMP, which may lead them to choose those more likely to give their product a favourable report (Garattini and Bertele' 2001). While efforts are being made to improve the infrastructure of the EMEA, with more staff for information technology and to create functional clinical trials and pharmacovigilance databases, there has been little discussion of the need for the scientific support (especially in terms of human resources, such as hiring epidemiologists or those in other scientifically based disciplines) to complement this.

With respect to transparency, Garattini and Bertele' (Chapter 4) argue that there is a need to disseminate information on both positive and especially negative application outcomes. New products should undergo a comparative assessment to demonstrate increased efficacy, safety and quality with existing therapies. These independent reviews and summaries of product characteristics should also compare the new product with current medicines on the market instead of discussing each product in isolation. Additionally, the renewal of application in the future could require the submission of an updated risk–benefit profile instead of simply administrative renewal on a 5-year basis. This has also been proposed elsewhere (Ray *et al.* 1993) and is currently a major gap in the licensing system. Finally, more interaction among the EMEA, companies and patient groups, and clinical pharmacologists on a national level might be beneficial for pharmacovigilance and post-market surveillance.

Measuring, monitoring and evaluating pharmaceutical policies

The intended effects of pharmaceutical policy include improved access to cost-effective medicines, minimization of health risks, reduced drug overutilization and containment of expenditure growth. If access to medicines is inhibited, however, unplanned effects can occur, including worsened health status and increased utilization of other health care services. Despite the abundance of cost-containment policies, there have been few rigorous investigations in Europe to analyse the economic and health impact of these strategies. This is because many important measurement and methodological issues emerge during these studies of the impact of pharmaceutical policy.

To measure and monitor any aspect of pharmaceutical policy, dependable and legitimate data on processes and outcomes must be collected and evaluated. Monitoring alone will not explain the trend in drug expenditures, nor will it determine whether the level of spending is suitable to meet reasonable goals in health outcomes. The focus of analysis must be on drug consumption driven by patient need, prescribing choice, dispensing practices and price. It is important to know whether data include both inpatient and outpatient consumption and over-the-counter medications.

Monitoring pharmaceutical expenditure over time is useful when observations are considered in terms of the target of the policy and the population characteristic, specifically the proportion of elderly and chronically ill that can drive up pharmaceutical costs. In addition, many factors influence pharmaceutical consumption beyond obvious policy interventions, such as changing demographics, therapeutic advances, marketing campaigns, seasonal effects, changes in eligibility for insurance and the habits of health practitioners. These non-interventional factors can undermine the internal validity of the investigation.

The correct unit of analysis must be selected for investigation. The patient is often not appropriate as the unit of analysis, since prescribing practices depend on the behaviour of the physician or health care facility (Divine *et al.* 1992). Moreover, since multiple providers often care for individual patients, research in the clinical setting is complicated by contamination problems of changing patient–prescriber pairs and the influence of informal communication between providers. Ideally, one would conduct randomized controlled trials or well-controlled quasi-experiments (e.g. interrupted time-series with comparison series data) to identify the efficiency and effectiveness of drug programmes before they are formally introduced, but these arc rarely feasible: equity and legal considerations emerge if sick people are deprived of effective treatments to allow them to form the control group, and control groups may be contaminated within a single institution (Soumerai *et al.* 1998).

A further methodological problem is how to detect whether changes in prescribing affect patient outcomes. Studies may not be constructed with appropriate sensitivity to measure the correct clinical outcomes and may not be long enough to detect changes in clinical patient outcomes. Furthermore, low patient adherence to the therapy recommended or losing patients to follow-up may compromise the study. Given these problems, the number of patients needed for statistically significant results may be enormous and thus impractical.

Observations should be made before and after the intervention. In theory, changes in policy cause a period of instability as providers and patients modify their behaviour to the new environment. They may discover how to evade reimbursement controls over time; thus, long-term stability and resilience to change must be examined in drug utilization. However, at this stage, most European studies focusing on administrative measures introduced to control expenditure are observational or at best quasi-experimental. This is because there is a lack of systematic collection of data and government reluctance to support policy-relevant research.

Goodhart's law of government policy indicators predicts that when policy performance is being evaluated, individuals and institutions will dedicate a disproportionate amount of time and effort to meet the targets, thus neglecting other aspects that are not under investigation (Mrazek and Mossialos 2002). In contrast, by monitoring too many variables, the increased complexity and contradictory outcomes may confound the observable outcomes and further result in an 'audit explosion'. Moreover, relevant indicators should be selected to illustrate effectively the policy context of the health care system under investigation, and not be chosen simply because they are easily observable or provide favourable outcomes.

Pricing and reimbursement policies

Regulating pharmaceutical prices in Europe

Supply-side cost-containment measures are primarily targeted either directly or indirectly at regulating the prices of pharmaceuticals. The primary measures include direct fixed price controls, profit controls and reference pricing. There is an incentive to ensure that the prices paid for pharmaceuticals either by public funds or directly by patients, are not more than one would be reasonably willing to pay on the grounds of public health, social solidarity and efficiency. Economic efficiency – that is, identifying the best use of resources and usually determined by economic evaluations – is more often being taken into account when determining reimbursement decisions; the strengths and weaknesses of this are considered later.

Fixed pricing attempts to secure pharmaceutical prices that are considered 'reasonable' for a given health system. There are many approaches to set the maximum prices: negotiated prices, price-caps, cost-plus, price comparisons to other countries or to similar products within the same country or price/volume trade-offs. Perhaps the least transparent of these is where prices are negotiated between a company and a government; the criteria for these negotiations, if defined at all, often include a subjective category leaving decisions very much to the discretion of the regulator. There has been some improvement in clarifying the criteria behind such negotiated decisions, thanks mainly to the EU Transparency Directive (Council of the European Communities 1989). However, few countries make publicly available pricing data from their schemes or produce annual reports on their performance.

Some countries have moved away from 'cost-plus' pricing, where the price of drugs is set according to the costs of manufacturing the drug, a method confounded by the problem of transfer pricing. Fixed prices based on the prices of equivalent or similar drugs already on the domestic market or available in other countries are popular, making the product launch strategy challenging for the industry. There are, however, a number of methodological considerations to making such price comparisons, including appropriate comparator product (i.e. formulation, pack size) and price conversion into national currency units. It is also open to manipulation by pharmaceutical companies.

Many countries have additionally applied cuts and freezes to fixed prices, usually resulting in a one-off and very short-lived decrease in pharmaceutical expenditures.

Reference pricing, or setting a maximum reimbursement level, aims to contain pharmaceutical expenditure by defining a fixed amount to be paid by the government (or other third-party payer). In theory, this creates an incentive for both physicians and patients to consider drug prices in decision making, since any cost beyond the reference price must be borne by the patient. Pharmaceutical products are clustered to encourage substitution by either a cheaper generic or therapeutic equivalent. When applied extensively, reference pricing can be effective at eliminating price gaps between therapeutically similar products and improving market transparency (Giuliani *et al.* 1998). In practice, these schemes result in a price decrease for those medicines priced above the reference price limit, as patients often ask to be switched to a drug at the reference price (Lopez-Casasnovas and Puig-Junoy 2000). However, if pharmacist payments do not motivate selection of a least-cost generic equivalent, price competition that could lower the reference price may not occur, thus resulting in an artificial price floor (Mrazek 2001). There have been concerns that patients' access to new drugs might be restricted when dictated by the ability or willingness to pay an additional cost over the reference price, although this was not an issue in Canadian studies (Schneeweiss *et al.* 2002a). Furthermore, in most countries, criteria for defining therapeutic equivalence of drugs are not clear-cut or agreed. As a result, this approach has been predominantly applied only to off-patent generic equivalent drugs. In Germany, reference pricing was somewhat successful in cost savings, which were partly offset by price rises for medicines still under patent and outside the scheme. Despite these problems in Europe, the experience in British Columbia in Canada suggests that reference pricing combined with other approaches may be a valuable means of containing costs without harm to patient well-being (Schneeweiss *et al.* 2002b). In North America, the presence or level of co-payment is often linked to the reference price of a product, as a package to try to contain cost, but this linkage is not used in Europe (see Chapter 13).

Indirect price control through profit or rate-of-return regulation considers the manufacturer's contribution to drug development and the economy when determining drug prices. The objective is to ensure that pharmaceutical firms are not making excessive profits, specifically on patent-protected products paid for by public health care systems, but at the same time to reward innovation. Currently, this regulatory mechanism is unique to the UK where pharmaceutical pricing at drug launch is free, but later is subject to a non-statutory profit control regulation called the Pharmaceutical Price Regulation Scheme (PPRS) (Department of Health UK 1999). At present, the allowable profit is set at 21 per cent return on capital employed (ROC); this is higher than most UK industrial sectors. Margins are allowed before excess profits trigger a rebate to the Treasury or underperformance may trigger permission to increase prices. The PPRS provides positive incentives for pharmaceutical firms by allowing R&D costs to comprise 20 per cent of UK National Health Service (NHS) turnover (3 per cent higher depending on the number of patented products on the market or 3 per cent lower if applying for a price increase), much higher than the 14 per cent worldwide average (Mossialos 1997); consequently, the PPRS encourages innovation and local investment in R&D. Companies are also allocated 6 per cent of NHS sales for sales promotion spending (reduced to 3 per cent when considering a price increase). Furthermore, an operational relationship is maintained between the Department of Health and the industry, which allows flexibility in negotiating company-specific profit margins and ensures no sudden policy changes, thus facilitating a favourable and stable business environment.

A major difficulty with rate-of-return regulation is weak incentives for cost-cutting, potentially leading to high prices. A company may have little incentive to operate efficiently because increased costs can be recovered through increased prices, albeit to a lesser degree for firms operating across several markets. Furthermore, companies may overinvest in capital (Averch and Johnson 1962),[3] artificially inflate their asset base, or shift production costs from non-regulated divisions to regulated ones if they operate in several markets, allowing them to price their drugs higher.

However, as the company's costs can be compared with its costs in previous years and with other similar firms, and targets may be set for future gains in efficiency, some of the problems inherent in profit regulation can be mitigated. Nevertheless, there is a lack of transparency in the private negotiations to set target profits, and regulatory capture may be a problem.

In general, empirical evidence suggests that strict direct price regulation schemes (e.g. fixed maximum pharmaceutical prices) may be more effective in controlling the rise in pharmaceutical prices when looking at measurements of price levels across countries, but they seem less effective in controlling overall expenditure, since any savings may be counteracted by large increases in volume. The cause of increases in the costs of drugs is not usually, in fact, prices, but increases in volume of prescribing and the introduction of new products (Nefarma 2002) (Table 1.2). Even where price–volume agreements have been negotiated as in Spain and Italy, budgets have regularly been exceeded (Donatini *et al.* 2001); although a sizeable repayment was required in Spain (Lopez-Bastida and Mossialos 2000).

Current price control systems do not provide an indication of (or incentive to reward) any added therapeutic value of the drug. McGuire *et al.* (Chapter 7) argue that the ideal would be a system of marginal pricing according to the increased therapeutic benefit of the drug, in order to award real innovation and gains in clinical effectiveness; the wide use of economic evaluations in the reimbursement process would go some way to achieve this. The strengths and weaknesses of this approach are considered in the next section.

A final relevant point is that local optimization for one country may contradict global optimization. In the UK, for example, where securing low-cost medicines and encouraging the pharmaceutical industry are concomi-

Table 1.2 Pharmaceutical expenditure growth in selected EU member states in 2002: contribution of different growth factors

Country	Price (%)	New product (%)	Volume (%)	Total growth (%)
UK	0.00	2.80	8.70	11.50
Spain	0.70	2.60	8.40	11.70
The Netherlands	0.00	1.00	8.30	9.30
Germany	−0.20	2.70	5.50	8.00
Italy	−0.50	2.50	3.20	5.20
France	−0.80	2.50	2.30	4.00

Source: Nefarma (2002).

tant policy objectives, cost containment is still possible due to relatively free pricing balanced by low volumes of brand prescribing and extensive generic prescribing. But because the UK is often used as a reference country in price-fixing systems based on international price comparisons, and companies prefer to launch their products in the UK first due to free pricing for new chemical entities, cost containment in pharmaceuticals may become more difficult for other countries.

Overall, price measures are best used in conjunction with other supply- and demand-side incentives if these are to contribute to cost control.

Reimbursement decisions

Reimbursement levels will reflect the outcome of negotiations between the pharmaceutical company with the new product (monopoly) and the payer, normally a government or health insurance fund (monopsony). The final reimbursement price will reflect the political and economic power of the two parties and their bargaining skills. Reimbursement decisions may also define the level of public subsidies and user charges (see Chapter 13). Reimbursement can be used as a means of rewarding innovation, with new products judged to be truly clinically valuable receiving premium prices.

Where there is flexibility in pricing, reimbursement prices can be used to send signals to industry about what price levels are acceptable for what clinical gain. In practice, reimbursement and pricing are often not sufficiently integrated within governments to allow this to happen to any great extent (Austria is an exception to this). Reimbursement might then be based on cost-effectiveness analysis or on criteria related to the product's clinical effectiveness and potential budget impact, the aim being to maximize efficiency in the use of health care resources (e.g. in Finland where pricing is related to economic evaluation and, to a lesser extent, in the UK where the prospect of an appraisal by the National Institute of Clinical Excellence can influence pricing decisions of industry while not actually setting a price; see Chapter 7). Evaluating the clinical benefit of a new drug for which there is little experience, especially in the long term, is difficult, particularly since the data to compute these comparative benefits are lacking in the public domain, because information on both effectiveness and costs is proprietary and closely guarded by the industry (Collier and Iheanacho 2002).

Although attractive in theory, there is controversy about the appropriateness of such economic evaluation in policy making, both in terms of its theoretical basis as well as its application. There are methodological problems, where questions of what to include in both costs and consequences (e.g. what costs, what perspectives, analytical periods of studies) are exacerbated by questions of how to include them (Drummond *et al.* 1997a). There are technical difficulties to ensuring a consistent application of guidelines across studies. Generalizability is also restricted due to questions about incremental effectiveness and chosen comparators, as well as context-specific factors such as population, availability of health care resources, relative prices or costs, and variations in clinical practice (Drummond and Pang 2001). In practice, economic evaluation is further constrained by the fact that there are limited resources to conduct it, so that it becomes nearly impossible to construct league tables with all the possible health interventions – economic evaluations are therefore rarely global but confined to limited areas.

While the mindset behind economic evaluation of 'value for money' has influenced health policy makers, the impact of economic evaluation itself as a measure to improve efficiency has been extremely limited for several reasons. There is often no effective linkage between economic evaluators and decision makers. Practitioners and decision makers may also lack the time and expertise to assess adequately the lengthy and technical economic evaluations that may not set out clear policy implications of the new technology. Economic evaluation could play only a part of the policy-making process, as other key determinants (e.g. how much a certain health improvement is valued, rewards to industry for innovation) vary from country to country (Drummond *et al.* 1997b). The difficulties in transferring the results from economic evaluations between health care systems undermine the relevance of externally produced data in countries with limited researcher capacity or the lack of necessary funds to carry out their own enquiries. Finally, the role of economic evaluation is to promote efficiency – not contain costs – and it would be seen as appropriate that a highly effective and efficient therapy should be used, even if overall costs were to rise as a result. Economic evaluation or a wider health technology assessment, which has to take into account other issues such as equity, affordability, and delivery and service implications, may become one of the drivers of health care costs (Oliver *et al.* 2004).

At present, therefore, there are few examples of marginal pricing founded on increased therapeutic benefit. One might assume that a manufacturer, aware of this fourth hurdle, has gone through a process of using economic evaluation as part of its internal price setting, although anecdotally this is exceptional at present. The possibility of using levels of innovation or therapeutic benefit in price negotiations, therefore, exists but would be difficult at present. In several European countries, it is becoming the norm to explicitly include economic concepts in applying for a reimbursement listing, although how the payer uses these is not always clear. Finland is the only EU country where a product's price and reimbursement is explicitly linked to the economic evidence. Italy, Portugal and Ireland also consider economic criteria and may use them to determine price for reimbursement. Austria, Belgium, Denmark and the Netherlands are also paying increasing attention to economic considerations.

In the UK, this role is taken by the National Institute of Clinical Excellence (NICE), which uses economic evaluation as part of its consideration in recommending a new technology or drug for use in the UK NHS. This has been criticized because its work may delay the introduction of medicines, and because its recommendations are simply a 'long-deferred catch-up in best practice' (Lynch 2003). Conversely, NICE is criticized because it is not responsible for the funding of new technologies and does not consider affordability – its decisions can therefore pose serious problems for health service managers with limited budgets. In practice, NICE recommendations have been one of the major drivers of the rise in NHS drug costs in recent years. Some health economists believe that it is politically difficult for these organizations to say 'no' to certain drugs, and that these institutions should genuinely challenge pharmaceutical companies to show the value of their new product (Cookson *et al.* 2001).

Nevertheless, even with these procedures to determine suitability of a drug for reimbursement, many drugs lack appropriate documentation of efficacy. There is also a large discrepancy among different countries regarding what should and should not be reimbursed, and efforts to reimburse drugs on cost-effectiveness criteria have not yet been employed at the supranational level. The prospect of a single agency, complementary to the EMEA, which would make recommendations for reimbursement across Europe – a sort of EuroNICE – is remote.

Selected lists, too, have been implemented with little uniformity across Europe. These may overlap in part with the selection of products for reference pricing. They are created by the health care funder and explicitly state whether or not a specific product may be adopted for reimbursement. To be placed on a 'positive list', a product must meet certain criteria that can be associated with therapeutic benefit, low risk factors, price and budget impact, and possibly cost-effectiveness analysis. These could decrease overall costs by decreasing the costs of prescription and the number of prescriptions, particularly if targeted at high-cost medicines where there is an effective lower-cost preparation available. But if the alternatives are not acceptable to the professionals or the patient, the result will be inappropriate use of higher-cost substitutes; for instance, the delisting of antacids in Ireland in the 1980s increased the use of drugs such as cimetidine and ranitidine, and increased overall expenditure (Ferrando *et al.* 1987).

Monitoring and influencing physician decision making

Since physicians are the key decision makers on the demand-side of the pharmaceutical market, there is much interest in ensuring that they are engaging in good prescribing practices. 'Good prescribing' should encompass the appropriate choice of medicine not only from the perspective of the physician but also that of the patient, while at the same time aiming to maximize effectiveness, minimize risk and minimize cost (Barber 1995). Prescribers, patients and payers in different health care systems may have different perspectives on what constitutes good prescribing.

There are significant differences in the prescribing habits of individual practitioners and across countries. For instance, only 62.9 per cent of consultations result in prescriptions in the Netherlands, whereas in Italy this figure is 94.5 per cent (Nefarma 2002). In 1996, only five medicines were common among the 50 most prescribed medicines of France, Germany, Italy and the UK (Garattini and Garattini 1998). It is, of course, premature to attribute these differences only to prescribing culture, but clearly discrepancies are significant (Nefarma 2002). Study of good prescribing is difficult: the patient's 'needs' are difficult to define and measure, and are not well captured by administrative databases (see Chapter 8). Disentangling the complex interaction of factors that lead to a decision to prescribe a particular drug for a particular patient is difficult.

Various approaches have been made to monitor prescribing quality, including the use of a medical appropriateness index and a review of detailed medical records. The medical appropriateness index assesses prescribing suitability for an individual patient based on 10 dimensions (see Chapter 8). The use of medical records is the most accurate measure of performance quality, although it is not a realistic option for most European countries. Financial incentives also have been used to influence prescribing behaviour (see Chapter 10).

Prescribing data are used, in the UK for example, to provide doctors with reliable, regular and prompt information on their current prescribing in an effort to improve cost-awareness, in theory leading to more effective and economical prescribing. In practice, the usefulness of such cost-focused prescribing data in initiating change is limited because change depends on the doctors' willingness to consider costs when prescribing. Although doctors are not necessarily averse to considering costs, other criteria such as clinical benefit, personal experience or opinion are valued more highly (Denig and Haaijer-Ruskamp 1995).

Clinical practice guidelines – specific criteria for how and when particular tests and treatments should be used – have also been employed in an attempt to standardize physician variation to management of diseases as well as control spending. While there is often no mechanism for monitoring or enforcement after dissemination of the guidelines, their introduction may be complemented with financial incentives (or disincentives) and educational efforts. Clinical practice guidelines appeal to policy makers as well as clinicians because their objectives are to improve, not simply ration, care. Sometimes these guidelines are used in utilization reviews (at times used to penalize doctors or hospitals) or to determine coverage policy, which makes them less acceptable to some health care professionals. In France, prescribing guidelines were poorly followed because of the volume of guidelines, a lack of information systems and limited capacity for monitoring, and physicians' concern that following the guidelines could negatively affect the quality of care being delivered (Durieux *et al.* 2000).

Studies on the effectiveness of clinical guidelines have been conflicting (Gundersen 2000). Some have shown little effect of clinical guidelines on physician prescribing behaviour (Hetlevik *et al.* 2000), while others suggest that evidence-based guidelines, if designed well and implemented consistently, can help to deliver 'best practice' (Garfield and Garfield 2000; Richman and Lancaster 2000; Perleth *et al.* 2001).

In general, adherence to evidence-based guidelines would be expected to improve the quality, efficiency and equity of care, but might increase or decrease total expenditure depending on previous practice – if patients were undertreated, increases in total expenditure are likely. Guidelines written with the explicit objective of cost containment are unlikely to be acceptable because of serious ethical and legal implications (Carter *et al.* 1995; Cheah 1998). Guideline development and implementation is expensive and like any other health technology must prove its value (Gandjour and Lauterbach 2001; Mason *et al.* 2001).

Another approach to influence physician prescribing is educational (Soumerai and Avorn 1990). There are many forms of educational interventions, including the simple distribution of educational bulletins or pamphlets, lectures and seminars, in all of which the prescriber can be a passive recipient. More participatory approaches to prescriber education include audit and feedback, and academic detailing. In general, there has been no good evidence showing effectiveness of the simpler, more passive measures such as circulation of educational materials, or even auditing and feedback (Freemantle 2000). These do, however, improve knowledge and while not securing change in themselves, may prepare the ground for more direct approaches, such as academic detailing.

Academic detailing, where a trained individual meets with a physician in their practice setting to modify their performance, can change practice (Avorn and Soumerai 1983), but it is expensive. Recent studies in the UK show a useful effect in general practices with small numbers of doctors, but less of an effect in larger practices with more doctors, where securing the 'buy in' to change practice from all the doctors is more difficult (Freemantle *et al.* 2002). An alternative method to directly assist in clinical decision making is the use of computerized decision support systems that use software to generate patient-specific assessments or recommendations. These two educational methods – academic detailing and computerized decision support – can be expected to bring about a 15 per cent change towards the desired behaviour by professionals (Freemantle 2000). Here, an important qualification to academic detailing is that the people chosen to educate professionals should not be seen as biased health managers. In the UK, for example, one problem with prescribing advisers in the early 1990s was that they were seen as agents of the government and thus were received with some antagonism by doctors. Finally, other methods such as socialization and instilling certain norms of behaviour for physicians have been attempted, but with much less success (Robinson 2001).

The changing doctor–patient relationship

Recently, the doctor–patient relationship has changed as patients become more involved in choice of treatment, and can easily access an abundance of detailed medical information through books, the media and the internet. Many patients seem less trusting of physicians. Furthermore, in an environment geared to containing health care spending, patients have an increased responsibility in paying for their medicines and may be encouraged to care for minor ailments with over-the-counter remedies, paid for out-of-pocket.

Research on doctor–patient relationships and medicine taking has revealed that patients have complicated agendas during general practitioner (GP) consultations (Barry *et al.* 2000). Patients are ambivalent and often averse to taking medicines and do not fully express these feelings to their GPs. At the same time, some patients want prescriptions that may not be medically indicated (see Chapter 9). These behaviours create communication difficulties between the doctor and patient that can lead to poor consultation outcomes, incorrect use of medicines and non-adherence with medicine taking. Exacerbating this situation is the fact that patients are often poorly educated by their doctors in terms of how to use their medication correctly, expected duration of treatment, possible side-effects, available alternatives (medical and non-medical) and indications to return (see Chapter 9).

Furthermore, national and regional populations differ in how they regard disease, thus influencing how illnesses are managed. Culture is defined as the socially transmitted beliefs, norms, values, religion, civilization and all other products of human work and thought of a population. Just as health care utilization differs between cultures and nations, so does the use of medicines. The influence of culture on pharmaceutical prescription and consumption must be considered in the context of the respective health care system structure and economy (Payer 1988). Rates of prescription differ enormously across Europe (Table 1.3).

The use of drugs in a society goes far beyond their chemical properties and considers the cultural definitions of disease, attitudes towards health and pain, and the perceived effects of the drug on the individual. The ritualistic nature of medicines is deeply embedded in the ethos of a group. Cross-national differences have been observed regarding the acceptance of generics, the sharing of medicines, patient compliance, self-medication and information seeking. In some societies, the very act of a physician prescribing a medicine may convey the message to a patient that the consultation is complete and the illness is in fact real. Thus, patients need to be educated about the benefits and limitations of specific pharmaceuticals by physicians in a clear, understandable and timely fashion.

Patient compliance is an important area for policy, since its implications are wide. Poor patient compliance can have adverse effects on the public health (e.g. low rates of childhood vaccination in parts of the UK; Meulemans *et al.* 2002). One of the reasons behind non-compliance may be a growing mistrust of the health care industry (Robertson 1985). Another may be that what patients view as a worthwhile personal benefit may not be the same as what the health professional considers useful. Better understandings of non-compliance and its consequences can lead to more effective strategies for improved concordance between doctors and patients and better adherence to medicines (Dardano 2000). Some non-compliance is not just due to misinformation or individual irresponsibility, but also to external factors outside the patient's control, such as

Table 1.3 Prescriptions dispensed per capita in European countries in 1995

Country	Prescriptions	Country	Prescriptions
Austria	11.5	Italy	5.2
Belgium	9.5	Luxembourg	26.0
Denmark	7.1	The Netherlands	11.0
Finland (1994)	5.7	Norway (1994)	6.9
France	52.2	Portugal	21.0
Germany	12.0	Sweden	6.1
Iceland	16.0	Switzerland	8.0
Ireland	11.0	UK	10.0

Source: Yuen (1999).

poverty and logistical problems (Fletcher 1989). Monitoring patient compliance may also be important to ensure that the potential therapeutic benefits are not wasted (Kaveh 2001). Financial incentives (cash, vouchers, lottery tickets, gifts) have also been used successfully in the USA to improve patient adherence (Giuffrida and Torgerson 1997). Recent initiatives in the UK show anecdotal evidence that patients can manage some of their own health conditions much more effectively than by simply depending on health care professionals (Donaldson 2002). In all cases, an ethos where patients begin to take more responsibility for their health has the potential to improve doctor–patient relationships and health gains.

The media can have a positive influence on health care issues through public health education campaigns, or a negative impact when exaggerating the benefits of breakthrough drugs or the disasters of adverse effects. Newspapers, television and, more recently, the internet can manipulate public beliefs, attitudes and behaviours pertaining to health care and medicines. Information from particular sources (such as the internet) can often be misleading or wrong, and can contribute to mistrust between doctor and patient (see Chapter 9). Incomplete information given by pharmaceutical companies, especially about the limits of clinical benefit, is a major concern (Woloshin *et al.* 2001).

Since 1997, direct-to-consumer advertising of prescription drugs has been allowed in the USA, thus influencing the consumption of medicines by raising public awareness. Direct-to-consumer advertising for prescription-only medicines is illegal in Europe and opposition to it generally remains widespread, both among health professionals and by most patient and consumer groups. Such opposition stems from uncertainty about any benefits of the system and its well-documented problems. The industry points to advantages in 'empowering the consumer through information', resulting in more autonomy and speedier access to medicines. This is to be weighed against the often dubious nature of the information provided. This is apparent from evidence that, in the USA, even over-the-counter advertisements – which the FDA regulates – often make inaccurate statements and neglect to mention potential side-effects (Sansgiry *et al.* 1999). The dividing line between information and advertising is therefore narrow.

Evidence from the USA and, to some extent, New Zealand suggests that direct-to-consumer advertising mainly benefits manufacturers, rather than simply reflects, consumer need (Hoffman and Wilkes 1999). Direct-to-consumer advertising (DTC) has thus been seen as an industry tool, not for the promotion of information, but rather to make further profit. While the pharmaceutical industry is hoping to receive DTC rights in Europe by claiming to share accurate and scientifically based information with consumers to help them become more involved in their own health care, strident opponents say that, as the goal of providing this information would be to increase sales, it is inevitable that the benefits are discussed more than the risks (Garlick 2003; Jones 2003).

Pharmaceutical companies can promote themselves in many other ways: in addition to indirect financial support to physicians, such as sponsoring drug lunches or dinners, giving industry gifts, or paying for travel and expenses to educational conferences (Moynihan 2003a), companies will use ostensibly neutral and independent sources (whether individuals, patients' groups or medical journals) (Smith 2003; Wager 2003) to promote new drugs. Another traditional route is through medical journals, which often depend on the large-volume reprint requests and advertisements of drug companies, and where editorial lines can be influenced. A new approach is through patients' organizations, which gain financial support from drug companies. Yet the unequal 'partnership' can allow pharmaceutical companies to misrepresent their own agendas or distort those of patient organizations (Herxheimer 2003).

Such potential conflicts of interest should be made more explicit (Burton and Rowell 2003). Recently in the UK and the USA, movements have been formed by medical students, professional associations and other groups to oppose intimate ties with pharmaceutical companies (Moynihan 2003b). 'Good publication practice', where drug companies are encouraged to publish negative results, would ameliorate the problem of publication bias (Singh 2003). Another idea is that of a 'blind trust', where pharmaceutical companies could contribute to a national pool of funding, to be allocated to educational providers (Moynihan 2003c).

The implications of these changes – where patients armed with increasing information of varying quality, as well as more alternatives in obtaining medications – are that new ways of engaging patients with health professionals must be found and encouraged to protect patients and prevent abuse of more convenient ways of finding treatment.

Financial incentives and prescribing

Prescribing budgets can be used at the level of the individual doctor, practice or region to limit the resources available for providing medicines. Hard budgets use penalties or rewards to motivate doctors to meet budgetary goals, while target budgets do not impose an immediate penalty but allow useful record-keeping of the costs incurred by the agent concerned. There may be rewards or fines for meeting or failing to meet treatment guidelines or quality targets, or staying within a cash-limited prescribing budget scheme.

Prescribing budgets have generated financial and ethical concerns. They risk reducing patients' confidence in their doctors, as they increasingly become aware of the financial incentives linked with prescribing behaviour. There is a risk that the quality of prescribing may deteriorate if the financial incentive becomes the driving force behind the prescribing decision. Should doctors be especially rewarded for doing a professional job, or perhaps depriving patients of the medicines they need? The use of cheaper medicines to meet budgetary constraints may not necessarily be cost-effective. Additionally, prescribing economies might be only short-term. Perverse incentives may cause cost shifting to other health services (e.g. improper use of the emergency room) thus decreasing prescribing spend but increasing overall health care costs. Moreover, there may be problems of 'cream-skimming' associated with physicians referring severely ill and expensive patients to hospitals (or at least making patients with chronic illnesses less of a priority) (Goodwin 1998) and the possibility of doctors denying appropriate but expensive treatments to patients. This suggests that extreme care should be taken in the design and implementation of these incentives.

The conflict doctors face between giving the best treatment to each patient and being responsible stewards of the health care system is felt more keenly with these new arrangements. Awareness of these risks and possible solutions (e.g. compensating physicians not only through financial incentives to decrease utilization but also through rewards for quality and productivity, providing regular information on approved ways of managing particular conditions) is crucial for policy makers hoping to design incentive systems that align interests of patients, providers and payers.

Although some suggest that drug budgets may not be necessary for containing costs, and that better data on cost-effectiveness would empower prescribers to make rational decisions regarding treatments (Laupacis *et al.* 2002; Levy and Gagnon 2002), others argue that budget constraint is essential to contain costs (Brougham *et al.* 2002). Moreover, it is argued that containing costs without budgets and exclusively depending on prescribers to make their own rational decisions based on evidence not yet collected is impractical (Fernandes 2002).

Financial incentives can be effective, but mostly in choice of drug as opposed to volume of prescribing. In other words, the decision of a doctor to prescribe is difficult to change but the type of drug chosen, however, is negotiable. Even so, these changes in prescribing (often simple shifts to generic medications) are usually one-off and cannot be repeated, although their benefits can be maintained. Punitive disincentives placed on physicians (as until recently in Germany and in France) appear less acceptable as well as being more difficult to enforce, and thus less successful. At the same time, weaker schemes that appeal to professionalism but hold no real positive or negative incentives have been shown (at least in the UK) to be relatively ineffective at changing behaviour (see Chapter 10). The types of incentives employed should be chosen according to particular circumstances, such as current practice patterns and levels of provision. Few studies have determined whether health outcomes are changed due to financial incentives. Most evidence does, however, imply that physicians prefer that their autonomy be protected (as in UK fundholding) and, when combined with simple and transparent appropriate incentives, can save money with no loss of quality (Chapter 10). Drawing on less visible yet still persuasive forms of regulation such as peer pressure through professional associations, as well as these other measures, may also be important in changing the culture of prescribing. In the end, while the effects of financial incentives may be more visible in the short term, they may also be less professionally and ethically acceptable and, in the long run, less effective at containing costs.

Regulating pharmaceutical distribution, retail and hospital pharmacy in Europe

Pharmaceuticals pass from the manufacturer to the patient through a distribution chain of wholesalers and pharmacists. The distribution of pharmaceuticals in the EU is governed by both supranational and national regulations in conjunction with professional bodies, health service providers and health care payers. The principal objective of regulating distribution is to protect the public's interest in safety and access to medicines; secondary objectives include ensuring the financial viability and integrity of wholesalers and pharmacies, promoting quality services, limiting overall drug costs and encouraging increased consumer choice. The specific details of regulation differ between member states.

There are many different types of wholesalers, each playing a particular role in the pharmaceutical distribution chain. Wholesalers may offer a full range of products, support the supply of bulk orders, provide selected product ranges or engage in parallel importation. The number of pharmaceutical wholesalers has decreased in the EU since the 1990s, and at present the market is dominated by a few key players in each member state. All European countries impose limits on drug wholesalers' margins (see Chapter 11).

In the past, the role of the community pharmacist was to dispense prescription medicines and sell over-the-counter products. This is now evolving throughout Europe because of rising awareness of their extensive knowledge about the appropriate use of medicines and their potential as independent providers of health care. Pharmacists are highly educated professionals and, in some countries, will have a more integrated clinical role in the future. In addition, the pharmacist can be instrumental in controlling pharmaceutical expenditure when given the freedom to engage in generic and therapeutic substitution, and when economical dispensing practices are promoted through financial incentives. There is much variation between the regulatory patterns related to pharmacists in EU member states. These include controlling community pharmacy ownership and location, setting allowable profit margins, and influencing drug distribution patterns and product selection through different incentives and remuneration methods.

How pharmacists are paid influences their product selection. In countries such as Ireland, the Netherlands, Sweden and the UK, pharmacists receive a fixed fee per item dispensed. In the UK, which also sets a fixed reimbursement price on unbranded generics, pharmacists have the incentive to dispense the cheapest suitable product and, in doing so, retain the difference between the purchase price and the reimbursement price; similar preferential margins to motivate dispensing choice operate in some other EU markets as well. Denmark has a unique approach applying a dispensing budget that introduces a collective incentive to dispense cost consciously. Most other countries (Austria, Belgium, Denmark, Germany, Greece, Italy and Portugal) pay pharmacists with regressive scaled margins or margins that are a fixed percentage of a product's price. Denmark, Finland, France, Norway and Spain allow a pharmacist to substitute a generic for a branded preparation, regardless of how the prescription was written.

The distinction between manufacturers, wholesalers and community pharmacies is becoming increasingly vague with more vertical integration (when permissible) that allows for consolidation of the distribution channel and increased margins for wholesalers. In addition, competition is growing with the introduction of mail-order and online pharmacies. Yet the evolution and further deregulation of the pharmaceutical supply chain in Europe may face countervailing trends: the continued demand for face-to-face pharmaceutical advice and care; divergent and deeply rooted regional histories of pharmacy services; the strength of the professional lobby of pharmacists; and lack of consistent public pressure and sound political vision for the future of the distribution sector. As a result, the likely future of pharmacy service regulation may be one characterized by slow evolution rather than radical change (see Chapter 12). One radically new role for pharmacists in the UK will be as prescribers, taking on responsibility for dose adjustment and monitoring in a range of chronic conditions where a doctor has made the diagnosis.

The role of hospital pharmacies has also been transformed dramatically over the past three decades. Hospital pharmacists are increasingly required to become comfortable with larger roles – not only their traditional responsibilities of drug preparation and verification, but also working as clinical pharmacists at the ward level. The international trend in hospital pharmacies has become to provide products to meet individual patient need, thus necessitating increased collaboration between hospital pharmacists and prescribers, nurses, dietitians, biochemists and laboratory scientists. On an institutional level, hospital pharmacies must support the safe, effective and economic use of medicines in hospitals in accordance with government rules and budgetary requirements. Carrying out these responsibilities requires medicines information services and clinical pharmacy services within the hospital to service outpatient care (see Chapter 12). In addition, specialized databases and medicine information services based in hospitals have been developed to facilitate drug treatment decision making by clinicians (Taggiasco *et al.* 1992).

Expanding the roles of hospital and community pharmacies also has the potential of reducing medical errors. In the USA, fatalities from prescription errors are claimed to have increased by 243 per cent between 1993 and 1998, outpacing almost any other cause of death, and also progressing faster than the increase in prescriptions (Phillips and Bredder 2002). In one study, errors in prescribing medications were the most common mistake made among family physicians (Dovey *et al.* 2003). Another study in an American teaching hospital reports finding four errors per 1000 medication orders, 70 per cent of which had the potential to be seriously harmful (Lesar *et al.* 1997). Preventable adverse reactions to drugs are claimed to be the single leading cause of hospitalization in the USA, where 2–7 per cent of hospitalized patients have avoidable adverse drug events and, consequently, have hospital stays 8–12 days longer than they should (Kohn *et al.* 2000). Studies performed in the UK have shown similar results, with one report of a 49 per cent error rate in the administration of intravenous drugs (Taxis and Barber 2003). Medical errors have been attributed to a number of causes: administrative and investigation failures, simple ignorance, lapses in treatment delivery, miscommunication, complications in payment systems, as well as many others (Dovey *et al.* 2002).

The United States Institute of Medicine and the Agency for Healthcare Research and Quality have both called for a systematic way of formulating and incorporating safety into the process of care. Drawing on examples outside of health care and considering such processes as incident reporting, root cause analysis and simulators, specific recommendations regarding certain clinical practices are mentioned, as well as the issue of how to promote safety practices on an institutional level (Shojania *et al.* 2001).

The idea of 'pharmaceutical care' (Cipolle *et al.* 1998) has changed the traditional role and function of hospital pharmacists from dealing solely with inpatient care to involvement in: the ambulatory care setting, working closely in treatment delivery; the patient care setting, regarding hospital risk management strategies; and the clinical setting, contributing information on adverse side-effects to national pharmacovigilance systems. In addition, hospital pharmacists play an important role in combating inaccuracies in transmitting patient drug information between community physicians and hospital specialists. Hospital pharmacists can and do work in conjunction with nurse specialists to improve patient education and, in special cases, provide follow-up visits in the patient's home. Furthermore, pharmacists serve a fundamental role in improving patients' self-management in diabetes and other chronic conditions that can potentially reduce hospital readmission rates and improve patient compliance to drug treatment regimes.

Influencing patient demand through co-payments

In all Western European countries, cost sharing for pharmaceuticals has been introduced to try to control pharmaceutical expenditure and influence the demand for prescription drugs. There are three different forms of cost sharing currently employed. Co-insurance, the most common form, requires the patient to be liable for some percentage of the total cost of a drug; flat-rate payments oblige the patient to pay a fixed fee per item or per prescription; and deductibles involve the individual paying the initial expense up to a specified amount. There is great variation across Western European countries with respect to the implementation of prescription drug charges or co-payments. Although co-payments are not usually linked to reference pricing in Europe as they are in North America, there has been linkage with variable co-payments for drugs on restricted lists in France and Italy, based on the perceived therapeutic value of that drug to the health service.

Advocates of cost sharing argue that it increases efficiency by reducing excessive demand and containing overall health costs. Individuals become price sensitive and will seek what is to them the least expensive treatment. If there is competition between providers, individuals' sensitivity to price may result in lower prices. Introducing the price mechanism in this way may also prevent unnecessary (or even potentially harmful) care, since individuals will select treatments and interventions that are of high value to them (see Chapter 13). Other supporters of cost sharing maintain that any additional revenue raised could be targeted at low-income people or used to confront inequality in the health care system. The ability of cost sharing to raise revenue, however, is limited by the prevalence of widely applied exemptions and high administrative costs. In many countries, significant groups within the population (based on age, income and clinical condition) are exempt from cost sharing in an attempt to protect the disadvantaged, satisfy need and ensure equitable access to drugs. Moreover, the existence of complementary voluntary health insurance in some countries (e.g. France, Croatia, Slovenia) effectively removes price signals for those who can afford to purchase a medicine and therefore negates the potential for cost sharing to reduce demand (see Chapter 13).

Critics argue that the theoretical case for using cost sharing as a means of reducing excess utilization is weak because health care markets are characterized by information asymmetry, proxy demand and heterogeneity. Furthermore, since demand for health care is largely provider-determined, policy tools that focus on the demand side may not be as effective in controlling demand as those that focus on supply. Cost sharing also has implications for equity in funding health, because it shifts the financial burden towards individuals and households and away from population-based risk-sharing arrangements. Equity in access to health care is also reduced by cost sharing, as those with low incomes (and likely to be in poorest health) are most likely to be discouraged from using health services. This decrease seems to be in essential as well as non-essential drug therapy (Evans *et al.* 1995).

In terms of macro-efficiency, the savings in drug costs may be outweighed by increased utilization of other health care services, which may, in fact, increase overall health care spending. In addition, the transaction costs of implementing prescription charges and exemption schemes limit the cost saving. Third, in cost sharing for pharmaceuticals, governments impose a risk on individuals for an intervention that is largely beyond their control; that is, where consumption depends on prescription by doctors. In other words, financial (dis)incentives are placed on individuals, who have less power to control drug spending than prescribers (see Chapter 13) and user charges can be seen as punishing the patient for following their doctor's orders. The use of co-payments is a blunt mechanism of controlling costs and must be applied cautiously so as not to be counter-productive to the overall objective of a health care system (see Chapter 21). Careful use of differential co-payments or co-payments with well-defined exemptions may be more acceptable.

The off-patent and over-the-counter pharmaceutical markets

Once the patent on a pharmaceutical product has expired, generic equivalents may come on the market, so increasing competition. A generic equivalent is a perfect substitute to the original brand and competes in price for market share. The new product must demonstrate bioavailability for the main active ingredient comparable to a brand leader. These virtual copies of the original branded medicine may be branded or unbranded and are also known as off-patent, post-patent or multi-sourced drugs. Because of their low cost compared with the brand leader, generic drugs potentially offer significant savings that can release funds to pay for innovative, patent-protected products.

The low cost of generics is due to supply-side factors such as market size and the number of suppliers. Equally important are the demand-side incentives that encourage prescribing, dispensing and consumption of generics. Financial incentives to increase generic prescribing may tie into physician budgets or guidelines. The selection of the least expensive multi-sourced drugs by the pharmacist and generic substitution where it is allowed are also motivated more effectively by financial incentives that give pharmacists higher margins or additional payments for dispensing a lower-cost generic medicine.

Differential or lower co-payments for generics over brands also encourage patients to ask for generic substitution, and are extensively used by managed care in the USA as part of reference pricing systems linked to co-payments, as described above. This has yet to take hold in the EU mainly because generic substitution for a branded prescription is not allowed in most EU countries. In the UK, the government's promotion of generic prescribing by doctors has been so successful that generic substitution may make little further saving. There are other opposing factors: the extent of use of branded generics and low priced original brands impede the extent of price competition. Although evidence suggests that price competition with the right combination of demand-side incentives does stimulate price competitiveness, many EU governments nevertheless choose to regulate the prices of generics directly (UK) or indirectly through reference price schemes.

Some EU member states have less explicit financial incentives for generic prescribing but do mandate responsibility to inform patients of cheaper generic alternatives to either physicians (as in Sweden) or pharmacists (as in Denmark) (see Chapter 14). Evidence seems to point to the finding that financial incentives for physicians, pharmacists and consumers towards demand-side cost-awareness may be more effective than regulating prices of generic products (see Chapter 14).

Medicines that can be obtained without prescription from a medical practitioner are termed over-the-counter (OTC) pharmaceuticals. This is already the largest sector of medicines use as measured by numbers of patients treated (see Chapter 15). The sale of OTC products might require pharmacist supervision or they may be for general sale. In the past, reclassifying medicines to OTC status required good reasons; the climate now is the reverse. There must now be good reasons not to reclassify medicines as OTCs, such as a need for medical supervision to prevent direct or indirect dangers to health, potential for misuse, lack of thorough scientific investigation, or a need to be parenterally administered (see Chapter 15). The motivation behind this reallocation is to enhance patient access to medicines; to shift drug distribution costs from governments to individual consumers; and to encourage greater public responsibility in self-medication. Product selection in this market has traditionally been based on experience of benefit and safety reported by customers, personal previous use, advertisements, lay advice, and professional advice from general practitioners, nurses and pharmacists.

There remain important economic and equity issues here. Achieving overall cost savings requires that the consumer can both diagnose the condition correctly as well as identify the correct treatment, whether it is an OTC product or not. Available data show that this may not always be the case (Brass 2001). Furthermore, the equity dimension is an essential consideration; if deregulation from prescription-only to OTC removes a drug from the list reimbursed, then those with low ability to pay or cope with these changes may suffer adversely and, again, cost the system overall more than intended.

Industry is often keen to promote OTC switches at a late stage of a product's life cycle, as it expands the market, especially at a time when a drug is coming off patent and facing generic competition, and allows direct-to-consumer advertising, perhaps reinforcing brand loyalty. This may increase pressure on general practitioners and other prescribers from patients as consumers demanding certain products, especially if the cost of a prescription charge is less than the price of the OTC product, or if the patient were exempt from the prescription charge. The impact of newly deregulated products has been observed in early health economics research to generate significant government savings in some but not all drug-associated costs (Berndt *et al.* 2000). Generally, patients have been receptive to deregulation of medicines to OTC status, even though one of the objectives in deregulation has, in fact, been to increase their financial burden. Doctors, too, seem amenable to this idea, especially in the area of medicines for 'social' decisions, such as emergency contraception or smoking cessation, although in other areas (e.g. dyspepsia treatments) deregulation has made little difference to prescribed drug use (see Chapter 15).

In some countries, the OTC market has extended the role of the pharmacist. For products requiring 'pharmacist supervision', community pharmacists must ensure compliance with the licensed indications of the OTC products, assessing the potential for drug interactions, and avoiding sales to patients with contra-indications. Difficulties arise when patients are not aware of this role for the pharmacists and are resistant to their professional advice. This may be exacerbated in cases where the patient wants a medication for a purpose outside the OTC licence (e.g. hydrocortisone 1 per cent is often purchased to be used on the face, although this is outside the OTC licence) (see Chapter 15).

Pharmaceutical products receive continuous monitoring even when fully deregulated to OTC status through the use of spontaneous reporting, event monitoring and specific surveillance. In spite of these measures, pharmacovigilance monitoring for OTC products is especially difficult because of the lack of detailed records on product users and the rationale for use.

Genetics and pharmaceuticals

The regulation, consumption and potential reimbursement of other areas of drug therapy pose problems for policy makers; one such area is the application of pharmacogenetics and pharmacogenomics. Pharmacogenetics is defined as the study of the variability of drug responses due to heredity (one gene, many drugs), while pharmacogenomics includes the study of all genes within the human genome that may determine drug response, and the effects of different compounds on gene expression (see Chapter 16).

Pharmacogenetics could be valuable in predicting likelihood of response or adverse effects to a drug therapy in an individual. Already, innovations in genetics have altered the medical landscape and have – at least in the field of screening – provided a significant amount of information about individuals, previously only available at the onset of disease. Yet advances and widespread accessibility of these tests may create further demands on health systems that may not be prepared (Jones 2000). The use of individual genetic information also raises problems of confidentiality, stigmatization and insurance, thus creating changes in the balance of responsibility between the individual, the family, the community and the medical practice. Most diseases are not single gene in origin but the result of an interaction between genetic profile and environment, so such tests for the most part will be predictive rather than completely diagnostic.

Pharmacogenomics can potentially enable the creation of medicines working from the gene to target protein to potential drug, rather than the more traditional approach of working backwards from pathophysiology. Examining the effects of different compounds on gene expression may ultimately lead to target identification and drug discovery, and will impact on pre-clinical drug development and clinical trials.

These advances may lead to drug development for well-defined but small populations, increasing drug effectiveness but also reducing the size of the market and increasing the burden of research and development onto fewer patients. At present, however, such therapies have only a minor role in clinical practice no matter how awesome their prospects in the laboratory environment. When examining any new technology, policy makers are concerned with the associated costs, benefits, and social and ethical issues. When considering genetics, these observations may be more uncertain. Regulatory agencies such as the EMEA and the FDA will have to establish new guidelines encompassing this new technology to govern the process of clinical trials, licensing and labelling of these products and related tests.

Lifestyle drugs and alternative medicines

Another contentious area is that of pharmaceuticals used for what is pejoratively termed 'lifestyle' benefits, and complementary and alternative medicines. Drugs used to tackle 'non-health' problems, to improve one's lifestyle, or to treat health problems caused by one's habits, then, can be termed 'lifestyle drugs'. These can include pharmaceuticals for erectile dysfunction (Sildenafil), obesity (Orlistat), smoking cessation (Bupropion) and other afflictions. A key issue here is the definition of disease and health need. While the World Health Organization defines health as a state of total physical, mental and social well-being, it is unclear if the mandate of governments is to operationalize this definition in allocating health care resources. Cultural and social norms also influence the point at which a health-related problem becomes a 'disease'. The distinction between 'pain avoiding' and 'pleasure seeking' may point to what governments should and should not be expected to provide. While 'pain-avoiding' measures may allow individuals to reach a social reference point of health or functioning (and is a collective rather than merely personal responsibility), 'pleasure-seeking' measures are those that individuals may desire that go beyond that social reference point (see Chapter 17). This would allow funding of, for instance, treatments for sexually transmitted diseases or impotence due to diabetes but not, for instance, for enhancement of sexual prowess, although all might be deemed in some way to be lifestyle issues.

Given the limited resources and the desire for cost containment of pharmaceutical expenditure by public health authorities, lifestyle drugs are necessarily rationed. To determine whether public funding should subsidize these interventions, prudent decision-making principles should be applied. Useful principles for establishing national criteria for priority setting were detailed by the Dutch government's Committee on Choices in Healthcare in the Dunning Report (Government Committee on Choices in Health Care 1992). These include the demonstration of effectiveness, efficiency (cost-effectiveness), necessary care and public responsibility. The first two criteria are technical and can be demonstrated in the licensing or reimbursement process; the latter two are based on value judgements, thus generating an ethical dilemma.

An outright ban on the reimbursement of lifestyle drugs is probably less effective than allowing some exceptions (Klein and Sturm 2002). Exclusions (no reimbursement) can still be made in paying for drugs when the patient both diagnoses their condition and demands their chosen medication; while exceptions (reimbursement) can be made when a physician has been involved in expressing a genuine need for the pharmaceutical product. Furthermore, when the medical profession is included in devising the criteria for rationing, they are able to maintain their decision-making autonomy while continuously under the constraints of capped budgets, as in the UK. Key issues are how to ensure that patients are well-informed consumers of such drugs, and how to engage the public in debate about defining the limits of (publicly funded) medical therapy.

Some of the same concerns apply to complementary and alternative medicines (CAM), which supplement or transcend conventional medical treatment, such as homoeopathy, or herbal medicine. In addition, there is a major problem in the poor evidence base to support the use of these products. The market for alternative medicines is significant and growing; for example, it was worth US$18 billion in the USA in 1997 (more than 50 per cent paid by patients directly; Morris and Avorn 2003) and £450 million in the UK in 1998 (more than 90 per cent purchased privately; Coulter 2003). While usage is difficult to quantify, some literature suggests that lifetime prevalence use of alternative and complementary medicines may be as high as 40–50 per cent in the UK. These trends are likely to be caused by patient discontent with mainstream medicine, anti-science attitudes, or desperation in the case of chronic illness. In Europe, most spending on CAM is by direct out-of-pocket payments by consumers and will likely remain this way given the lack of organized evidence of efficacy and the focus on cost containment.

Alternative medicine in many countries has often not involved the medical profession, as in the UK, although this is less the case in Germany. This makes integration into the UK NHS a challenge, even though this is part of the official NHS agenda (House of Lords Select Committee 2000). In fact, this separation from the medical profession may be precisely what gives CAM its appeal, as CAM practitioners offer more holistic (and less time-limited consultations) approaches to illness (Coulter 2003). Because CAM encompasses such a sweeping number of interventions, the ability to reach consensus on its effectiveness and efficacy is limited. It seems that while the public has been eager and sometimes politically assertive in pushing for greater acceptance, the scientific community and mainstream medicine have been much more cool towards CAM due to the lack of systematic evidence (Ernst 2002, 2003a,b). Reviews of data both from laboratory research and randomized controlled clinical trials show that some homeopathic remedies are extremely questionable in terms of efficacy, and that existing data are largely plagued with weak or poor evidence (Jonas *et al.* 2003). Here again, acceptance of CAM varies widely in different countries, and courses in unconventional medicine are obligatory in many medical faculties across Europe (Baberis *et al.* 2001).

A second reason for the diminished enthusiasm for CAM from the traditional scientific community may be fear of loss of medical dominance. While doctors have traditionally been the final arbiters of medicine and health care, the potential role of CAM to acquire more authority is a barrier to its acceptance (Coulter 2003). Inherent in this process is a changing dynamic in the doctor–patient relationship, where patients may feel that doctors are trying to limit the use of potentially effective treatments. Doctors, however, may feel that they are protecting patients' interests by prescribing only those medications and therapies that have been rigorously tested (Ernst 2003a).

The regulation of alternative medicines has been piecemeal. Herbal medicines can currently be licensed through the conventional procedures for drug approval; in 2004, however, EU regulation on traditional herbal medicines is expected to be implemented. To achieve a European traditional use licence, an applicant must demonstrate through bibliographic or expert evidence the medicinal use of the product in the EU for 30 years. The Committee for Herbal Medicinal Products (Commission of the European Communities 2002) is expected to be set up within the EMEA to create a positive list of approved products, require similar standards for quality and labelling as conventional pharmaceutical products, and outline the relevant information on therapeutic indications, strength, route of admission and safety of the traditional use herbal medicines. Systematic labelling with phrases such as 'efficacy not proven' will also be required (Barnes 2001). For homeopathic medicines, the EU does not require details on safety or efficacy if the product is amply diluted, but does regulate the quality of these products. In the long run, maintaining high requirements for CAM as well as the same amount of scrutiny (as well as consideration) given to other, more traditional therapies can only serve patient, doctor and payer interests.

With regard to the public funding of these medicines, the picture is variable: many are available over the counter and are so inexpensive that there is little public provision. In some countries like Germany, these therapies are widely provided from public funds. In others, the lack of a strong evidence base for their efficacy has discouraged their provision.

Conclusions

There are many different approaches to regulating pharmaceuticals in Europe that affect public policy objectives to control costs while improving efficiency, quality of care and equity. International comparisons may contribute to a better understanding of how different measures and policies are implemented. However, there are significant limitations to the relevance and transferability of lessons and policies across countries. Contextual factors such as the social, economic, medical, health care and political environment, as well as constraints of history and institutional frameworks, play a major role in how policies are developed and implemented in practice. This is particularly important for EU member states, not only because of national regulation but also supranational regulations. A policy adopted in one country, therefore, may not necessarily work, or at least not to the same extent, in another and may need to be modified to the new context. As described before, it is often difficult to be clear on which component of a diverse range of measures undertaken was most successful. Given these two factors, deriving any sense of which of the many possible interventions are most effective is difficult. A further complication is that governments must consider those policies already in place and their effects before new policies are adopted. Trade-offs between competing policy objectives (health versus industrial) or the needs of different stakeholders (patients, health professionals, industry) are inevitable.

Governments in Europe are all faced with rising pharmaceutical expenditures but have taken widely divergent approaches to tackling these. Some government policies that enhance quality of care, efficiency or access may decrease the ability to contain expenditures. Rising expenditures of themselves may not be a problem if they are accompanied by health gain or by a similar rise in government revenues. In practice, the added health gain for added expenditure is often unclear, and the rate of rise of expenditure often exceeds revenue, so governments are forced to act. At the same time, they must aim not just to contain costs but to improve the efficiency and quality of the health service, and preserve or enhance equity. Any approach to cost containment, therefore, has to be evaluated in terms of its effects in these four dimensions.

From the review presented here, it is clear that no single policy approach acts without a trade-off on the impact along these four dimensions, in addition to competing trade-offs between the objectives of the policies themselves. Therefore, a policy maker needs to be clear what primary impact is desired, but conscious of where a subsequent negative impact of any policy may arise in other dimensions; if the impact of the trade-off along the other evaluative areas outweighs the gains in the primary indicator, a policy must be reconsidered.

Considering these four dimensions, it is clear that most of the measures intended to contain costs do have an impact; however, the extent of any cost savings or their sustainability over the longer term is variable – for example, GP fundholding and associated incentives in the UK (Chapter 10) or reference pricing in Germany (Chapter 6). In fact, in most cases the cost savings generated by any one policy are either limited or short-term. The most effective approaches work best when combined with other policy measures. For instance, price controls alone have a limited effect, but are more successful when policy measures are applied to the volume side of the expenditure equation as well.

In general, few of the measures demonstrate a clear efficiency gain, in part due to a lack of rigorous studies. This is often, however, a key aim of government polices – containing costs without any diminution in quality. One that does succeed in this regard is generic prescribing or substitution (Chapter 14). Academic detailing (Chapter 8) might increase quality, equity and effectiveness by encouraging the application of evidence-based medicine. It might increase costs by encouraging appropriate treatment where previously there was undertreatment, or decrease costs where there was overtreatment or waste. Of the interventions considered here, it is probably the most professionally acceptable. The use of economic evaluation or wider health technology assessment may improve efficiency, but may increase overall costs (see Chapter 7). Some policies might inadvertently seriously decrease efficiency – for example, if saving money on drugs leads to more hospital admissions, as has been clearly seen in one case in the USA (Soumerai *et al.* 1991) and as allegedly happened in Germany in the early 1990s in response to GP budgets. This illustrates the need to consider the broader effects, including efficiency, in evaluating any intervention.

Policies aimed solely at cost containment might reduce equity, but if the aim of cost containment (e.g. increasing prescribing of generics) is to reduce unnecessary expenditure so as to allow access to other therapies, then cost containment could increase equity. In general, policies for the rational use of medicines would be expected to result in improvements in equity at an aggregate level. Policies such as reference pricing and prescription co-payments (Chapter 13) may reduce equity, unless there are exemptions to protect more vulnerable patients; used carefully (e.g. differential user charges), these interventions can increase efficiency and decrease cost, without damaging quality and with minimal disruption to equity.

The quality of care dimension is usually raised as a primary objective of some measures that target the rational use of medicines (Chapter 8). In these, cost is secondary and in fact some measures may increase costs. This raises the difficult balance faced by policy makers in this sector to secure quality, maintain equity and improve efficiency, but yet contain costs.

It is clear that there is no perfect solution to balancing these four dimensions in the pharmaceutical sector. Even if one is sure where the balance should lie, no one policy or policy combination is right for all countries. Different countries will need to meet their own objectives and needs through policy approaches that reflect their particular environment.

Nevertheless, there are some general principles of best practice that policy makers should keep in mind. First, the objective of the policy must be clear from the outset, and consideration must be given to its possible impact on all of the evaluative dimensions of efficiency, equity, quality and cost. Rigorous price control schemes seem to have an impact on controlling prices, but controlling price alone, if this can be achieved, does not necessarily improve efficiency, nor does it necessarily control total expenditures (see Chapter 6). Attention to the demand side and the promotion of rational drug use is vital if efficiency, equity and quality are also to be improved. New drugs and changes in product mix will certainly drive drug expenditure in the future. The policy community at large needs to consider how we define and reward clinically valuable innovation, so that drug expenditure reflects the value of the drug's benefits for society. The future will require a greater partnership between all stakeholders if the solidarity of socialized pharmaceutical care is to be maintained despite greater needs and constrained resources.

Notes

1 The stabilization (or reduction, in the case or Ireland) of pharmaceutical expenditure as a percentage of GDP in some countries may not reflect success in controlling growth in pharmaceutical spending but rather may be a function of economic growth. For example, pharmaceutical expenditure in Ireland grew by an annual average of 6.4 per cent from 1990 to 2000 and the economy grew by 7.3 per cent. Conversely, in Denmark, Finland, France and Italy, pharmaceutical expenditure grew faster than GDP between 1990 and 2000.
2 Available from http://www.emea.eu.int.
3 This may, in some cases, include higher expenditure on R&D, which may be a positive factor.

References

Abel-Smith, B. and Grandjeat, P. (1978) *Pharmaceutical Consumption*. Brussels: Commission of the European Communities.

Averch, H. and Johnson, L. (1962) Behaviour of firms under regulatory constraint, *American Economic Review*, 52: 1052–69.

Avorn, J. and Soumerai, S. (1983) Improving drug-therapy decisions through educational outreach: a randomized controlled trial of academically based 'detailing', *New England Journal of Medicine*, 308: 1457–63.

Baberis, L., de Toni, E., Schiavone, M., Zicca, A. and Ghio, R. (2001) Unconventional medicine teaching at the Universities of the European Union, *Journal of Alternative and Complementary Medicine*, 7(4): 337–43.

Barber, N. (1995) What constitutes good prescribing?, *British Medical Journal*, 310: 923–5.

Barnes, J. (2001) Developments in the regulation of herbal medicinal products: requirements and features of the 'traditional use' directive (2nd draft), *Pharmaceutical Journal*, 266(7151): 794.

Barry, C.A., Bradley, C.P., Britten, N., Stevenson, F.A. and Barber, N. (2000) Patients' unvoiced agendas in general practice consultations: qualitative study, *British Medical Journal*, 320: 1246–50.

Berndt, E.R., Ling, D., Kyle, M.K. and Finkelstein, S.N. (2000) The long shadow of patent expiration: do Rx to OTC switches provide an afterlife? Paper presented at the *National Bureau of Economic Research Conference on Research in Income and Wealth*, September, Arlington, VA.

Brass, E.P. (2001) Changing the status of drugs from prescription to over-the-counter availability, *New England Journal of Medicine*, 345(11): 810–16.

Brougham, M., Metcalfe, S. and McNee, W. (2002) Our advice? Get a budget!, *Healthcare Papers*, 3(1): 83–5.

Burton, R. and Rowell, A. (2003) Unhealthy spin, *British Medical Journal*, 326: 1205–7.

Carter, A.O., Battista, R.N., Hodge, M.J. *et al.* (1995) Proceedings of the 1994 Canadian Clinical Practice Guidelines Network Workshop, *Canadian Medical Association Journal*, 153: 1715–19.

Cheah, T.S. (1998) The impact of clinical guidelines and clinical pathways on medical practice: effectiveness and medico-legal aspects, *Annals of the Academy of Medicine, Singapore*, 27(4): 533–9.

Cipolle, R.J., Strand, L.M. and Morley, P.C. (1998) *Pharmaceutical Care Practice*. New York: McGraw-Hill.

Collier, J. and Iheanacho, I. (2002) The pharmaceutical industry as an informant, *Lancet*, 260: 1405–9.

Commission of the European Communities (2002) *Proposal for a Directive of the European Parliament and of the Council: amending the Directive 2001/83/EC as regards traditional herbal medicinal products*. Brussels: 2002/0008 (COD).

Cookson, R., McDaid, D. and Maynard, A. (2001) Wrong SIGN, NICE mess: is national guidance distorting allocation of resources?, *British Medical Journal*, 323: 743–5.

Coulter, A. (2003) Killing the goose that laid the golden egg?, *British Medical Journal*, 326: 1280–1.

Council of the European Communities (1989) Council Directive 89/105/EEC of 21 December 1988 relating to the transparency of measures regulating the prices of medicinal products for human use and their inclusion in the scope of national health insurance systems, *Official Journal*, L40, 11.02.1989: 8–11.

Dardano, K.L. (2000) Contraceptive compliance, *Obstetrics and Gynecology Clinics of North America*, 27(4): 933–41.

Davis, P. (1996) *Contested Ground: Public Purpose and Private Interest in the Regulation of Prescription Drugs*. New York: Oxford University Press.

Davis, P. (1997) *Managing Medicines: Public Policy and Therapeutic Drugs*. Buckingham: Open University Press.

Denig, P. and Haaijer-Ruskamp, F.M. (1995) Do physicians take cost into account when making prescribing decisions?, *Pharmacoeconomics*, 8(4): 282–90.

Department of Health UK (1999) *The Pharmaceutical Price Regulation Scheme*. London: Department of Health (available from http://www.doh.gov.uk/pprs.htm).

Divine, G.W., Brown, J.T. and Frazier, L.M. (1992) The unit of analysis error in studies about physicians' patient care behaviour, *Journal of General Internal Medicine*, 7: 623–9.

Donaldson, L. (2002) Expert patients usher in a new era of opportunity for the NHS, *British Medical Journal*, 326: 1279.

Donatini, A., Rico, A., D'Ambrosio, M.G. *et al.* (2001) *Health Care Systems in Transition: Italy*. Copenhagen: European Observatory on Health Care Systems.

Dovey, S.M., Meyers, D.S., Phillips, R.L., Jr. *et al.* (2002) A preliminary taxonomy of medical errors in family practice, *Quality and Safety in Health Care*, 11(3): 233–8.

Dovey, S.M., Phillips, R.L., Green, L.A. and Fryer, G.E. (2003) Types of medical errors commonly reported by family physicians, *American Family Physician*, 67(4): 697.

Drummond, M. and Pang, F. (2001) Transferability of economic evaluation results, in M. Drummond and A. McGuire (eds) *Economic Evaluation in Health Care: Merging Theory with Practice*. Oxford: Oxford University Press.

Drummond, M., O'Brien, B., Stoddart, G. and Torrance, G. (1997a) *Methods for the Economic Evaluation of Health Care Programmes*. Oxford: Oxford University Press.

Drummond, M., Jonsson, B. and Rutten, F. (1997b) The role of economic evaluation in the pricing and reimbursement of medicines, *Health Policy*, 40(3): 199–215.

Dukes, G., Haaijer, F., Joncheere, C. and Rietveld, A. (2003) *Drugs and Money: Prices, Affordability and Cost Containment*. Amsterdam: IOS Press.

Durieux, P., Chaix-Couturier, C., Durand-Zaleski, I. and Ravaud, P. (2000) From clinical recommendations to mandatory practice, *International Journal of Technology Assessment in Health Care*, 16(4): 969–75.

Ernst, E. (2002) A systematic review of systematic reviews of homeopathy, *British Journal of Clinical Pharmacology*, 54(6): 577–82.

Ernst, E. (2003a) Panel discussions about CAM and research: science and friction, *Complementary Therapies in Nursing and Midwifery*, 9: 81–2.

Ernst, E. (2003b) Weighing the homeopathic evidence, *Homeopathy*, 92(6): 67–8.

Evans, R.G., Barer, M.L. and Stoddart, G.L. (1995) User fees for health care: why a bad idea keeps coming back, *Canadian Journal on Aging*, 14(2): 360–90.

Fernandes, R. (2002) Managing healthcare costs within an integrated framework. *Healthcare Papers*, 3(1): 70–6.

Ferrando, C., Henman, M.C. and Corrigan, O.I. (1987) Impact of a nationwide limited prescribing list: preliminary findings. *Drug Intelligence and Clinical Pharmacy*, 21: 653–8.

Fletcher, R.H. (1989) Patient compliance with therapeutic advice: a modern view, *Mount Sinai Journal of Medicine*, 56(6): 453–8.

Freemantle, N. (2000) Implementation strategies, *Family Practice*, 17(suppl. 1): S7–S10.

Freemantle, N., Nazareth, I., Eccles, M., Wood, J. and Haines, A. (2002) A randomised controlled trial of the effect of educational outreach by community pharmacists on prescribing in UK general practice, *British Journal of General Practice*, 52: 290–5.

Gandjour, A. and Lauterbach, K.W. (2001) A method for assessing the cost-effectiveness and the break-even point of clinical practice guidelines, *International Journal of Technology Assessment in Health Care*, 17(4): 503–16.

Garattini, S. and Bertele', V. (2001) Adjusting Europe's drug regulation to public health needs, *Lancet*, 358: 64–7.

Garattini, S. and Bertele', V. (2002) Efficacy, safety, and cost of new anticancer drugs, *British Medical Journal*, 325: 269–71.

Garattini, S. and Garattini, L. (1998) Discrepancy remains in pharmaceutical prescriptions in four European countries, *British Medical Journal*, 317: 947.

Garfield, F.B. and Garfield, J.M. (2000) Clinical judgment and clinical practice guidelines, *International Journal of Technology Assessment in Health Care*, 16(4): 1050–60.

Garlick, W. (2003) Should drug companies be allowed to talk directly to patients? NO, *British Medical Journal*, 326: 1302–4.

Giuffrida, A. and Torgerson, D.J. (1997) Should we pay the patient? Review of financial incentives to enhance patient compliance, *British Medical Journal*, 315: 703–7.

Giuliani, G., Selke, G. and Garattini, L. (1998) The German experience in reference pricing, *Health Policy*, 44: 73–85.

Goodwin, N. (1998) GP fundholding, in J. Le Grand, N. Mays and J. Mullligan (eds) *Learning from the NHS Internal Market: A Review of the Evidence*. London: King's Fund.

Government Committee on Choices in Health Care (1992) *Report*. The Hague: Ministry of Welfare, Health and Cultural Affairs.

Gundersen, L. (2000) The effect of clinical practice guidelines on variations in care, *Annals of Internal Medicine*, 133: 317.

Hetlevik, I., Holmen, J., Krüger, O. *et al.* (2000) Implementing clinical guidelines in the treatment of diabetes mellitus in general practice, *International Journal of Technology Assessment in Health Care*, 16: 210–27.

Herxheimer, A. (2003) Relationships between the pharmaceutical industry and patients' organisations, *British Medical Journal*, 326: 1208–10.

Hoffman, J. and Wilkes, M. (1999) Direct to consumer advertising of prescription drugs: an idea whose time should not come, *British Medical Journal*, 318: 1301–2.

House of Lords Select Committee on Science and Technology (2000) *6th Report*. London: HMSO.

Jacobzone, S. (2000) *Labour Market and Social Policy*. Occasional Papers No. 40. Pharmaceutical Policies In OECD Countries: Reconciling Social and Industrial Goals. Paris: OECD.

Jonas, W.B., Kaptchuk, T.J. and Linde, K. (2003) A critical overview of homeopathy, *Annals of Internal Medicine*, 138: 393–9.

Jones, S. (2000) *Genetics in Medicine: Real Promises, Unreal Expectations*. Report of the Milbank Memorial Fund. New York: Milbank Memorial Fund.

Jones, T. (2003) Should drug companies be allowed to talk directly to patients? YES, *British Medical Journal*, 326: 1302.

Kaveh, K. (2001) Compliance in hemodialysis patients: multidimensional measures in search of a gold standard, *American Journal of Kidney Disease*, 37(2): 244–66.

Klein, R. and Sturm, H. (2002) Viagra: a success story for rationing?, *Health Affairs*, 21(6): 177–87.

Kohn, L.T., Corrigan, J.M. and Donaldson, M.S. (eds) (2000) *To Err is Human: Building a Safer health system*. Washington, DC: National Academy Press.

Laupacis, A., Anderson, G. and O'Brien, B. (2002) Drug policy: making effective drugs available without bankrupting the healthcare system *Healthcare Papers*, 3(1): 12–30.

Lesar, T.S., Briceland, L. and Stein, D.S. (1997) Factors related to errors in medication prescribing, *Journal of the American Medical Association*, 277(4): 312–17.

Levy, A.R. and Gagnon, Y.M. (2002) Getting the cat back in the bag: reforming the way provinces manage drug expenditures to make them manageable, *Healthcare Papers*, 3(1): 32–7.

Lopez Bastida, J. and Mossialos, E. (2000) Pharmaceutical expenditure in Spain: cost and control, *International Journal of Health Services Research*, 30: 597–616.

Lopez-Casasnovas, G. and Puig-Junoy, J. (2000) Review of the literature on reference pricing, *Health Policy*, 54(2): 87–123.

Lynch, B. (2003) Capecitabine [National Institute for 3-Year Delay?] Rapid response, *British Medical Journal* (available from http://bmj.com/cgi/eletters/326/7400/1166-d#32783).

Mason, J., Freemantle, N., Nazareth, I. *et al.* (2001) When is it cost-effective to change the behavior of health professionals?, *Journal of the American Medical Association*, 286(23): 2988–92.

Meulemans, H., Mortelmans, D., Liefooghe, R. *et al.* (2002) The limits to patient compliance with directly observed therapy for tuberculosis: a socio-medical study in Pakistan, *International Journal of Health Planning and Management*, 17(3): 249–67.

Morris, C.A. and Avorn, J. (2003) Internet marketing of herbal products, *Journal of the American Medical Association*, 290: 1505–9.

Mossialos, E. (1997) An evaluation of the PPRS: is there a need for reform? in D. Green (ed.) *Should Pharmaceutical Prices be Regulated?* London: Institute of Economic Affairs.

Mossialos, E. and Le Grand, J. (1999) *Health Care and Cost Containment in the European Union*. Aldershot: Ashgate.

Mossialos, E., Kanavos, P. and Abel-Smith, B. (1994) *Policy Options for Pharmaceutical Research and Development in the European Community*. Brussels: European Parliament.

Moynihan, R. (2003a) Who pays for the pizza? Redefining the relationships between doctors and drug companies. 1: Entanglement, *British Medical Journal*, 326: 1189–92.

Moynihan, R. (2003b) Who pays for the pizza? Redefining the relationships between doctors and drug companies. 2: Disentanglement, *British Medical Journal*, 326: 1193–6.

Moynihan, R. (2003c) Drug company sponsorship of education could be replaced at a fraction of its cost, *British Medical Journal*, 326: 1163.

Mrazek, M. (2001). The impact of different regulatory frameworks on competition in post-patent pharmaceutical markets in the United Kingdom, Germany and the United States, 1990 to 1997. PhD thesis, London School of Economics, London.

Mrazek, M.F. and Mossialos, E. (2002) Methods for monitoring and evaluating processes and outcomes, *International Journal of Risk and Safety in Medicine*, 15(1–2): 55–66.

Nefarma (2002) *Market Data: Drugs Use in International Perspective*. Annual Report. The Hague: Nefarma.

OECD (2002) *OECD Health Data 2002*. Paris: OECD.

Oliver, A., Mossialos, E.A. and Robinson, R. (2004) Health technology assessment and its influence on health care priority setting, *International Journal of Technology Assessment in Health Care*, 20(1): 1–10.

Payer, L. (1988) *Medicine and Culture*. New York: Henry Holt & Co.

Perleth, M., Jakubowski, E. and Busse, R. (2001) What is 'best practice' in health care? State of the art and perspectives in improving the effectiveness and efficiency of the European health care systems, *Health Policy*, 56(3): 235–50.

Phillips, D.P. and Bredder, C.C. (2002) Morbidity and mortality from medical errors: an increasingly serious public health problem, *Annual Review of Public Health*, 23: 135–50.

Ray, W.A., Griffin, M.R. and Avorn, J. (1993) Evaluating drugs after their approval for clinical use, *New England Journal of Medicine*, 329: 2029–32.

Richman, R. and Lancaster, D.R. (2000) The clinical guideline process within a managed care organization, *International Journal of Technology Assessment in Health Care*, 16(4): 1061–76.

Robertson, W.H. (1985) The problem of patient compliance, *American Journal of Obstetrics and Gynecology*, 152(7 Pt. 2): 948–52.

Robinson, J. (2001) Theory and practice in the design of physician payment incentives, *Milbank Quarterly*, 79(2): 149–77.

Rosian, I., Antony, K., Habl, C., Vogler, S. and Weigl, M. (2001) *Benchmarking Pharmaceutical Expenditure: Cost Containment Strategies in the European Union*. Vienna: Osterreichisches Bundesinstitute fur Gesundheitswesen (ÖBIG).

Sansgiry, S., Sharp, W.T. and Sansgiry, S.S. (1999) Accuracy of information on printed over-the-counter drug advertisements, *Health Marketing Quarterly*, 17(2): 7–18.

Schneeweiss, S., Walker, A.M., Glynn, R.J. *et al.* (2002a) Outcomes of reference pricing for angiotensin-converting-enzyme inhibitors, *New England Journal of Medicine*, 346: 822–9.

Schneeweiss, S., Maclure, M., Dormuth, C. and Avorn, J. (2002b) Pharmaceutical cost containment with reference-based pricing: time for refinements, *Canadian Medical Association Journal*, 167: 1250–1.

Shojania, K.G., Duncan, B.W., McDonald, K.M. and Wachter, R.M. (eds) (2001) *Making Health Care Safer: A Critical Analysis of Patient Safety Practices, Agency for Healthcare Research and Quality*. Evidence Report/Technology Assessment No. 43. Washington, DC: US Department of Health and Human Services.

Singh, D. (2003) Drug companies advised to publish unfavourable trial results, *British Medical Journal*, 326: 1163.

Smith, R. (2003) Medical journals and pharmaceutical companies: uneasy bedfellows, *British Medical Journal*, 326: 1202–5.

Soumerai, S.B. and Avorn, J. (1990) Principles of educational outreach ('academic detailing') to improve clinical decision-making, *Journal of the American Medical Association*, 263: 549–56.

Soumerai, S.B., Ross-Degnan, D., Avorn, J., McLaughlin, T. and Choodnovskiy, I. (1991) Effects of Medicaid drug-payment limits on admission to hospitals and nursing homes, *New England Journal of Medicine*, 325: 1072–7.

Soumerai, S.B., McLaughlin, T.J., Ross-Degnan, D., Casteris, C.S. and Bollini, P. (1998) Effect of local medical opinion leaders on quality of care for acute myocardial infarction: a randomized controlled trial, *Journal of the American Medical Association*, 279: 1358–63.

Taggiasco, N., Sarrut, B. and Doreau, C.G. (1992) European survey of independent drug information centres, *Annals of Pharmacotherapy*, 26: 422–8.

Taxis, K. and Barber, N. (2003) Ethnographic study of incidence and severity of intravenous drug errors, *British Medical Journal*, 326: 684.

Wager, E. (2003) How to dance with porcupines: rules and guidelines on doctors' relations with drug companies, *British Medical Journal*, 326: 1196–8.

Woloshin, S., Schwartz, L.M., Tremmel, J. and Welch, H.G. (2001) Direct-to-consumer advertisements for prescription drugs: what are Americans being sold?, *Lancet*, 358: 1141–6.

Yuen, P. (1999). *Compendium of Health Statistics*, 11th edn. London: Office for Health Economics.

two

The politics of pharmaceuticals in the European Union

Govin Permanand and
Christa Altenstetter

Introduction

This chapter is an overview of the 'politics' of the pharmaceutical sector in the European Union (EU). By focusing on how medicines policy is achieved within the context of having to serve three often competing inputs – public health, health care and industrial policy – we consider the political factors at stake in regulating the EU pharmaceutical sector in both national and supranational environments. We have two complementary objectives. The first is to understand the complex issues at stake at both national and supranational levels. This involves not just capturing the nature of the policy conflict but also the interests and roles of several vested interests. The second and underlying objective is to show the difficulty in achieving a European single market in medicines. More specifically, we argue that the conflicting policy inputs and the differences between the member states in addressing them, the actors and political elements involved, combined with the uncertainty over what a fully harmonized market would mean for the member states, result in the continuing lack of a single market in medicines. In this chapter, therefore, we offer a general discussion of the politics of medicines within the EU context, rather than a detailed explanatory discourse on an as-yet unrealized unified market.

The discussion is divided into four sections. The first outlines the challenge in serving the three policy inputs, identifying the conflict between health care and industrial policy priorities (most notably over medicine pricing) as the most politically exigent issue for policy makers; especially given the interests of other important players. So although all member states seek to maximize allocative efficiency in the health care versus industrial policy challenge, they have different priorities and different regimes. The next section looks at member state and EU regulatory prerogatives – where pharmaceutical regulation is a joint competence – and considers the dissonance between national and supranational designs for the sector. The third section highlights the diverse nature of government–industry (power) relations and stresses the highly politicized nature of the sector, particularly in relation to the issue of cost containment. Here the roles and impact of other actors are highlighted against that of industry. The final section recaps the main issues, summarizing how these factors currently impede the emergence of a single European pharmaceuticals market.

Balancing multiple policy interests

In light of the three policy inputs, policy makers face overlapping and at times competing regulatory tasks (Table 2.1). Foremost is a responsibility to the consumer in terms of guaranteeing that only safe, good-quality and efficacious medicines make it to market. Next is the balancing of health care budgets with regard to controlling health expenditures and drug costs. And third, in many countries, given the economic contribution of the sector, is to promote a regulatory environment conducive to business. Additionally, pharmaceuticals reflect several market features that necessitate further government intervention. These include the unique demand structure whereby the patient neither chooses nor

Table 2.1 Competing pharmaceutical policy interests*

Health care policy	Industrial policy	Public health policy
• Cost containment and improving efficiency in health services and care • Cost-effective medication • Regulating doctor and consumer behaviour *vis-à-vis* medicines • Generic promotion and/or substitution • Improving prescribing • Ensuring access to medicines	• Promoting local research and development capacity • Intellectual property rights protection • Supporting local scientific community • Generating and protecting employment • Promoting small and medium enterprise policies • Contributing to positive trade balance • Sustaining the university research base	• Safe medicines • High-quality preparations • Efficacious treatments • Innovative cures • Patient access to medicines

* A simple listing; does not indicate priority.
Source: Permanand (2002).

pays for the medicines they consume – doctors prescribe and a third party (generally via some form of medical scheme) tends to bear most of the cost – and the nature of competition where, in some sub-markets, one or two leading companies can dominate therapeutic categories. The world market for statins,[1] for instance, is dominated by just two products: Pfizer's Lipitor and Merck's Zocor account for 42 and 32 per cent of the global market, respectively (Simons 2003). Such market concentration, when combined with unusually strict and extended patent rights[2] – particularly in the EU through the 1992 Supplementary Protection Certificate legislation (Council of the European Communities 1992) – means that governments intervene also to prevent the emergence of monopolies. Although such concentration does not on its own differentiate medicines from other markets, the inextricable link to public health means that the regulatory imperative is very different.

A central element when considering the politics of pharmaceuticals is the widely acknowledged conflict between health care and industrial policy priorities; how to provide the best quality medicines possible at prices that are concurrently affordable and serve wider economic interests. In Europe, this is particularly difficult as the state generally bears the cost of health care. Although pharmaceutical spending as a share of gross domestic product has remained fairly stable in most countries since the 1980s, as a percentage of total health expenditure it has risen sharply from the early 1990s (Jacobzone 2000). Thus, even in countries such as the UK and Germany, which support strong local pharmaceutical industries, cutting back on drug spending has become a priority. Government intervention in the UK is concerned with keeping prices affordable within the wider sustainability of the health care system, while in Germany the aim is not simply cost containment but also to promote efficiency. Each member state has evolved its own approach based on a host of country-specific factors, including: the structure of the health care system and financing mechanisms; medical requirements (member states have differing patterns of disease, for example); ethnic and cultural factors *vis-à-vis* medicine consumption and prescribing; macroeconomic performance; demography; and relative wealth. In addition, medicines involve or impact upon a plethora of further actors and interests beyond the state (Table 2.2).

Even within the generalized designations of 'industry', 'consumer' and 'health service', Table 2.2 shows the diversity of issues at stake and the conflicts of interest, such as between innovative and generic producers, between health care providers and pharmacies, or between insurers and patients. Medicines are clearly a politically charged sector.

In looking at the policy balancing act, it is important to disaggregate national and supranational priorities. While the manner in which the policy conflict is reconciled may be seen as the defining characteristic of any national regime, in terms of EU policy it is manifest in a dissonance between the rules of the single European market and the principle of subsidiarity as enshrined under the European Union Treaties. The former, as for all industrial goods, demands the free movement of pharmaceuticals between member states; the latter, in delimiting policy competence to the lowest level at which it can be effectively undertaken, undermines the European Commission's authority – member states have used subsidiarity to defend their right to set their own health care priorities. This

Table 2.2 National actors and policy objectives in the pharmaceutical sector*

Sector	Entity	Policy objectives
State	*Ministries*	
Regulation	Health	Adequate supply of safe, quality and effective drugs
Funding	Finance	Minimize tax-funded health expenditure
Delivery	Service	Maximize access to care for those most in need
Economic	Trade, industry	Encourage local industry, employment and exports
Industry	*Firms*	
Innovation	Research	Maximize profits and safeguard research base
Reproduction	Generic	Improve competitive position
Distribution	Wholesalers	Improve margins
Insurance	Insurers	Segment market to best advantage
Professions	*Associations*	
Prescribing	Medicine	Maximize autonomy and meet patient needs
Dispensing	Pharmacy	Enlarge professional role and meet client needs
Health Service	*Organizations*	
Primary	Practices	Maintain local visibility and community support
Secondary	Hospitals	Maintain market share and organizational visibility
Regional	Health systems	Meet requirements of key stakeholders
Other	*Various*	
Consumers	Associations/patient groups	Ensure access to safe and effective drugs
Scientific community	Journals	Advance knowledge and academic freedom
Media	Firms	Enhance or maintain market segment

* A simple listing; does not indicate actors' strength of influence or importance of interest.
Source: adapted from Davis (1997).

often means opposing aims between national and supranational policy makers (i.e. cost containment versus market liberalization). Furthermore, it has meant that despite a lengthy history of Community involvement in the arena of medicines regulation (predating the single European market),[3] there is still no single market for medicines.

At EU level, therefore, the list of priorities reflected in Table 2.1 is broadly the same if not identical. First, the EU has a public health mandate, both with regard to a wide-ranging Community Action Programme for Public Health,[4] and in having set the safety, quality and efficacy criteria for the market approval of new medicines.[5] However, its role is limited by Article 152 of the Amsterdam Treaty, which stipulates that 'Community action in the field of public health shall fully respect the responsibilities of the Member States for the organisation and delivery of health services and medical care'. And while this does not mean that national health care systems are immune from EU influence – indeed, the European Court of Justice has been involved in several important cases concerning the compatibility of national health care arrangements with EU law (Mossialos and McKee 2001) – it does mean that the Commission's capacity is restricted. So although a Community-wide market authorization system for pharmaceuticals has been in place since the mid-1970s, it has evolved mainly towards promoting their free movement. This helps to contextualize why the European Agency for the Evaluation of Medicinal Products (EMEA), which, since 1995, has been responsible for granting EU market approval, is limited to the issuing of recommendations and has no power of sanction (see Chapter 4).

Second, given the lack of health care policy competence, EU policy makers have no say over pharmaceutical pricing and reimbursement. Not that the Commission has not sought influence here. Indeed, the 'Transparency Directive' of 1989 established Community-wide guidelines for national authorities when setting their own pricing and reimbursement policies (Council of the European Communities 1989). But this remains the only EU initiative in the pricing arena (see Chapter 3).

In yielding to member state governments' health care competence, the EU's main goal for the pharmaceutical sector has thus been the deregulation of national markets. But this has proven problematic. The sensitivities involved mean that governments are keen to retain a firm regulatory hand. Moreover, it has resulted in an EU framework that is decidedly industrial policy-leaning – that is, the EU has a strong regulatory remit over issues pertaining to the promotion of the single market (e.g. common packaging requirements, advertising rules, EU product licensing, wholesale distribution, patent protection), but no ability to affect countries' choices *vis-à-vis* pricing and reimbursement. So while the member states' own regulatory systems developed primarily to protect patients in the aftermath of the Thalidomide tragedy, the underlying concern of the EU regime has been to liberalize the pharmaceutical market within the context of the single European market. In pursuit of price deregulation as required under a single market, the Commission has thus been restricted to pushing for convergence of national measures and, more recently, promoting the competitiveness of the European pharmaceutical industry (European Commission 2003).

National versus supranational interests and competencies

Profiling the member states' regulatory regimes is beyond the scope of this chapter. But as many seek to balance the priorities already mentioned, some generalizations can be made. First, with regard to public health regulation, each country requires drug producers to demonstrate the quality and safety of new substances in terms of delivering a therapeutic benefit to patients under specific conditions and at a particular dosage. Known as 'new drug applications', these are assessed by public bodies (generally a medicines agency) before market authorization is granted.

A second generalization is that most governments support the industry for the economic rewards it brings – particularly where a manufacturing sector is present – and thus regulate also to pursue industrial policy goals. Not only are medicines highly profitable and investment-intensive, but the industry is also a significant employer. Over 500,000 people are directly employed in the EU pharmaceutical industry (EFPIA 2002), with many more jobs indirectly generated. Adequate incentive structures are thus sought to ensure continued industry presence. Policies often include favourable tax incentives, strict intellectual property rights and *quid pro quo* pricing arrangements.

Next, as all EU governments share concerns over cost containment, all regulate the demand and supply sides of the market to control overall drug expenditures (see Chapter 1). Demand-side measures aim to affect the behaviour of patients and health care providers. User charges and financial incentives for doctors attempt to engender price awareness and sensitivity to prevent induced demand and increase cost-efficiency. Supply-side measures are the more favoured, however, with most states controlling medicine prices; whether as direct controls on individual products or average or reference pricing schemes. Industry generally disputes the value of price controls, claiming that they impede innovation, are difficult to manage and that they have no clear impact, as drug costs are more dependent on prescribing and consumption patterns. But from the policy makers' perspective, price controls carry with them the added benefit of ensuring for governments a strong say in the market, enabling them also to pursue other aims. So while price regulation in France has been used to protect the domestic industry, in the UK the Pharmaceutical Price Regulation Scheme (PPRS) seeks to boost local investment. As to a pattern, countries with a strong industrial base tend to allow somewhat freer pricing (UK, Germany) – France being an exception, although this is changing – while those with a comparatively weak base employ a variety of price controls (Spain, Italy). That said, the variance in national approaches stems from other (political) factors beyond simply the market.

In Italy, for instance, freer pricing might be favoured by policy makers, but it is opposed by the medical profession, traditionally a strong voice in the Italian health care context. As part of the 2003–2006 agreement between the industry and government in France, aimed primarily at reducing approval times, free pricing is to be applied only to innovative drugs (SNIP 2002). This has been agreed as a counter-weight for the industry as the government concurrently seeks to improve generic uptake in France. The methodology of the (much-reformed) German reference price system, and the government's continued inability to implement a positive list, reflects the strength of the country's industry. Meanwhile, the Irish and Dutch governments' preference for average pricing can be seen as something of a politically correct manner of promoting price controls. Since average pricing schemes are based on international comparisons of drug prices, governments cannot then be accused of price-fixing. That said, companies often develop strategies to overcome these, such as launching products in higher-priced markets first, markets that other countries look to when averaging their own prices.

The type of health care system also has an influence on the type of policies that can be agreed. Countries with a national health service such as the UK and Sweden, where the state is regulator and payer, are better able to agree control measures than social insurance-based systems such as in Austria and Germany. The dispersal of power between the regulator and third-party payer within the latter means that control of health care budgets and decision making falls to several bodies beyond the public administration. This is not to say that the former are necessarily more efficient. Indeed, Portugal, which operates a national health service, has much direct government regulation, but numerous reforms over the past three decades have failed to control costs (EOHCS 1999).

The decision-making structure within countries also impacts on policy. The UK Department of Health exercises control over most elements of pharmaceutical policy. *Inter alia*, it regulates prescribing guidelines (including drug classification), reimbursement, dispensing, patient information and prices. Because of the strong involvement of the Department, priorities and policies tend to be based around a wider view of the sustainability of the National Health Service as a whole. In Germany, as with the political system itself, health care policy is more diffuse and efficiency remains a key goal. The federal government sets the overall direction of policy; the *Länder* are responsible for most aspects of health within their own territory; and (statutory health insurance-contracted) corporatist bodies representing the payers (sickness funds) and providers (physicians' and dentists' associations) exercise operational control. This type of fragmentation may create difficulties, as in Spain, where the considerable power accorded the autonomous regions, including over pharmaceutical policy, has seen regional authorities often oppose policies at the central level.

Moreover, it is not always the equivalent body in the member states that exercises the same role. For example, while in Italy and France the responsibility for setting medicine prices lies within the Ministry of Health, in the latter it is in fact the purview of a special Economic Committee within the Ministry. In Austria meanwhile, the Federal Ministry for Social Security and the Generations has responsibility for setting drug prices, but in keeping with the country's corporatist traditions, it consults with a pricing committee made up of representatives from other ministries, together with the Austrian Economic Chamber and Federal Chamber of Labour. Prices in the UK are indirectly regulated via the PPRS (managed by the Department of Health), in Portugal via the Directorate-General for Trade and Competition, while the Federal Standing Committee of Physicians and Sickness Funds groups drugs under Germany's reference pricing system, thereby indirectly setting prices. Responsibility for reimbursement also differs among the member states, though most do have separate pricing and reimbursement competencies.

The regulatory brief at supranational level is more limited. First, with regard to the EU's institutional structure, the pharmaceutical sector suffers from what Hancher (1991) has termed 'horizontal multi-regulation' – that is, there are several Commission Directorates-General (DGs) with an interest in related matters, whether health, research or competition. Furthermore, the European Court of Justice enjoys an unusually prominent role in pharmaceutical policy, particularly in relation to 'free movement' cases (see Chapter 3). In delivering rulings on issues such as intellectual property rights, competition policy and public health requirements, it has helped to set the EU's pharmaceutical agenda. Nevertheless, primary responsibility has traditionally fallen to the DG account-able for industrial affairs (DG Enterprise). The health and consumer affairs DG (DG Sanco), which, within its wider brief, is responsible for public health policy, has comparatively little input. Consequently, EU priorities and policies for medicines reflect both the uncoordinated nature and inherent industrial policy leanings of the decision-making structure. Even the EMEA is in many ways more a licensing office than a patient protection agency.

Chapter 4 looks at the EMEA in some detail, but it should be mentioned here that the agency has been accused of favouring industry in its work. Speed of approval rather than stringency of assessment has been criticized by numerous commentators as the agency's prime function (e.g. Abraham and Lewis 2000; Garattini and Bertele' 2001). So while industry is generally happy with the agency's quicker and less bureaucratic approval processes, consumer and patient interests remain concerned about a lowest-common-denominator approach to assessment. The specific criticisms raised in Chapter 4 regarding the extent to which the agency cooperates with the companies, and the lack of transparency that characterizes its decision-making processes, stem in large part from the manner of its establishment. As Permanand (2002) has shown, the impetus for a pan-European licensing authority came from the Commission during the late 1980s; in fact, it convinced the industry as to the merits of centralized approval, specifically because of a concern that the pharmaceutical sector was well behind schedule *vis-à-vis* the 1992 deadline for the single European market. The aim was to make the approval process more efficient, so as to promote the 'free movement' of medicines. It is perhaps unsurprising, there-fore, that the EMEA does not have an equivalent mandate to national agencies.

A second reason for the limited EU brief is that the health care policy void has meant that EU policy makers' primary designs – ultimately a single medicines market – have generally been restricted to measures to liberalize the market. With the divergent national pricing regimes posing the major hindrance, the Commission has traditionally sought policies that circumvent its lack of com-petence. In this way, price deregulation rather than outright convergence of national markets has become the aim. Instigating more competition in the sec-tor, price transparency and collaboration with global regimes such as the Inter-national Conference on Harmonization,[6] have been seen as ways of promoting price competition, lessening government control and thereby serving the aims of the single market. From the perspective of patient and consumer groups, however, this is a somewhat tenuous line of argumentation. Their fear is that price deregulation will lead to convergence at higher prices, and groups such as the European Consumers' Organization have traditionally not favoured out-right harmonization in a European context.

More importantly, the member states remain unwilling to give the Commis-sion the equivalent regulatory authority it exercises in other industrial sectors. Most fear a loss of autonomy over health care under a single medicines market.

Equally, they also have economic concerns, as harmonization would involve industry rationalization and the probable collapse of less competitive industries. Despite criticisms of over-capacity,[7] it is something of an open secret that member states have used subsidiarity as a means of protecting their industry (jobs in particular). Some countries' pricing (UK) and reimbursement (France, Greece) systems are also designed to serve industrial policy goals. Moreover, there appear to be too many uncertainties as to what a single medicines market would bring or require. Beyond some countries losing out, it is not clear, for instance, what would really happen to manufacturing in the EU. Already industry points to the fact that domestic research and development (R&D) investment in Europe has been decreasing over the past 10 years, down from 73 per cent in 1990 to 59 per cent in 1999, with the USA being the main beneficiary of this shift in spending (EFPIA 2002). In addition, eastwards expansion to bring in the accession countries presents a host of further uncertainties given the nature of their pharmaceutical sectors and health care requirements (see Chapter 19). In other words, full harmonization implies 'winners' and 'losers', such that even those member states with more established industries are simply unwilling to gamble over what a single market might mean. And this makes support for a single medicines market difficult to secure.

The Commission is caught in a quandary here, for it too wants to see a successful European sector in both productivity and employment terms. Hence it has often – even if unsuccessfully – tried to bargain with industry and the member states, trading-off industrial policy measures in exchange for movement on market (price) deregulation. The most notable case was in agreeing the 1996 Resolution on the 'Outlines of an Industrial Policy for the Pharmaceutical Sector in the European Community' (Council of the European Communities 1996), in which all references to price harmonization had been removed from earlier drafts at member state (and industry) insistence.

A tangible example of differences between (and among) member states' and EU interests lies in the controversial practice of parallel trade. This is particularly vexing within the context of the single European market, as it stems from price differentials for the same medicines between member states; it also exposes the extent to which governments' regulatory priorities diverge. Although parallel imports already comprise a significant market share in the UK, the government is unlikely to promote the practice to a greater extent, as it is inevitably its own innovative industry that 'suffers' (Germany opposes the practice for the same reason); Spain and Portugal are net parallel traders, deriving considerable revenues via the practice, while for the Dutch and Danish governments, it is an integral element of their cost containment measures. Parallel importation finds support among consumer groups and the Commission's Competition DG for the cost savings it generates, while wholesalers who engage in the practice can make considerable profits. Industry opposes it and, in some cases, so do health care professionals who have safety concerns about the re-imported products. Parallel trade remains a much-contested issue, where the European Court of Justice has delivered several rulings generally sanctioning the practice on free movement grounds (see Chapter 3).

Finally, since the 1999 restructuring of the Commission, the focus has been on improving the competitiveness of the EU industry. Medicines is one of the few highly research-intensive industries where Europe has traditionally been able to compete with the USA and Japan, and European policy makers are desperate to retain this. This means balancing the industry's (global) concerns with the member states' (domestic) requirements, as well as with the process of European integration. EU officials are thus especially concerned over the industry's claims of declining competitiveness in terms of the number of new chemical entities being discovered, new medicines placed on the world market and, as mentioned, R&D investment in Europe. In this way, both the (price and market) liberalization and competitiveness approaches are ultimately aimed at achieving a single market, but represent different paths. And both run into difficulties in light of the member states' interest in retaining a firm regulatory hold. Thus, despite the harmonization efforts pursued at EU level, numerous factors (e.g. divergent member state priorities, continued pressures on health care budgets, changing drug consumption and lifestyle patterns, industry strategies *vis-à-vis* differing national pricing measures, the inadequacy of current controls in managing costs) have led to the differences between member states' regulatory systems increasing rather than decreasing since the beginning of the 1990s.

Government–industry relations

Turning now to government–industry relations in the sector, these generally stem from each country's own regulatory traditions – for example, interventionist/statist (France), non-interventionist and market-dominated (UK), middle-ground *Soziale Marktwirtschaft* (Germany) – and are where political culture and bargaining style can shape preferences and outcomes. Indeed, as Hancher and Moran (1989) note with regard to the UK: 'many of the most important regulatory arrangements . . . were evolved in a political culture marked by a deferential attitude on the part of mass publics towards authority, and by a preference for informal and private regulation on the part of élite groups'. Relations are thus embedded in the political economy and state tradition, leading to considerable variations among member states. As Wilks and Wright (1987) have noted, 'industrial culture' helps to define state intervention.

More importantly, understanding government–industry relations is crucial to grasping the nature of policy in any sector, for industry cannot be seen simply as a recipient of (government-imposed) regulation. This is nowhere more the case than in the pharmaceutical sector, where the relationship between government and industry is shaped by the nature and scope of a country's dominant approach to securing health protection and equitable access to health services and prescription drugs. Moreover, given that EU governments exercise regulatory competencies that define the prices at which drugs will be sold and how long they might remain profitable (via patent legislation), industry lobbying is a key feature of what is generally a close relationship.

The relationship between government and the industry in the UK has been described as a case of 'clientele pluralism' (Macmillan and Turner 1987), where the state has a high concentration of power but, because of a lack of expertise and/or resources, effectively little autonomy. Here, the Ministry of Health agrees to 'trust' the industry to produce new and safe medicines in what then becomes a relationship of mutual dependence (Lexchin 2001). Profits (so-called 'margins of tolerance') are thus agreed in negotiation with individual companies under the PPRS, and industry – often represented by its trade organization, the Association of British Pharmaceutical Industry (ABPI) – is assured a considerable say. The centrality of the ABPI's role stems from the relationship forged with the Ministry of Health in the mid-1950s over a strategy for cutting drug spending. Moreover, industry representation may be sought on government committees or expert groups. Thus, the ABPI is generally regarded as the most successful national association in terms of its influence. Many members of staff in the Department of Health's Medicines Division, which issues product licences, and most members of the Committee on Safety of Medicines which comprises scientific experts and advises the Medicines Division, have financial interests in the industry (often with more than one company); and there has been a strong 'revolving-door' syndrome, with industry officials moving to the Medicines Division for a period and then back to industry (Abraham and Lewis 2000).

In Italy, government–industry relations have to a considerable degree shaped the current regulatory framework. Following a series of scandals in which several high-ranking Ministry of Health officials (including an ex-minister) were in 1992 found to have accepted bribes from individual companies, regulatory responsibilities were reformed to relieve the Department of Health of its central role (Fattore and Jommi 1998). An independent expert committee (albeit under the auspices of the ministry) was established, with price-setting as one of its key functions. Prices are agreed in negotiation with companies, but unlike in the UK they are agreed on individual products rather than at company level. In Spain, the relationship between the industry's association, *Farmindustria*, and the Ministry of Health has long been antagonistic over cost-containment measures. An element of the Spanish system, whereby companies agree to a percentage limit on their annual profit growth from sales to the health service (to ensure the government a certain level of cost savings), has been an especially sore point.

Differing health care and industrial goals mean that the strength of industry in influencing policy differs by member state. The centrality of the ABPI's role (and the nature of the PPRS) thus reflects the UK government's industrial policy goals. In Germany, where the industry is strong in both research and generic segments, the federal government's position is more nuanced. Not only that, but several of the larger research-based firms have forged their own representative body, the *Verband Forschender Arzneimittelhersteller*, separate from the *Bundesverband der Pharmazeutischen Industrie*, which represents the industry as a whole.

Differences in member states' priorities are also reflected in the relationship companies have with the respective national medicines agencies. For although the agencies are generally responsible for ensuring new medicines meet strict guidelines, their mandates differ. These differences reflect, among other things, the political tradition in each country, the nature of government–industry relations, and specific national interests and requirements *vis-à-vis* medicines policy. In Germany, for instance, the licensing of new drugs via the Federal Institute for Pharmaceuticals and Medical Devices is a lengthy affair, on average taking well over a year following EMEA approval. While this may be a result of the Thalidomide tragedy, and in part stems from the fragmented nature of policy making, it results in a sometimes hostile relationship with the industry. In contrast, the Swedish medical products agency, the *Läkemedelsverket*, and its UK counterpart the Medicines Control Agency,[8] have traditionally worked towards speeding market approval. The Spanish medicines agency, the *Agencia Espaniola del Medicamento*, was only established in 1997, primarily because of poor Spanish participation in the EMEA regime. A key function is to convince companies to carry out their clinical trials in Spain.

As mentioned at the outset, beyond industry there are a host of other actors with vested interests in the pharmaceutical sector, contributing to policy in various ways. The scope of this chapter precludes an analysis of their roles, but it is to be noted that doctors, patient groups, pharmacists, importers and whole-salers have often organized to voice their interests at both national and EU levels. Here, too, differences between member states are apparent. While doctors have traditionally been a strong voice in German health care policy, medical groups in France are divided and more concerned about preserving their auton-omy than policy setting. And while consumer advocacy is prevalent in the UK, it is considerably less so in Germany. The UK Consumers' Association has also been very active at EU level, pushing for many issues including generic substitu-tion. That said, as balancing health care and industrial policy priorities is most governments' primary concern, consumers are in general a marginalized stake-holder. This is mirrored at EU level where there is no consumer representation on the Committee on Proprietary Medicinal Products, the body within the EMEA responsible for assessing market applications; the Commission consults almost exclusively with industry; and DG Sanco is rarely involved directly in pharmaceutical policy decisions.

Indeed, at EU level the industry's influence is strong, and it is the research-based industry's relations with the Commission and EMEA that are particularly noteworthy. There are several reasons for this. First, cost containment is not a direct policy competence; the Commission may support member state efforts (e.g. generic substitution), but it cannot influence them directly. Second, the Commission's industrial policy goals are not dissimilar to the interests of pharmaceutical companies. Next, through a strong trade association created in 1978, the European Federation of Pharmaceutical Industries and Associations (EFPIA), companies have successfully lobbied on many issues (Greenwood and Ronit 1994), such as patent-term extension.[9] That Commission officials and members of the European Parliament who are involved in decision making regarding pharmaceutical policy are not necessarily experts in the field, has meant that they are reliant on the industry for their information. And this has also contributed to EFPIA's access to the EU policy-making arena. The industry's insider status is further strengthened by representation on all relevant policy committees; most notably the EMEA's Committee on Proprietary Medicinal Products and the 'G10 Group', which was created by the European Commission in 2001 to devise a new agenda towards meeting Europe's health care and indus-trial policy goals. The close nature of the relationship was identified as early as the late 1970s; as noted by Stenzl (1981), European officials were reluctant to discuss how the Commission consulted or cooperated with the industry.

This lack of transparency over industry involvement, while widely criticized by groups such as the International Society of Drug Bulletins,[10] has continued in many respects: EMEA experts are not named; decisions on negative applications are not published; companies are involved in writing the product summaries for proposed drugs; and they may choose who carries out assessments on their EU applications. And recently, under its review of Community pharmaceutical legislation, the Commission's proposal for industry representation on the EMEA management board was approved by the European Parliament on first reading (European Commission 2002). Unless the Council of Ministers rejects the proposals, it is therefore likely that two of the board's 15 members will now come from 'industrial associations'. It is, of course, in part because industry's (global) priorities correspond broadly with DG Enterprise's competitiveness and industrial policy goals, that the EFPIA and the research industry wields considerable influence. But it is at least equally the case that through consistent and well-organized lobbying strategies, the EFPIA has been able to play a central role in shaping the EU regulatory framework as it currently stands. And there are other reasons as well.

One of the most important is that the sector's other actors have a much weaker voice. The views of groups such as the European Consumers' Association (BEUC) or the Standing Committee of European Doctors have traditionally not been heeded by European policy makers (Orzack 1996), nor do they enjoy equivalent degrees of representation in the policy-making machinery. A lack of resources means that consumer interests in particular have had a diminishing role in the European pharmaceutical arena; for instance, there are no dedicated EU-level consumer pharmaceutical groups. The BEUC has medicines policy as only one of its areas of focus – and even here it is less active than during the 1980s and early 1990s in the run-up to the single market – while Health Action International is involved in advocacy on an international scale. Other groups, such as the European Public Health Alliance, also do not have pharmaceuticals as a priority area. While recently the Commission appears to be giving prominence to the views of patient groups in the review of Community pharmaceutical legislation, it is the case that many of these groups are financed by the industry. Although cooperation between patient groups and the industry may be seen as inevitable given not only their shared interest in seeing the release of new and better therapies but also the latter's lack of resources, it ought also to be a cause for concern among policy makers. For not only can it lead to patient groups organizing around specific companies' products, but industry-financing may compromise their integrity and independence more widely. Thus, larger and better-financed groups are better placed to lobby for their interests. It is worth noting, as Herxheimer (2003) has done, that the European Commission prefers to deal with these larger groups and patients' federations such as the International Alliance of Patients' Organizations and the Global Alliance of Mental Illness Advocacy Networks Europe (both financed directly by industry) rather than voluntary or more 'grass-roots' groups; the justification being that it is easier to deal with multinational associations representing European patients in general.

As something of a counterweight to the comparative marginalization of consumer and other interests versus that of industry, the unique nature of the EU polity offers additional tiers that non-industry actors can target in pressing their case. The 'multi-level governance' literature of community decision making (e.g. Christiansen 1997), characterized especially by committee-based decision making and a central role for the European Parliament, means a considerable dispersal of authority between the national and supranational levels. National, sub-national and EU actors are involved in a policy process that is both horizontal and vertical, and there is no single pattern of governance. There is an extensive literature on so-called 'euro-lobbying' (e.g. Mazey and Richardson 1993; Greenwood 2003) that acknowledges and analyses the multiplicity of lobbying conduits available within the EU policy-making dynamic. Moreover, with the EU being a continuously evolving polity, many of the path-dependencies that characterize national administrations and state–society relations do not yet exist as rigidly. Not just the EFPIA, therefore, but other groups with an interest in EU pharmaceutical policy – and with strong voices at national level – such as the pharmacists' association (Pharmaceutical Group of the European Union) and the European Association of Pharmaceutical Wholesalers, are seeking to influence EU policy.

Conclusions: the continuing lack of a single medicines market

In this chapter, we have sought to outline the complexity of making pharmaceutical policy in Europe with regard to the political elements involved at both the national and supranational levels. This is in terms of the need to reconcile public health, health care and industrial policy interests, while also meeting the interests of a host of vested interests. The discussion has shown medicines to be an area of shared competence between the member states and the Commission and, given the competing interests at stake, the number of actors with an immediate interest/involvement, and the regulator's multi-faceted task, has hinted at the extremely politicized nature of policy making. Moreover, the discussion has shown how this contributes to both an industrial policy leaning at EU level and the continuing lack of a single medicines market. By way of summary, two main points bear recapping.

First, because of the subsidiarity principle, the EU lacks the necessary competencies to force the harmonization agenda as it has in other industrial sectors. Due to differing national requirements and interests, the member state governments remain unwilling to defer regulatory oversight to EU policy makers. This has resulted in the Commission seeking to reduce intra-Community tariffs and promote the competitiveness of the EU industry, both as a means of breaching the impasse and to ensure a strong European presence in the pharmaceutical arena. The emphasis has been on liberalization and the securing of an interventionist regulatory role with regard to ensuring the free movement of goods underpinning the single market, rather than outright harmonization *per se*. Here the Commission is supported by a considerable body of European law, which, in the case of pharmaceuticals, is mainly concerned with freeing impediments to inter-EU trade.

Second, although the reasons behind the member states' insistence on regulatory control may stem from similar interests (e.g. cost containment), they in fact reflect specific national requirements. The member states have different regulatory regimes in place to balance the affordable provision of safe, effica-cious and high-quality medicines, with policies to maintain jobs, promote industry and ensure a favourable trade balance. These, in turn, stem from their own political traditions and relations with industry. Thus, not only are there inherent differences between the *vis-à-vis* medicines and their regulation, but also national and supranational priorities often do conflict. The result, as iden-tified in this chapter, is that a host of (primarily political) factors combine to hamper completion of a single pharmaceutical market in the European Union.

Notes

1 A group of drugs prescribed to lower cholesterol and prevent coronary ailments.
2 A single medicinal product may carry in excess of 20 patents, covering everything from substance and compound, through to application and use.
3 The first piece of Community pharmaceutical legislation was Directive 65/65/EEC, which defined what a medicinal product represented in the European Community and established guidelines for market authorization. See *EudraLex, Vol. 1: Medical Products for Human Use* for a listing of all EU pharmaceutical legislation (available from http://dg3.eudra.org/F2/eudralex/vol-1/home.htm).
4 The latest programme (2003–2008) was adopted on 23 September 2002, and focuses on the better provision of health information, rapid reaction to health threats (including creating an EU centre for disease prevention/control) and tackling health determinants. It builds on eight previous multi-year programmes.
5 See Council of the European Communities (1965).
6 The International Conference on Harmonization seeks the elaboration of common European, American and Japanese regulatory standards for pharmaceuticals in order to speed market approval.
7 Comparing statistics from the EU and US trade associations shows that the US indus-try has similar output to the combined EU industry, but with just under half the number of full-time employed (EFPIA 2002; PhRMA 2002).
8 Now the Medicines and Healthcare Products Regulatory Agency after merging with the Medical Devices Agency in April 2003.
9 The generics industry has been far less successful, in part because of the Commission's priorities and competencies, but also because generics companies lacked EU level representation until 1992.
10 The International Society of Drug Bulletins promotes exchange of information on drugs to encourage the development of and cooperation between professionally independent drug bulletins in all countries.

References

Abraham, J. and Lewis, G. (2000) *Regulating Medicines in Europe: Competition, Expertise and Public Health*. London: Routledge.
Christiansen, T. (1997) Reconstructing European space: from territorial politics to multi-level governance, in K.-E. Jorgensen (ed.) *Reflective Approaches to European Governance*. Basingstoke: Macmillan.
Council of the European Communities (1965) Council Directive (65/65/EEC) of 26 January 1965 on the approximation of provisions laid down by law, regulation or

administrative action relating to proprietary medicinal products, *Official Journal of the European Communities*, L22, 09.02.1965: 369.

Council of the European Communities (1989) Council Directive (89/105/EEC) of 21 December 1988 relating to the transparency of measures regulating the pricing of medicinal products for human use and their inclusion within the scope of national health insurance systems, *Official Journal of the European Communities*, L40, 11.02.1989: 8.

Council of the European Communities (1992) Council Regulation (EEC) No. 1768/92 of 18 June 1992 concerning the creation of a supplementary protection certificate for medicinal products, *Official Journal of the European Communities*, L182, 02.07.1992: 15.

Council of the European Communities (1996) Council Resolution of 23 April 1996 designed to implement the outlines of an industrial policy for the pharmaceutical sector in the European Community, *Official Journal of the European Communities*, C136, 08.05.1996.

Davis, P. (1997) *Managing Medicines – Public Policy and Therapeutic Drugs*. State of Health Series. Buckingham: Open University Press.

EFPIA (2002) *The Pharmaceutical Industry in Figures – Key Data (2002 Update)*. Brussels: European Federation of Pharmaceutical Industries and Associations.

EOHCS (1999) *Health Care Systems in Transition: Portugal*. Copenhagen: European Observatory on Health Care Systems.

European Commission (2002) 735 final. Modified proposal for a regulation of the European Parliament and of the Council laying down Community procedures for the authorisation and supervision and pharmacovigilance of medicinal products for human and veterinary use and establishing a European agency for the Evaluation of Medicinal Products.

European Commission (2003) Communication from the Commission to the Council, European Parliament, the Economic and Social Committee, and the Committee of the Regions: a stronger European-based pharmaceutical industry for the benefit of the patient – a call for action, COM (2003) 383 Final of 01.07.2003.

Fattore, G. and Jommi, C. (1998) The new pharmaceutical policy in Italy, *Health Policy*, 46: 21–41.

Garattini, S. and Bertele', V. (2001) Adjusting Europe's drug regulation to public health needs, *Lancet*, 358: 64–7.

Greenwood, J. (2003) *Interest Representation in the European Union*. Houndmills: Palgrave Macmillan.

Greenwood, J. and Ronit, K. (1994) Interest groups in the European Community: newly emerging dynamics and forms, *West European Politics*, 17: 31–52.

Hancher, L. (1991) Creating the internal market for pharmaceutical medicines – an Echternach jumping procession, *Common Market Law Review*, 28: 821–53.

Hancher, L. and Moran, M. (1989) *Capitalism, Culture and Economic Regulation*. Oxford: Clarendon Press.

Herxheimer, A. (2003) Relationships between the pharmaceutical industry and patients' organisations, *British Medical Journal*, 326: 1208–10.

Jacobzone, S. (2000) *Pharmaceutical Policies in OECD Countries: Reconciling Social and Industrial Goals*. OECD Labour Market and Social Policy Occasional Paper No. 40. Paris: OECD.

Lexchin, J. (2001) Pharmaceuticals: politics and policy, in P. Armstrong, H. Armstrong and D. Cohen (eds) *Unhealthy Times: Political Economy Perspectives on Health and Care*. Oxford: Oxford University Press.

Macmillan, K. and Turner, I. (1987) The cost-containment issue: a study of government–industry relations in the pharmaceutical sectors of the United Kingdom and Germany, in S. Wilks and M. Wright (eds) *Comparative Government–Industry Relations: Western Europe, the United States and Japan*. Oxford: Clarendon Press.

Mazey, S. and Richardson, J. (1993) *Lobbying in the European Union*. Oxford: Oxford University Press.

Mossialos, E. and McKee, M. (2001) Is a European healthcare policy emerging? Yes, but its nature is far from clear, *British Medical Journal*, 323: 248.

Orzack, L. (1996) Professionals, consumers, and the European Medicines Agency: policy-making in the European Union, *Current Research on Occupations and Professions*, 9: 9–29.

Permanand, G. (2002) Regulating under constraint: the case of EU pharmaceutical policy. PhD dissertation, London School of Economics and Political Science, London.

PhRMA (2002) *PhRMA Industry Profile 2002*. Washington, DC: Pharmaceutical Research and Manufacturers of America.

Simons, J. (2003) The $10 billion pill, *Fortune Magazine*, 6 January.

SNIP (2002) *Propositions pour une nouvelle politique du médicament en France. Syndicat National de l'Industrie Pharmaceutique*. Paris: SNIP.

Stenzl, C. (1981) The role of international organisations in medicines policy, in R. Blum, A. Herxheimer, C. Stenzl and J. Woodcock (eds) *Pharmaceuticals and Health Policy: International Perspectives on Provision and Control of Medicines*. London: Croom Helm.

Wilks, S. and Wright, M. (eds) (1987) *Comparative Government–Industry Relations: Western Europe, the United States and Japan*. Oxford: Clarendon Press.

three

The European Community dimension: coordinating divergence

Leigh Hancher

Introduction

National schemes, with attendant rules and regulations to control the level of public expenditure on pharmaceutical products, continue to proliferate alongside repeated government efforts and attempts to rationalize both consumption and control related health budgets. National divergence across Europe as opposed to convergence seems to be the rule, both in terms of approach and effect. A concern to keep levels of public expenditure on pharmaceuticals under control is not necessarily such a direct or pressing matter on a European level, given that the Community institutions are not themselves responsible for funding health care to any significant extent. This does not, however, mean that the Community has not, or should not, take an interest in this complex area. In particular, the European Commission has made repeated attempts to address the issues and, indeed, the problems raised by the divergence of national approaches. The Commission's involvement revolves around two primary axes: first and foremost, concern as to the fragmentation of the 'internal' or single European market and the related concern as to the implications of national intervention for the overall competitiveness of the European research-based industry, second, a concern to ensure a high level of health provision across the Community. Community policy and Community law are not only of vital relevance for national governments and their various cost-containment strategies, but are also of direct relevance to the various actors involved in the production, distribution and consumption of pharmaceutical products. The commercial strategies of the industry – whether research-based, generic or parallel traders – as well as those of wholesalers and health insurance providers cannot and do not operate in isolation from the European legal and policy environment, even if their primary target is often national policy and implementing instruments. In turn, pharmacists, the medical profession and patients are also affected by European developments and may also invoke European law to counter national strategies which they consider might adversely affect their own interests.

In this chapter, I examine the legal and policy dimensions of Community intervention in national pricing and reimbursement control strategies. A report, entitled *Global Competitiveness in Pharmaceuticals: A European Perspective*, commissioned by the Directorate-General for Enterprise in 2000, hereafter the Pammolli Report (Gambardella *et al.* 2000), confirmed that the European industry has declined in competitiveness compared with the USA, albeit that there are large differences and trends across the member states. The report puts forward a number of explanations to support its finding that as a whole Europe is lagging behind its ability to generate, organize and sustain innovation processes that are increasingly expensive and organizationally complex. Significantly, it stresses that many national European markets are not competitive enough, and that the nature and intensity of competition in final based markets is too weak to nurture efficiency and innovation. It is self-evident that the publication of this report, which also coincided with the review of the Community regime for market authorization for pharmaceutical products, raises many complex issues. Several of these issues have been addressed by the so-called 'G10 process', instituted in March 2001 (G10 2002) with a mandate to review the extent to which current Community and national pharmaceutical, health and enterprise policies can achieve the twin goals of both encouraging innovation and competitiveness and ensuring satisfactory delivery of public health and social imperatives. This chapter examines the outcome of the G10 process – a series of recommendations – and its further implications for Community policy and the nature and direction of Commission intervention. The G10 process may mark a departure from the traditional approach of Community-led harmonization of national rules and regulations. The G10 recommends a preference for coordination of national results, not of the underlying rules themselves.

An important question, but one that does not seem to have been posed at all in this process, is how this new approach to pharmaceutical pricing policy would co-exist with the traditional Community approach, which has been based essentially on the removal of national disparities arising from divergent rules and regulations. In this context, I will also examine the continuing importance of the EC Treaty rules for the organization of the Community pharmaceutical market – the rules on free movement and the competition rules, and relevant secondary legislation designed to uphold and reinforce the application of the principles espoused in the Treaty. I also consider the implications of increasingly harmonized marketing authorization procedures, the centralized Community authorization procedure and the role of the European Medicines Evaluation Agency (EMEA), parallel trade and related aspects of intellectual property law and will consider whether they can be seen to contribute to or to conflict with the new objectives of coordination of results.

Can a new approach that appears to reinforce disparity be reconciled with the Commission's own related legal duties to uphold and enforce the principles of

European law – including the principles of free movement of goods and undistorted competition – the same principles that serve to protect and promote the processes of inter-brand and intra-brand competition from, respectively, generics and from parallel imports?

In practice, this legal framework implies that even if the Commission were to choose to support wholeheartedly the research-based industries' frequent requests to abolish certain forms of national price regulation, it could not necessarily immunize or protect that industry from intra- and inter-brand competition, especially in the form of parallel imports from low priced countries. It is noteworthy that these legal restrictions on the Commission's room for manoeuvre have not been addressed directly or dealt with by the G10 process. Before turning to each of these sets of issues, it is necessary to recall briefly the general institutional framework in which Community law and policy towards the sector has evolved.

Community competence and instruments

The division of legal competences between member states and the Community differs depending on whether industrial policy or public health and social security are at stake. The latter areas remain, from a legal as well as a political perspective, very much the preserve of the member states.[1] Article 152 of the EC Treaty, as amended by the Treaty of Amsterdam, extends Commission competence on health care only to a limited extent in relation to health policy. Before the introduction of a specific Treaty competence on health, the Community slowly developed a complex, sophisticated system of pharmaceutical regulation on the basis of its general powers under Articles 100 and 100A EEC (now 95 EC) to promote the internal market. The Commission's executive competence to launch policy initiatives and eventually propose binding rules or take other action (including enforcement action) has encompassed three areas:

- national prices and profit regulation, reimbursement regulation, rational use and advertising;
- free movement and competition issues; and
- market access through harmonized and eventually centralized authorization procedures.

An increasing dilemma for Community policy, especially in relation to pharmaceutical pricing and reimbursement issues, but also with regard to classification of products and their advertising ('rational use'), is whether its point of departure should remain rooted in the industrial policy perspective, or is this increasingly to be viewed as a health policy issue or a social security and consumer protection issue? Price controls on pharmaceuticals have implications for the entire pharmaceutical distribution chain. Consumers purchase a combination of pharmaceutical services (provided by the pharmaceutical manufacturer) and pharmacy services (provided by the pharmacist). It is of course impossible to ignore the fact that these issues are intertwined and, indeed, that the costs of the distribution chain are a significant part of the total costs (OECD 2002), but the point of departure remains important, as does the eventual level of intervention. If the industrial policy perspective is taken to be the predominant focus, this may imply that higher wholesale prices are deemed prima facie acceptable if this is what is required to reward the research-based industry. Consumer protection issues, including the need to guarantee the supply of requisite products to patients at a fair price, may then be dealt with by other (predominantly national) measures – for example, controls on retail prices and/or measures that are designed to enhance the promotion and prescribing of generics by doctors, and/or by taking measures to ensure that the costs advantages of generic substitution are passed on to patients and, where relevant, their insurers. These measures may, in turn, include limitations on the profits earned by pharmacists; for example, through deep discounting on certain patented as well as generic products. A combination of wholesale and retail price control may also prove to be desirable; indeed, this is national practice in many European countries. Nevertheless, setting the appropriate margin for retail price control is particularly difficult, given that pharmacy costs differ considerably from one member state to another, as do the methods of retail price control (OECD 2002). Unsurprisingly, the Commission has never proposed any form of legislative measure to address retail price control and has viewed this to be primarily a national concern.

The Community's powers to intervene in and impose greater convergence on national practice are not limited to its powers to adopt harmonizing legislation. Nor are the Commission's concerns only directed at the actions of governments and regulatory authorities. Traditionally, in the quest to create a single or internal European market, the Community legal framework has provided its institutions, citizens and industry with two sets of instruments: (1) so-called 'positive' harmonization instruments such as regulations and directives; and (2) the potential to enforce the primary Treaty rules – particularly on competition and free movement – often known as 'negative' harmonization, under which member states should amend their legislation and related rules, if these operate as a barrier to free movement of goods and services. The Treaty competition rules provide for the removal of essentially similar restrictions imposed through industry cartel arrangements or by dominant firms. The Commission as 'legal guardian' must guarantee the proper enforcement of the Treaty rules on free movement of goods and competition, two of the major pillars on which the single market edifice is constructed. Hence, the Commission may effectively promote intra-brand competition via parallel importation through a judicious enforcement of the Treaty competition rules – rules which are addressed to companies: it can and has ruled that companies who seek to impose export bans or other restrictions on wholesalers operating in low priced countries to supply their products for parallel trade into higher price markets infringe Article 81(1) EC, which outlaws cartels and agreements restricting competition.[2]

The Treaty provisions on competition are, of course, equally applicable to the demand side of the market, with the added proviso that national regulatory measures may be justified on grounds of social solidarity. Much can depend on the mechanics of the national scheme in question and whether responsibility for setting prices or drawing up reimbursement reference lists rests with governmental authorities or is entrusted to market actors such as health care or insurance funds. By way of example, the German federal association of sickness funds was initially actively involved in the national reference pricing system, as amended in 1999, and set the upper price limits for certain reference profits. This system was estimated to lead to savings of, on average, DM3 billion per year – almost 9 per cent of the total pharmaceutical expenditure of these funds. Early in 1999, however, a German court ruled that price setting by the sickness funds violates Article 81 EC.[3] In his opinion of 22 May 2003 in Joined Cases C-264/01, C-306/01, C-354/01 and C-355/01 AOK Bundesverband (ECJ 2003a), Advocate General Jacobs has advised that although the actions of the sickness funds in jointly determining the highest price at which they will purchase and pay for medicinal products is, in principle, subject to Community competition rules, as this action is a result of a state-imposed requirement, it cannot be attributable to the autonomous conduct of the sickness funds. It is required by national law and hence the conduct of the sickness funds, as such, does not infringe Article 81 EC. At the same time, given that the prices and reimbursement levels result from a statutorily imposed requirement on the funds, the measure in question would be capable of exemption under Article 86(2) EC.

The processes of intra-brand (i.e. parallel trade) and inter-brand competition (i.e. generics) are considered in general by the European Commission, and in particular by the Directorate-General for Competition, as essential if not inevitable for the eventual realization of a single market across the European Union. If the original manufacturer attempts to protect a high priced market from parallel importation, for example through seeking to enforce its intellectual property rights, it may well find that it has infringed the Treaty rules on free movement. Attempts to reach contractual agreements with wholesalers/distributors to restrict supplies to a particular territory and cut off the very source of parallel trade may also infringe the Treaty competition rules. At the same time, the Commission does not have the monopoly on enforcement of these provisions; all these Treaty principles, enshrined in the directly effective Articles 28, 30, 81 and 82 EC, can be enforced by the party claiming injury through local courts in each member state.

Although Commission intervention by virtue of competition law powers occurs on an *ad hoc* basis, usually as a result of a complaint of a parallel trader, the Commission can use these occasions to give clear guidance as to how it interprets the Treaty rules in individual cases. This, in turn, can provide guidance to national courts and authorities entrusted with the enforcement of both national and European competition law. As discussed in greater detail below, the Commission's interpretation of its competition-based powers to prevent dual pricing regimes and export bans is now under direct legal challenge before the European Courts.

The importance of the application of the basic Treaty principles on free movement and competition is not only apparent in relation to parallel trade or intra-brand competition. They have played an important role in the evolution of the case law of the Court of Justice in interpreting secondary legislation on product licensing, as well as intellectual property rights.

From harmonization to coordination?

Harmonization practice to date

Extensive use of secondary legislation, through Community directives and regulations, has been made with regard to the licensing of pharmaceutical products, leading to a high degree of harmonization of national practices and, indeed, the gradual centralization of the licensing (also known as market authorization) of biotechnology and high-technology products, under the auspices of the EMEA (see Chapter 4). The centralized system will be extended to a wider category of products, including some generic products, once the proposed amending legislation, now before the European Parliament, has entered into force.

In the field of pricing and reimbursement, however, very little progress has been made through harmonization. The only existing measure in this field, the so-called Price Transparency Directive in 1989 (Council of the European Union 1989), was originally intended as a first, but retrospectively is perhaps the last, step in the direction of Community regulation of national price and profit control. Despite subsequent reviews of its impact and effectiveness, the Commission could not establish sufficient consensus among the member states to move towards a stricter Community level regime. The 1989 measure is limited in its aims: neither does it harmonize the levels at which national price controls or profit caps are fixed, nor does it seek to harmonize rules on reimbursement. It merely endeavours to ensure that the relevant national procedures are efficient, transparent and fair.[4] Moreover, if the process of setting prices and profit caps becomes more transparent, it becomes easier for the Commission as well as stakeholders to establish whether or not the Treaty rules on free movement and competition are being properly respected, particularly if these processes favour domestic production over and above imports. An attempt by the UK parallel trade organization for judicial review of the modulation provision in the UK Pharmaceutical Price Regulation Scheme (PPRS) is a case in point.[5]

The emergence of soft law instruments?

The conclusions of the Pammolli Report on Global Competitiveness, as well as the work of the G10 Group set up by the Commission to examine the various issues raised by the report, has provided renewed stimulus for Community action on the very national price regimes that insulate the sector from competitive forces. National price and profit regulation was criticized in the Pammolli Report as having essentially protective effects on European industry and reducing the incentive to innovate. Following on from the December 2000 'Competitiveness Round Table', the so-called 'G10 Group', comprised of health and industry ministers, pharmaceutical company and patient representatives was to report by April 2002 to Commission President Romano Prodi on key objectives that reconcile the needs of patients and industry. From the outset, the Commission expressed the hope that the Group would agree on policy approaches that would not necessarily require the Commission to take legislative action.[6]

The G10 process

The G10 Group's deliberations have departed from past practice and have instead followed the 'Lisbon Method' of open coordination – that is, the Commission was expected to play only a facilitative role to allow the members of the Group to develop their own practical recommendations. Consultation with, and the involvement of, a wider group of stakeholders was facilitated through a special website and a series of workshops based around an initial discussion paper setting out the major issues identified by the Group for the completion of its report (European Commission 2001b). This commitment to transparency resulted in a large number of critical and usually conflicting responses, many of which have been posted on the G10 website. The aim of G10's own working practice was to arrive at consensus on future action, a process that has led to the presentation of a package of 14 recommendations for future action, all of which were agreed by its members to have equal value and which should be considered as an integrated whole that represents, as a package, an acceptable balance between competing interests and a practical framework for future action.

Indeed, in addressing the twin goals of encouraging innovation while ensuring satisfactory delivery of public health, the Group was mandated to arrive at a 'benchmarking' exercise of competitiveness and performance indicators, which would capture not only the individual factors affecting the competitiveness of the EU-based industry but also its ability to contribute to the delivery of European health objectives. Two facets of this 'benchmarking exercise' have been emphasized in the Group's final report. First, the report claims that currently there is no set of agreed EU indicators on which to make comparisons between the EU and its major competitors as a basis for establishing best practices within the EU. Second, this same exercise has to extend to public health objectives, given that the assessment of competitiveness indicators alone could not allow a full assessment of the value and role of the Community's pharmaceutical industry. Hence the G10 (2002) recommended (see Recommendation One) that the Commission itself should develop a comprehensive set of indicators covering the performance of the industry, the performance of its products and, importantly, the relationship between the various EU and member state regulatory structures (licensing, pricing and reimbursement) and availability (time to license and time to market), access and uptake. This 'benchmarking process' and the subsequent 'best practices' recommendations and guidelines, all of which clearly are the Commission's preserve, would presumably be used to encourage member states to take unilateral initiatives and action to align their own regulatory practice with those of the country that performed best. Hence, the Group recommends that each national government should review its current regulatory structure and find ways to make it more efficient to ensure better access to markets and availability of products. Aligning regulatory practice is not necessarily the same thing as aligning regulation. Divergence of regulation is not so much the problem, but diversity of result. If the output of the divergent national regulatory processes were similar, this would seem to be sufficient. The Group recognized that this would not be a straightforward exercise, given regulatory divergence, but has argued that it is necessary if existing and subsequent policies in this area are to be assessed effectively.

This general approach clearly informs the remaining, substantive recommendations that will be considered briefly here. Recommendation Two centres on access and availability of innovative medicines and stresses the link between the effective operation of the Community and national licensing systems as central to the development of a comprehensive research-based industry.

Recommendation Three is linked to this theme – regulatory procedures should be effective and ensure speed of access to the market. Importantly, it states that pricing and reimbursement procedures are national competencies.

Recommendation Four deals with generic competition, which should be promoted through improvements in the licensing process, by achieving an appropriate balance between providing sufficient intellectual property protection for the research-based industry and generic market access via a Bolar provision.[7] It is, however, for member states to determine the requisite degree of generic penetration of their markets.

Recommendation Five suggests that national regulatory 'switch mechanisms' should be put in place to ensure ease of reclassification of certain products from prescription to non-prescription status, and at the same time to allow the continued use of the same trademarks. Furthermore, Recommendation Six suggests that 'the Commission and Member States should secure the principle that a Member State's authority to regulate prices in the EU should extend only to those medicines purchased by or reimbursed by the State. Full competition should be allowed for medicines not reimbursed by State systems or sold into private markets' (p. 16). In addition, all restrictions or bans on advertising of non-prescription medicines should be abolished and such products should only be subject to general rules against misleading advertising, together with sharing of information and development of common approaches to the regulation of such advertising. This approach should eventually provide an opportunity for a genuine EU-wide market for such products and even a pan-European price. The related Recommendations Ten and Eleven deal with access to information and standardization of patient information – matters to be dealt with in any event under the Community's review of the marketing authorization systems. While recognizing that advertising of prescription medicines was not desirable, the Group felt that patient access to product information should be improved by means of guidelines emanating from collaborative public–private partnerships involving a range of interested parties.

Recommendation Seven concerns national mechanisms to establish relative cost and clinical effectiveness of medicines and while recognizing this as a matter of national competence, suggests that the Commission could facilitate exchange of information and data on this issue. Stricter pharmacovigilance mechanisms and funding of patient groups are also recommended.

Inevitably, a major factor determining the future success of the Group's proposed approach and recommendations will be whether the Commission can succeed in convincing national governments to accept coordination, by means of intervention through 'soft law' mechanisms such as guidelines, and benchmarks, not only in industrial policy matters but also for sensitive health policy issues, which the Group itself recognizes to be primarily matters of national competence. But an important – and indeed difficult – part of the process will be how appropriate 'benchmarks' are to be designed. This in itself is a complex issue but from a legal perspective it will also be crucial to examine how such benchmarks, which are to be developed to measure and assess the effectiveness of national systems governing market access, can function within the existing legal framework as supplied by the Treaty and related secondary legislation. A system of coordination based on benchmarking will not necessarily eliminate diversity of approach and disparity in regulatory instruments; rather, it could endorse disparity and diversity. Each national system's chosen method of achieving an adequate balance between industrial and health policy objectives may well be deemed appropriate in the light of the particular national trade-offs that have to be made. These trade-offs will inevitably vary depending on whether the member state in question is (or intends to be) an important home market for research-based products or whether it is primarily an importer of such products. It will obviously depend on whether trade-offs have traditionally been made between high volumes of consumption and low-priced medicines or higher prices and lower consumption. A key question, then, is whether a particular national trade-off that results in a particular set of prices being granted for pharmaceutical products can effectively be 'insulated' from external factors such as parallel trade and, to a lesser extent, generic competition. Can industry based in a high-price country legitimately claim that competing imports should be prohibited? Can industry based in a low-priced country, where different trade-offs have been agreed, impose restrictions on exports of these low-priced products to markets where they have been awarded higher prices? In this respect, the final Recommendation Fourteen on enlargement deserves particular attention: the Group recommends that the differences in marketing and economic conditions between member states and candidate countries should be taken into account and a derogation governing parallel imports should be included in the accession Treaties. It is to these issues of diversity and disparity within the Community legal framework to which I now turn.

National disparities and the Community legal framework

Free movement

In its case law relating to the application of the rules on free movement of goods and services in the health care sector, the European Court of Justice has been notably cautious in applying the relevant Treaty rules (Articles 28 and 48 EC) and have recognized that it is for the individual member states to determine their requisite standard of product safety and health care and to organize their social security schemes, subject to the proviso that the Treaty rules should be respected. In the absence of harmonization measures (i.e. secondary legislation), the Court has been generally reluctant to strike down national rules and regulations on price and profit regulation as well as on positive and negative lists designed to control the types of medicines admitted for reimbursement. Member states remain in principle free to determine selling methods of pharmaceutical products pursuant to Article 28, provided that imported products are not discriminated against in an arbitrary or disproportionate way (ECJ 1995a).

As most of this case law has been directed at national regimes aimed at controlling prices (and reimbursement levels), attempts to use the Treaty rules on free movement to attack national price regimes resulting in low prices have not proved successful. Thus these same rules, which are often regarded as an important contributing factor to the process of parallel trade, can remain intact. At the same time, however, the European Court has been keen to guarantee the process of parallel trade and the rights of parallel traders and to strike down what it regards as unnecessary obstacles to free movement resulting from the exercise of nationally divergent intellectual property rights (IPRs). It has also proved willing to tackle what it considers unnecessary burdens imposed through national licensing regimes on parallel imports. In this way, parallel traders who source their products in a low-priced country can often re-brand or re-name a particular product and market it in a high-priced country, while at the same time relying on the product authorization obtained by the producer who first obtained authorization to market the product in the high-priced country as a 'reference product'.

The early case law of the Court firmly established the principle that the owner of an IPR, such as a patent, trademark or copyright, could not invoke it to prevent the importation and sale of a medicinal product, which had been placed on the market with his consent in another member state. The so-called principle of 'exhaustion of rights' was prompted by the desire to eliminate any risk of the use of intellectual property rights to establish artificial divisions within the common market. The principle balanced the idea that the owner could hold or enjoy the national rights in question – that is, that the rights in question continued to exist in national law – against the idea that the exercise of those rights was controlled by Community law. As with any principle, its limits were quickly put to the test.

The recent case law reviewed below indicates that the European Court of Justice has been unwilling to reverse its traditional pro-internal market and hence pro-parallel import approach, especially in the field of intellectual property law even if, as the G10 Report has underlined, intellectual property rights are of vital importance to the research-based pharmaceutical industry.

As already noted, generic or inter-brand competition between products whose patent protection has lapsed is another important source of price competition. Barriers to increased market entry for generics abound, however. These include not only difficulties in obtaining market authorization without generating all the requisite data, but may also relate to the workings of national price and profit control regimes.

Article 28 EC and intellectual property rights

Article 28 prohibits all measures that have an equivalent effect to quantitative restrictions on the free movement of goods, including, in principle, national IPR laws. Article 30 offers a limited exemption from this strict prohibition and provides that Article 28 shall not preclude prohibitions or restrictions on imports, which are justified by the protection of industrial and commercial property rights as long as these rights do not constitute a means of arbitrary discrimination or a disguised restriction on trade between member states.

The European Court was offered its first opportunity to reverse its traditionally pro-parallel trade approach to IPRs in *Merck* v. *Primecrown* (ECJ 1996a). Merck argued that pharmaceutical companies did not choose where to market their products, but that they were under an ethical and sometimes even a legal obligation to supply their products to a particular national market. They could not discontinue existing supplies to a market and were forced to put up with national price controls. The Advocate General strongly recommended that the Court should reconsider the earlier case law, and should recognize that a patent holder should be able to prevent parallel imports from member states (Spain and Portugal) where it could not have obtained adequate IPR protection. The Court, however, ruled that the original manufacturer had 'consented' voluntarily to putting its products on the market in the knowledge that full patent protection could not be obtained. While acknowledging the problems created by national price differentials as being the fuelling force for parallel trade, as discussed above, the Court firmly placed responsibility for resolving them with the Commission and the Council. It resolutely refused to water down the rights of free movement as guaranteed by the European Community Treaties. The judgment has, however, been criticized as failing to take on board the realities of the situation confronting the industry, which are, of course, that national price regulation schemes still divide the common or single market. This issue is now put before the Court of First Instance in the Glaxo Wellcome case, which is discussed below.

The Court's insistence on a strict application of the 'exhaustion doctrine' has led the research-based industry to lobby for strict safeguards in the accession treaties with those new member countries that have also traditionally denied strong patent protection to pharmaceuticals. The precedent of such safeguard measures in the earlier accession agreements with Spain and Portugal indicate that a transitional period preventing importation of non-patented products is possible, but that these safeguard measures must be properly drawn up to be effective in practice.

Repackaging

Complex litigation has arisen with regard to the reliance on IPRs by the original manufacturer to defend its trademarks where parallel importers have repackaged a product sold under a particular trademark in Country B in order to resell it under the trademark current in Country A. Once again the doctrine of exhaustion is of importance here, although the problem is further complicated by the fact that national trademark law has been subject to a certain degree of harmonization as a result of the adoption of secondary legislation in 1989. Has the manufacturer exhausted his trademark rights by putting the product on the common market under different trademarks in the first place? The answer to this question lies in the nature of the specific subject matter of the trademark right. The Court has recognized that trademarks have as an essential function, a guarantee to the consumer or end user of the identity of the trademarked product's origin (ECJ 1978a). Nevertheless, in its early case law, the Court added an important proviso: it was still necessary to consider whether the exercise of an IPR could constitute a disguised restriction on trade, contrary to Article 28 (ex 30) EC (ECJ 1978b).

Three cases decided in 1996 – *Paranova* (ECJ 1996b), *Eurim-Pharm* (ECJ 1996c) and *Rhône-Poulenc* (ECJ 1996d) – raised the issue of whether the trademark holder could rely upon the First Trade Marks Directive[8] to prevent importation of repackaged parallel-imported products. The parallel importers had repackaged the goods, either by removing the blister packs from their original external packs and placing them in new packs or by severing the blister strips and repackaging them. The key issue before the Court in these 'repackaging cases' was whether any of these actions impaired or changed the conditions of the products. However, the Court was also asked to address the relevance of the trademark owner's intention to partition markets. In essence, it was asked to determine whether this test should be a subjective or an objective one: was it necessary to demonstrate that the trademark owner actually planned this result, or was it sufficient to demonstrate that this was the inevitable result of its action in using different marks in the first place?

The Court took a strict approach to the question of intention.[9] The power of the owner of trademark rights protected in a member state to oppose the marketing of repackaged products under a different trademark could be limited where the repackaging undertaken by the importer is necessary for the importer to market the product in the member state of importation. It was not up to the importer to demonstrate that the trademark owner had deliberately sought to partition the markets between member states by using different marks in different countries. Only if the action of the parallel importer affected or was likely to affect the product itself, could the trademark owner oppose the repackaging as an infringement of his legitimate trademark rights. In the Court's view: 'trade mark rights are not intended to allow their owners to partition national markets and thus promote the retention of price differences which may exist between Member States' (paras 42 to 45 of the *Paranova* ruling).

Numerous disputes before national courts have arisen as a result of these rulings and in particular there appears to be considerable variation as to how national courts apply the 'necessity' test, which the Court introduced in the *Paranova* cases. In Case C-433/99 *Merck, Sharp & Dohme* (ECJ 2002), the Court was asked to deal with a situation in which a trademark proprietor had opposed repackaging consisting in replacement of the original packaging by new packaging designed by the importer, and had required that the importer restrict itself to relabelling by means of self-adhesive stickers.

The Court recalled that it had already clarified what may constitute artificial partitioning of the markets between member states. In certain circumstances, where repackaging is necessary to allow the product imported in parallel to be marketed in the importing member state, opposition of the trademark proprietor to the repackaging of pharmaceutical products is to be regarded as constituting artificial partitioning of markets. Hence it was necessary to take account of the circumstances prevailing at the time of marketing in the importing member state, which make repackaging objectively necessary in order that the pharmaceutical product can be placed on the market in that member state by the parallel importer. The trademark proprietor's opposition to the repackaging is not justified if it hinders effective access of the imported product to the market of that member state.

Such an impediment exists, for example, where pharmaceutical products purchased by the parallel importer cannot be placed on the market in the member state of importation in their original packaging by reason of national rules or practices relating to packaging, or where sickness insurance rules make reimbursement of medical expenses depend on a certain packaging or where well-established medical prescription practices are based, *inter alia*, on standard sizes recommended by professional groups and sickness insurance institutions. In contrast, the trademark proprietor may oppose the repackaging if it is based solely on the parallel importer's attempt to secure a commercial advantage. Furthermore, a trademark proprietor may oppose replacement packaging where the parallel importer is able to re-use the original packaging for the purpose of marketing in the member state of importation by affixing labels to that packaging.

Thus, while the trademark proprietor may still oppose the parallel importer's use of replacement packaging, this is conditional on the relabelled pharmaceutical product being able to have effective access to the market concerned. Patient resistance to relabelled pharmaceutical products does not always constitute an impediment to effective market access such as to make replacement packaging necessary, within the meaning of the Court's case law. However, there may exist on a market, or on a substantial part of it, such strong resistance from a significant proportion of consumers to relabelled pharmaceutical products that there must be held to be a hindrance to effective market access. In those circumstances, repackaging of the pharmaceutical products would not be explicable solely by the attempt to secure a commercial advantage. The purpose would be to achieve effective market access.

In this light, the Court concluded that replacement packaging of pharmaceutical products is objectively necessary if, without such repackaging, effective access to the market concerned, or to a substantial part of that market, must be considered to be hindered as the result of strong resistance from a significant proportion of consumers to relabelled pharmaceutical products.[10]

The Court has attempted, however, to ensure that the trademark owner could exercise some degree of control over how products were repackaged. The parallel importer must indicate who has repackaged the product; the importer must indicate on the packaging that it has not manufactured the product and must not wrongly attribute any responsibility for any additional articles added to the packaging of the trademark owner. In addition, the importer must give the trademark owner advance notice of the product being put on sale, and the owner can require that it is supplied in advance of sale of a specimen of the repackaged product (ECJ 1996b).

Re-branding

A related issue concerns the right of a parallel importer to affix different trademarks to parallel imported products. The original trademark owner may have been compelled for reasons of national law to register its product under different marks in different member states. This may be because certain similar marks had already been registered at national level or because of simple language differences. Again, the basic question arises, should the trademark owner be allowed to take advantage of a situation that has arisen as a result of circumstances outside his control and rely on his trademark to exclude parallel imports even though the exclusion of such imports is not necessary on grounds of trademark protection. In Case C-379/97 *Upjohn* v. *Paranova* (ECJ 1997), the Court confirmed that the factors which led the trademark owner to use different marks in the importing and exporting member states are not relevant. It was necessary to examine the question of when it might be necessary for parallel importers to re-brand products in order to lawfully import and market them in another member state. In principle, if various practices or rules in the member state of import have the effect that the importer cannot market the products under the mark they bear in the member state of export, the trademark owner will not be able to rely on the trademark rights to prevent importation of identical goods. Indeed, there may be an even greater necessity for the importer to re-brand to avoid confusion with other marks currently used in the state of import.

The circumstances that led the original trademark owner to use different marks should be regarded as historical and there is no good reason for the Court to use them as defining criteria for determining the lawfulness of subsequent conduct. The decisive test is whether in a given case prohibiting the importer from re-branding would constitute an obstacle to effective access to the markets of the importing member state (ECJ 1997).

Free movement of goods and licensing issues in relation to generics and parallel imports[11]

Parallel imports

According to the principles laid down in Directive 65/65 (Council of the European Union 1993), no medicinal product may be placed on the market for the first time in a member state unless a marketing authorization has been issued in accordance with the Directive by the competent authority of that member state. Applications for marketing authorizations must contain extensive information, and must be accompanied by the documents listed in Article 4 of the Directive, even where the medicinal product concerned is already the subject of an authorization issued by the competent authority of another member state (ECJ 1999). However, those principles are subject to exceptions resulting, on the one hand, from the Directive itself and, on the other, from the rules of the EC Treaty relating to the free movement of goods. Thus, an operator who has bought a medicinal product lawfully marketed in one member state under a marketing authorization issued in that member state can import that medicinal product into another member state where he already has a marketing authorization without having to obtain such an authorization in accordance with Directive 65/65, and without having to provide information about the verification, prescribed by the Directive, of efficacy and non-toxicity of the medicinal product. It is not necessary for the protection of public health to subject parallel importers to such requirements, as the competent authorities of the member state of importation already have all the information necessary to carry out that verification.[12] In such a case, the parallel import is authorized in the member state of importation by reference to the marketing authorization issued in accordance with Directive 65/65 ('marketing authorization of reference').

In recent months, the Court has been asked to deal with a number of cases involving market authorization of a parallel imported product into a country where the original 'reference' product has either been modified or withdrawn. In Case C172/00 *Ferring* (ECJ 2000b), a medicinal product known as 'Minirin Spray' ('the old version') – an antidiuretic consisting of an active substance known as Desmopressin – was being marketed in Germany on the basis of an implied authorization issued under the then applicable German legislation. As of June 1996, Eurim-Pharm, a parallel trader, imported that medicinal product from another member state and marketed it in Germany. In July 1999, Ferring waived the implied authorization, by notification to the Bundesinstitut für Arzneimittel und Medizinprodukte, on the grounds that it was now marketing a medicinal product known as 'Minirin Nasenspray 5 ml' ('the new version') under a marketing authorization obtained in accordance with the new German legislation. The new version contains different excipients. Subsequently, Ferring brought proceedings against Eurim-Pharm before the courts of Köln for an order restraining it from importing and marketing the old version, claiming that Eurim-Pharm was marketing the 'old' product without authorization. That court made an interim order restraining Eurim-Pharm from importing the old version and placing it on the German market. In the absence of a marketing authorization, the parallel importer has no basis on which to operate, and Ferring argued that as a consequence of the cancellation of the marketing authorization that it held for the old version, Eurim-Pharm should have applied for a new parallel import licence by reference to the new marketing authorization. In the course of this procedure, the competent authority in the member state must ascertain whether the old and new versions have different therapeutic effects. Until that authority reaches a decision, the old version cannot be marketed. The German courts, in turn, turned to the European Courts for guidance on the interpretation of the Treaty rules on free movement in this situation. Would a national legal rule requiring a parallel importer to obtain a new licence run counter to Article 28 EC?

Giving judgment in favour of Eurim-Pharm, the Court observed that in accordance with German law it is no longer possible for the parallel importer to continue to import the old version of the medicinal product, as the mere fact that the marketing authorization of reference has been withdrawn entails the automatic withdrawal of the parallel import licence. Thus it was important to ascertain whether Articles 28 EC and 30 EC would preclude national legislation which had such effect. The Commission supported the parallel trader in its observations before the Court, and argued that as the competent authorities of the member state of importation have the necessary documents and, in particular, those concerning the manufacturing process and the qualitative and quantitative composition of the medicinal product of reference, then the withdrawal of the marketing authorization for that product at the request of the holder is a purely formal act, which changes nothing in relation to the medicinal product concerned. The Commission emphasized that a parallel import licence cannot depend on the wishes of the holder of the marketing authorization for the medicinal product of reference. An arbitrary withdrawal entailing the lapse of the parallel import licence would lead to a compartmentalization of the market and would be contrary to the proper functioning of the internal or single market.

The Court held first that the cessation of the validity of a parallel import licence following the withdrawal of the marketing authorization of reference constitutes a restriction on the free movement of goods contrary to Article 28 EC, unless it is justified by reasons relating to the protection of public health, in accordance with the provisions of Article 30 EC. It is for the national authorities responsible for the operation of the legislation governing the production and marketing of medicinal products – legislation that, as is made clear in the first recital of Directive 65/65, has as its primary objective the safeguarding of public health – to ensure that it is fully complied with. Nevertheless, the principle of proportionality, which is the basis of the last sentence of Article 30 EC, requires that the power of the member states to prohibit imports of products from other member states should be restricted to what is really necessary to achieve the aims concerning the protection of health that are legitimately pursued.[13] Thus, national legislation or practice cannot benefit from the derogation laid down in Article 30 EC when the health and life of humans can be protected equally effectively by measures less restrictive of intra-Community trade.

The Court further reasoned that, although adequate monitoring of the old version remains necessary and may in certain cases mean that information is requested from the importer, it must be pointed out that pharmacovigilance satisfying the relevant requirements of the Community Directives can ordinarily be guaranteed for medicinal products that are the subject of parallel imports, through cooperation with the national authorities of the other member states by means of access to the documents and data produced by the manufacturer or other companies in the same group, relating to the old version in the member states in which that version is still marketed on the basis of a marketing authorization still in force. While it was not open to the Court to rule on the question relating to the existence and reality of a risk to public health linked to the co-existence of the two versions of the medicinal product in question on the German market, it is conceivable that the risk to public health which the original manufacturer had warned against could have been averted satisfactorily by appropriate labelling.

The Ferring case, and the more recent ruling in Case C-113/01 *Paranova* (ECJ 2003b), confirm earlier case law which ensures that parallel imports can rely upon the protection of the Treaty principles on free movement, and further confirms that the Court is not averse to reviewing the decisions of national licensing authorities on sensitive public health issues.

Generics

Generic versions, which are 'essentially similar' to the original patented product, can also benefit from a special, fast-track licensing procedure. The so-called 'abridged procedure' is set out in Article 8(a)(iii) of the codified Directive. It is intended to ensure that, by allowing generic products to 'piggy back' on the data submitted by the licence holder for the original product, there is no unnecessary duplication of tests on humans or animals, which would be required if a full application had to be submitted. The need to ensure that innovative firms are not placed at a disadvantage is also recognized, and is dealt with by the requirement in point 8(a)(iii) that the reference product must have been authorized in the Community for a period of between 6 and 10 years, otherwise access by the national authority to the data submitted by the original licensee is precluded. Unfortunately, the relevant provisions of the Directive have given rise to substantial litigation – particularly, in relation to the exact meaning of the term 'essential similarity' – in circumstances where the generic and the original version of a particular product may exhibit certain differences with regard to dosage, form and indications.

As is clear from the Court's previous case-law, in particular Case C-368/96 *Generics* (ECJ 1998), the starting point when interpreting the meaning of essential similarity, as with the other requirements of the Directive, must be to ensure that the requirements of safety and efficacy are at all times maintained in respect of 'abridged' applications, through the specification of standards that are sufficiently precise and detailed to ensure a harmonized level of protection. In *Generics*, the Court adopted a definition of essential similarity drawn from the minutes of the meeting of the Council in December 1986 at which the 'abridged procedure' was originally adopted.[14] This specifies bioequivalence together with pharmaceutical form and qualitative and quantitative composition as criteria, which the competent authority of a member state may not disregard when determining whether two products are essentially similar.

In Case C-106/01 *Novartis* (ECJ 2001c), the research-based company had submitted to the Court that bioequivalence is a necessary requirement for essential similarity. The relevant licensing authority, the UK government and SangStat (the generic company) asserts that bioequivalence is not an invariable requirement for a finding of essential similarity. They submitted also that bioequivalence will not always be a relevant criterion to determine whether two products are equally safe and efficacious, and that therefore it should not constitute an inflexible requirement of essential similarity. They also argued that in respect of certain types of product, the criterion of bioequivalence is inapplicable because they owe their therapeutic effect to topical application rather than transmission via systemic circulation. To date, the Advocate General has rejected all these arguments and has stated that in his opinion bioequivalence is a necessary requirement of essential similarity (ECJ 2003b). Hence for two products to be essentially similar for the purposes of the abridged procedures, they must be bioequivalent.

In a further case, Case C-2203/01 *AstraZeneca* (ECJ 2001d), the exact scope of the abridged procedures have again been the subject of dispute, this time in relation to the use of the abridged procedures for a product where the original reference product had been withdrawn from the market of the member state in question before the application under the abridged procedure was lodged. In this case, the applicant, Generics, claimed that the procedure can be applied where the reference product has been at least some time previously authorized prior to the filing of the generic application in the member state concerned. The

Advocate General has preferred the interpretation favoured by the Danish government and the Commission that if, in accordance with the procedures, the applicant has to demonstrate that the reference product 'is marketed', he cannot do so by demonstrating that it 'has been marketed' at some time but no longer is marketed: the two are not synonymous (see ECJ 2003c). He did not, however, accept the even more restrictive interpretation advocated by Astra-Zeneca, namely that for a marketing authorization to be valid in accordance with point 8(a)(iii), the reference product must be covered by a marketing authorization both when the application is made and when the authorization is actually granted.

The Advocate General noted that in practice his approach would enable the manufacturer of a branded product to prevent generic manufacturers from using the abridged procedure by withdrawing that product from the market, a consequence stressed by several of the parties submitting observations. Even if a particular product to which reference could otherwise be made under point 8(a)(iii) has been withdrawn from the market in a member state, a generic company will in many cases still be able to obtain authorization to market the generic product in that member state. If a variant of the reference product is marketed in the member state in question, the Court's decision in *Generics* will often mean that reference can be made to the newer version, even if its authorization was obtained within the 6–10 year period of data protection.

AstraZeneca also argued that if its interpretation is not endorsed by the Court, the competent authority of the member state for which the application is made will be unable to discharge its duties of pharmacovigilance. The Advocate General found this argument to be unacceptable. It still remains open to the competent authority of the member state where an application under the abridged procedure is made, if it considers it appropriate, to approach the company that holds the marketing authorization for the reference product in another member state before issuing an authorization for the generic product. Furthermore, the person responsible for placing the product on the market is required to record and promptly report to the competent authorities all suspected serious adverse reactions brought to his attention by a health care professional and to maintain detailed records of all other suspected adverse reactions so reported. Those records are to be submitted to the competent authorities at once. These pharmacovigilance obligations will, however, continue to apply for so long as the reference products have marketing authorizations in other member states.

In this respect, the Advocate General drew an analogy with the case of a parallel importer where the marketing authorization for the reference product is withdrawn for reasons unconnected with the safety of the product. Although it is clear from the case-law of the Court that the parallel import of medicinal products is not governed by Directive 65/65, the question has arisen of whether in such circumstances, adequate pharmacovigilance may be ensured by the competent authority of the member state of import in the absence of a marketing authorization for the reference product. The Court stated in *Ferring* (ECJ 2000b) that, although adequate monitoring of the old version remained necessary in the member state of import, satisfactory pharmacovigilance could ordinarily be guaranteed through cooperation with the national authorities of the other member states by means of access to the documents and data produced by the manufacturer or other companies in the same group, relating to the old version in the member states in which that version was still marketed on the basis of a marketing authorization still in force.

The Court's approach in these various cases, as confirmed and developed by its Advocate Generals in the latest Opinions reviewed here, illustrate the continuing importance of the Treaty principles as well as the willingness of the Courts to review and strike down national licensing decisions. These rulings are of considerable importance given the frequent criticism that many manufacturers devote considerable resources to modifying older products with a view to extending their effective monopoly long after the underlying patents have expired.

Competition law (Articles 81–82)

Even if the parallel trader can take advantage of weak patent protection to obtain supplies of imitation products in some countries, the more usual source of this trade is through wholesalers supplied through official distribution channels by the original manufacturers in low-priced member states. The most obvious defensive strategy for such manufacturers is in turn to try to limit the available supplies to the volumes required to serve the relevant national markets or to attempt to persuade wholesalers not to supply parallel traders. Both these tactics can involve the risk of infringement of the Community competition rules, and with it the risk of a heavy fine. In this respect, pleas to the effect that the internal market is divided along national lines as a result of national pricing rules and that original manufacturers should be able to defend their position accordingly, have so far fallen on deaf ears at the Community's Competition Directorate. This argument was run, without success, by Organon in 1995 to defend its attempts to limit supplies of cheap contraceptive drugs from finding their way from the UK into the Netherlands (ECJ 1995b).

A similar fate befell Bayer in its attempts to stem the flow of parallel imports of its product Adalat, which could be purchased in France at up to 50 per cent less than the UK market price. A straightforward ban on export by wholesalers can lead to breach of Article 81(1) EC, which prohibits, *inter alia*, anti-competitive agreements between manufacturers and distributors. Bayer's approach was more subtle. Wholesalers were requested to provide regular information on their onward supplies. No contractual agreements were entered into, however. The Commission took action against this strategy, claiming that a quasi-contractual agreement existed between Bayer and the suppliers, and that these bilateral arrangements infringed Article 81(1). It should be noted that the Commission could not have condemned Bayer's apparent plan to control supplies as an abuse of a dominant position under Article 82, as it found that Bayer only held a relatively small share of the relevant market (European Commission 1996). Bayer challenged the Commission's decision on the ground that its behaviour was purely unilateral, and so could not be caught by Article 81(1) EC.

The Court of First Instance (CFI) has confirmed that the Commission had erred in law in its interpretation of Article 81(1) EC and has quashed the Commission's decision. The CFI ruled that the Commission cannot hold that apparently unilateral conduct on the part of a manufacturer adopted in the context of the contractual relations which he maintains with his dealers in reality forms the basis of an agreement between undertakings within the meaning of Article 81(1) if it does not establish the existence of an acquiescence by the other partners, express or implied, in the attitude adopted by the manufacturer. The Court appears to have imposed a high standard of proof on the Commission in such a case (para. 72), especially as the Commission will usually not have access to documentary evidence to support the conclusion that there is agreement or acquiescence on limiting or reducing exports. Much of the circumstantial evidence put forward by the Commission to support its claim that parties had agreed to an export ban was held to be irrelevant. Importantly, the Court ruled that 'the right of a manufacturer faced, as in this case, with an event harmful to his interest, to adopt the solution which seems to him to be the best is qualified by the Treaty provisions on competition only to the extent that he must comply with the prohibitions referred to in Articles 85 (now 81) and 86 (now 82EC). Accordingly, provided he does so without abusing a dominant position, and there is no "concurrence of wills" between him and his wholesalers, a manufacturer may adopt the supply policy which he considers necessary, even if, by the very nature of its aim, for example, to hinder parallel imports, the implementation of that policy may entail restrictions on competition and free trade between the Member States' (Court of First Instance 2000: para. 176). Contrary to the assertions of the Commission, the Court has never recognized in its jurisprudence that parallel imports must be protected in all circumstances. The Commission lodged an appeal against this ruling, not least because the CFI's approach now appears to offer manufacturers numerous possibilities of hindering parallel imports through restricting supply volumes on low-price markets and has effectively deprived the Commission of a meaningful way of dealing with them. The European Court of Justice on appeal, confirmed the ruling of the Court of First Instance.

A decision of 8 May 2001 prohibiting Glaxo Wellcome from maintaining a dual-pricing scheme in respect of its supplies to the Spanish market indicates that the Commission is not yet prepared to accept the research-based industry's argument that it should be entitled to take appropriate action to respond to differences in national price control regimes.[15] Glaxo Wellcome had notified the Commission of new conditions for the sale of all its products to wholesalers in Spain (where maximum regulatory prices prevail). These wholesalers would have to pay higher prices for products which they would export than for products which they would resell for consumption on the domestic market. Glaxo Wellcome's dual-pricing system was found to limit parallel trade from Spain to other member states for the vast majority of its products, therefore interfering with the Community's objectives of integrating national markets, and it restricted price competition for its products to a significant extent. The Commission was not convinced by the 'consumer welfare' claims that losses incurred by Glaxo Wellcome due to parallel trade would seriously affect its R&D budget, which it uses to develop innovative drugs. This argument was not corroborated by the facts.

Glaxo Wellcome's dual-pricing scheme was seen by many as an important test case – the Commission was confronted for the first time with a set of agreements which explicitly sought to restrict parallel trade but which the company sought to justify on economic grounds.[16] The policy implications are clear: the Commission considers that companies will have to continue to live with national regulatory divergences. Importantly, the Commission stressed that the R&D budget of most pharmaceutical companies only represents around 15 per cent of their total budget: losses stemming from parallel trade could equally be deducted from the companies' other budget items such as marketing costs (European Commission 2001c).

The findings of the Pammolli Report may have encouraged the Commission's competition services to make such a bold statement. Parallel trade, as the Commission emphasizes in the Glaxo Wellcome decision, is a major source of competition for products still in patent. Glaxo has appealed against this decision before the Court of First Instance. This will require the Court to consider the legitimate scope available to companies to deal with disparities arising from national price regulatory schemes. In its earlier ruling in Cases C-267/95 and C-268/95 *Merck and Beecham* (ECJ 1996f), the Court of Justice had ruled that such divergence did not justify any derogation from the principle of the free movement of goods and the possibility of preventing parallel imports entailed an undesirable partitioning of national markets. In the *Bayer* case, discussed above, the CFI noted that the Merck judgment confirms that 'it is not open to the Commission to achieve a result, such as the harmonization of prices in the medicinal products market, by enlarging the scope of the ... [competition rules], especially since the Treaty gives the Commission specific means of seeking such harmonization where it is undisputed that large disparities in the prices of medicinal products in the Member States are engendered by the differences between the state mechanisms for fixing prices' (para. 179). It went on to note that the case-law of the Court indirectly recognizes the importance of safeguarding free enterprise when applying the competition rules where it expressly acknowledges that even an undertaking in a dominant position may change its supply policies without falling under the prohibition of Article 82.

The question now before the Court is whether companies are entitled to react to the disparities in national laws and protect their legitimate commercial interests. In this context, the actual scope available to the Commission to address the very national disparities in question, which do not appear in themselves to conflict with the Treaty principles of free movement, appears limited. If, on the basis of the recommendations put forward by the G10 Group, coordination is preferred to harmonization, it is all the more likely that such disparities will remain.

Conclusion

The fact that European pharmaceuticals markets are still not a single 'internal' market, but 15 separate national markets, is something of a truism. Divergence and diversity in national approach to many fundamental issues is still the order of the day, despite four decades of Community-led attempts towards convergence. The G10 process may mark the beginning of a departure away from attempts to remove disparity between the rules and regulations governing national markets – and towards a new approach based on convergence of results. This is perhaps on one level the best that can be hoped for, given the entrenched differences between the member states in matters of health care and, to a lesser extent, industrial policy. In this chapter, I have tried to highlight that this new approach must still be situated in the existing Community legal framework. National divergences, which result in conflict with the basic Community principles of free movement and competition, may well prove vulnerable to successful legal challenge, not only by parallel traders but also by generic producers.

It is unfortunate that the G10 Group did not consider this important dimension in any detail in its deliberations. Its recommendations with regard to the new 'nearly' member states, which will become official members in May 2004, and which could be an important source of generic production as well as parallel trade, indicate that its preferred solution is to exclude their markets from the process of integration, even if on a temporary basis. No doubt creative entrepreneurs will still find ways to avoid continuing restrictions on parallel trade and generic competition, thus generating further complex case-law before the European courts. In the meantime, the viability of the benchmarked, individual national trade-offs eventually endorsed by the Commission along the lines recommended by the G10 Group for the current 15 member states remains open to question. As long as the Courts continue to uphold the rights of parallel traders to source their products in low-price markets, to repackage and even re-brand those products and, at the same time, allow these traders and generic manufacturers to benefit from fast-track licensing or abridged authorization processes, hence profiting from better margins in high-priced markets, this will surely erode market share for the research-based industry. Whether this process will take place on such a scale as to defeat the very purpose of the benchmarking exercise remains to be seen.

Notes

1 In its judgment in Case C-157/99 *Smits and Peerbooms* of 12 July 2001 (ECJ 2001b), the Court recalled that 'according to settled case law, Community law does not detract from the power of the Member States to organize their social security systems. In the absence of harmonization at Community level it is therefore for the legislation of each Member State to determine the conditions concerning the right or duty to be insured with a social security scheme. Nevertheless, the Member States must comply with Community law when exercising that power' (paras 44–46 of the judgment).

2 The judgment of the Court of First Instance in Case T-41/969 Bayer of 26 October 2000 (CFI 2000) illustrates the limits of its powers in this respect; however, see below.

3 This resulted in a reference for a preliminary ruling to the European Court of Justice from the German Federal Court on 4 July 2001. In early 2001, the German Health Ministry put reference prices on a new legal footing by means of an ordinance.

4 For a fuller discussion of the Directive, see Hancher (1990: 170–5).

5 Parallel importers claimed, unsuccessfully, that this scheme allows manufacturers to introduce deep discounts for prices of products under competition from parallel trade

while maintaining high prices for other products. See further, the Sixth PPRS Report to Parliament (Department of Health 2002). The research-based industry has also used the Directive to challenge national schemes that use imported product prices as a benchmark, thus in their view discriminating against domestic products; see the complaint filed by the Danish pharmaceutical industry association, LIF, 'Danish LIF complains to ECJ' Scrip no. 2612, 16 January 2001, p. 3. The Commission launched infringement proceedings against the Greek government in relation to its so-called confirmation price system and with regard to its failure to respect the timetables for price approval as imposed in the Directive, 'Commission threatens Greece with Court proceedings', Scrip no. 2589, 3 November 2000, p. 7. Infringement proceedings were also initiated against Finland for its failure to provide for reimbursement procedures for certain categories of drugs, 'Finnish Scheme Challenged', Scrip no. 2558, 19 July 2000, p. 6.

6   See European Commission (2001a) for list of members of the new group.

7   A 'Bolar' provision provides exemptions to exclusive patent rights which permit the testing, using, making (not selling) of patented pharmaceuticals for the purpose of submitting information required for obtaining marketing approval prior to the date of patent expiration.

8   European Commission (1989) Article 7(1) of the First Trade Mark Directive enshrines the principle of exhaustion of rights, but Article 7(2) introduces an exception so that the owner of the trademark may oppose further marketing of a repackaged product 'where there exists legitimate reasons for doing so especially where the conditions of the goods is changed or impaired'. The Directive has led to a number of competing interpretations, ranging from a narrow concept of exhaustion, where only if the imported product was in the very form in which it had been marketed could the trademark owner not oppose its use, to a broader approach whereby the trademark owner could only oppose the use if the product was put on the market and was substantially changed.

9   For a discussion of the earlier case law and the question of subjective versus objective intention, see Castillo de la Torre (1997).

10 See also the recent repackaging issues which arose in Case C-143/00 *Boehringer Ingelheim* (ECJ 2000a) and Case C-433/00 *Aventis* (ECJ 2001a).

11 For a detailed discussion of the earlier case law in this area, see Hancher (2002).

12 See, in particular, Case 104/75 *De Peijper* [1976] ECR 613, paras 21 and 36 (ECJ 1976) and Case C-201/94 *Smith & Nephew and Primecrown* [1996] ECR I-5819, para. 26 (ECJ 1996e).

13 See Case 174/82 *Sandoz* [1983] ECR 2445, para. 18 (ECJ 1983).

14 The formulation contained in the Council's minutes and reproduced at para. 25 of the Generics judgment states that 'the criteria determining the concept of essential similarity between medicinal products are that they have the same qualitative and quantitative composition in terms of active principles and the same pharmaceutical form, and, where necessary, bioequivalence of the two products has been established by appropriate bioavailability studies'.

15 The European Court of Justice had already made it eminently clear that divergent national price regulations in the pharmaceutical sector do not exclude the operation of the Treaty rules on free movement – *Merck and Primecrown* 1996.

16 Glaxo Wellcome has recently announced its intention to appeal this decision to the Court of Justice.

17 Rulings by the European Court of Justice (ECJ) and Court of First Instance can be read in full at http://www.europa.eu.int/eur-lex/en/index.html.

References[17]

Castillo de la Torre, F. (1997) Trade marks and free movement of pharmaceuticals, *European Intellectual Property Review*, 304: 304–12.

Council of the European Union (1989) Directive 89/105/EEC of 21 December 1988 relating to the transparency of measures regulating the pricing of medicinal products for human use and their inclusion within the scope of national health insurance systems, OJ L40, 11.02.1989: 8.

Council of the European Union (1993) Directive 65/65/EEC of 24 August 1993 on the approximation of provisions laid down by law, regulation or administrative action relating to proprietary medicinal products (OJ L22, 09.02.1965), as last amended by Directive 93/39/EEC: OJ L214, 24.08.1993; Bull. 6–1993, point 1.2.11

Court of First Instance (2000) Case T-41/969, Judgment of 26 October 2000, *Bayer* v. *Commission of the European Communities*.

Department of Health (United Kingdom) (2002) *Pharmaceutical Price Regulation Scheme: Sixth Report to Parliament*, December. London: Her Majesty's Stationery Office (available from http://www.doh.gov.uk/pprs.htm).

European Commission (1989) Notice on Article 7(1) of the First Trade Mark Directive, OJ, L140, 1989: 1.

European Commission (1996) Decision 96/478/EC of 10 January 1996 relating to a proceeding under Article 85 of the EC Treaty, OJ, L201, 1996: 1.

European Commission (2001a) Pharmaceuticals: high level group established to look at medicines for Europe, *Press Release* IP/01/444, Brussels, 26 March 2001.

European Commission (2001b) G10 Medicines Group reviews progress and announces new transparency initiatives, *Press Release* IP/01/1323, Brussels, 26 September 2001.

European Commission (2001c) Commission prohibits Glaxo Wellcome's dual pricing system in Spain, *Press Release* IP/01/661, Brussels, 8 May 2001.

European Court of Justice (1976) Case 104/75, *De Peijper* [1976] ECR 613.

European Court of Justice (1978a) Case 3/78, *American Home Products* [1978] ECR 1823.

European Court of Justice (1978b) Case 102/77, *Hoffman La Roche* [1978] ECR 1139.

European Court of Justice (1983) Case 174/82, *Sandoz* [1983] ECR 2445.

European Court of Justice (1995a) Case C-391/92, *Commission* v. *Greece* [1995] ECR I-1621.

European Court of Justice (1995b) Case IV/M.555, *Organon* [1995] OJ C65/4.

European Court of Justice (1996a) Joined Cases C-267/95 and C-268/95, *Merck* v. *Primecrown* [1996] ECR I-6285.

European Court of Justice (1996b) Joined Cases C-427/93, C-429/93 and C-436/93, *Bristol-Myers Squibb* v. *Paranova* [1996] ECR 1–3457.

European Court of Justice (1996c) Joined Cases C-71/94, C-72/94 and C-73/94, *Eurim-Pharm* [1996] ECR 1–3603.

European Court of Justice (1996d) Case C-232/94, *MPA* v. *Rhône-Poulenc* [1996] ECR 1–3671.

European Court of Justice (1996e) Case C-201/94, *Smith & Nephew and Primecrown* [1996] ECR I-5819.

European Court of Justice (1996f) Joined Cases C-267/95 and C-268/95, *Merck and Beecham* [1996] ECR I-6285.

European Court of Justice (1997) Case C-379/97, *Upjohn* v. *Paranova* at recital 43.

European Court of Justice (1998) Case C-368/96, *Generics* [1998] ECR 1–7967.

European Court of Justice (1999) Case C-94/98, *Rhône-Poulenc Rorer* and *May & Baker* [1999] ECR I-8789.

European Court of Justice (2000a) Case C-143/00, Judgment of 23 April 2002, *Boehringer Ingelheim*.

European Court of Justice (2000b) Case C-172/00, Judgment of 10 September 2002, *Ferring*.

European Court of Justice (2001a) Case C-433/00, Judgment of 19 September 2002, *Aventis*.

European Court of Justice (2001b) Case C-157/99, Judgment of 12 July 2001, *Smits and Peerbooms*.

European Court of Justice (2001c) Case C-106/01, *Novartis*.

European Court of Justice (2001d) Case C-2203/01, *AstraZeneca*.

European Court of Justice (2002) Case C-433/99, Judgment of 23 April 2002, *Merck, Sharp & Dohme*.

European Court of Justice (2003a) Advocate General's Opinion of 22 May 2003. Joined Cases C-264/01, C-306/01, C-354/01 and C-355/01, *AOK Bundesverband*.

European Court of Justice (2003b) Case C-113/01, Judgment of 8 May 2003, *Paranova*.

European Court of Justice (2003c) Advocate General's Opinion of 26 January 2003. Case C-106/01, *Novartis*.

European Court of Justice (2003d) Advocate General's Opinion of 23 January 2003. Case C-2203/01, *AstraZeneca*.

G10 High Level Group on Innovation and Provision of Medicines (2002) *Medicines*. Consultation Paper. Brussels: European Commission (available from http://www. entr-g10medicines@cec.eu.int).

Gambardella, A., Orsenigo, L. and Pammolli, F. (2000) *Global Competitiveness in Pharmaceuticals: A European Perspective*. Report for Directorate-General for Enterprise, European Commission. Brussels: European Commission.

Hancher, L. (1990) *Regulating for Competition: Government, Law and the Pharmaceutical Industry in the UK and France*. Oxford: Clarendon Press.

Hancher, L. (2002) The pharmaceuticals market: competition and free movement actively seeking compromises, in M. McKee, E. Mossialos and R. Baeten (eds) *The Impact of EU Law on Health Care Systems*. Brussels: P.I.E.-Peter Lang.

OECD (2002) *The Cost of Pharmaceuticals*. Paris: OECD.

four

The role of the EMEA in regulating pharmaceutical products

Silvio Garattini and Vittorio Bertele'[1]

Introduction

Established in 1995, the European Medicines Evaluation Agency (EMEA) in London amounted to a revolution in European pharmaceutical regulation. As one of the European Union's (EU) regulatory agencies, the role of the EMEA is to coordinate the scientific resources in EU member states to evaluate and supervise medicinal products for both human and veterinary use. Based on the EMEA's formal recommendations ('opinions'), the European Commission authorizes the marketing of new drugs. Thus, since 1995 the approval of a pharmaceutical product authorized centrally is binding in all of the 15 member states. Moreover, any opinion expressed on old or new products relating to changes in therapeutic indications or any part of the summary of product characteristics (SPC),[2] or suspension or withdrawal of a product by the EMEA, has to be accepted by all members of the EU.

In addition to this centralized procedure for the approval of new drugs, which is compulsory for biotechnology products, there is an alternative (decentralized) procedure for approving pharmaceutical products at the member state (national) level. Essentially, the decentralized procedure involves an applicant going directly to one member state's marketing authority to obtain marketing permission for its product, and if successful, then seeks to have other member states recognize the approval and grant their own marketing authorizations. The EMEA's Mutual Recognition Facilitating Group (MRFG) helps national agencies to overcome possible disagreements on the authorization of new products. Therefore, within the EU, there is currently a two-track authorization system and companies may choose either the centralized or decentralized procedure to gain marketing approval for their products in more than one EU member state. Figures 4.1 and 4.2 illustrate the various stages and time-frames followed in the two procedures. However, the EMEA's main evaluation group, the Committee for Proprietary Medicinal Products (CPMP), still has a formal role in the decentralized procedure by arbitrating between member states in cases

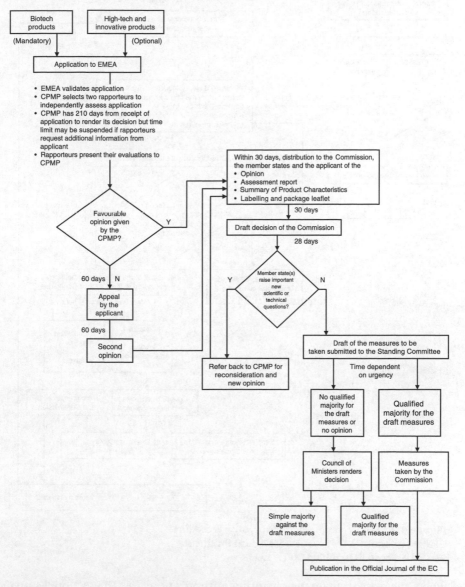

Figure 4.1 EU centralized drug approval procedure.
EMEA = European Medicine Evaluation Agency; CPMP = Committee for Proprietary Medicinal Products.
Source: US General Accounting Office (1996).

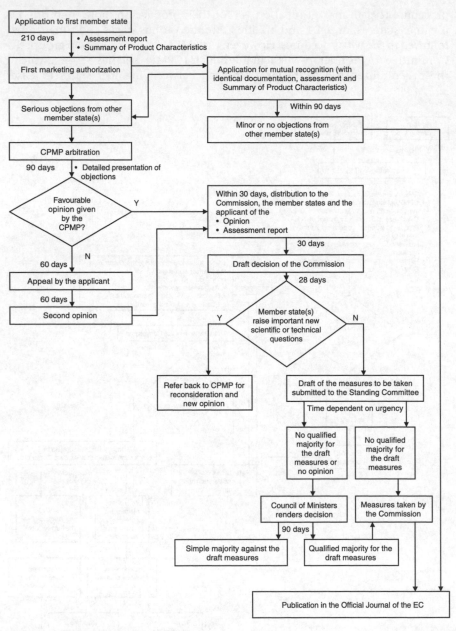

Figure 4.2   EU decentralized drug approval procedure.
CPMP = Committee for Proprietary Medical Products.
Source: US General Accounting Office (1996).

where there are disputes over granting authorizations (see the section 'Mutual recognition').

The activities of the EMEA are closely regulated by European law (Council of the European Communities 1993), which establishes a number of rules and procedures for the organization. After 8 years, these rules need some adjustment, and these are currently being discussed at the political level. The revision process will involve the European Parliament and the European Council, which both have a role in discussing and agreeing on proposals drafted by the European Commission. In this chapter, we review the structure and procedures of the EMEA and, within the context of current reform proposals, offer some suggestions for substantial modifications to the present legislation.

Organization

The EMEA has a management board and a technical group that operates in an advisory capacity for the scientific evaluation of medicinal products. The board comprises two representatives per member state, two representatives from the European Commission and two representatives appointed by the European Parliament. The technical group, the CPMP, is made up of 30 members, two for each country, appointed by their governments. A general director acts as the interface between the board and the CPMP and a staff of about 300 provides technical services. One of the CPMP's tasks is to provide scientific advice to help industry cope with authorization requirements when guidelines are not available for particular therapeutic areas. The CPMP evaluates the application dossiers and delivers an opinion to the European Commission on whether or not it should approve a product.

Several working parties (Table 4.1) and *ad hoc* groups for specific problems help the CPMP to undertake its complex duties. Special mention should be made of the Committee on Orphan Products, made up of one member from each country, two representatives of the CPMP, one from the management board and three from patients' associations. This committee is independent of the CPMP and its task is to make decisions on granting orphan drug status according to a law designed to foster the development of drugs for rare diseases (European Parliament and Council 2000). The advantages of a product being designated an 'orphan drug' include the conferral of 10 years of market exclusivity even after the patent has expired, as well as a reduction in the dossier examination fee. However, the responsibility for evaluating the dossier and giving a negative or positive opinion remains with the CPMP.

Table 4.1 CPMP-associated working parties

- Biotechnology
- Blood products
- Efficacy
- Pharmacovigilance
- Quality
- Safety
- TSE (transmissible spongiform encephalopathies)
- Herbal medicinal products

Procedures

The procedure for evaluating dossiers must be completed within 210 days (Figure 4.1) and begins with the EMEA Secretariat checking the dossier to ensure it is complete (the validation stage). Two members of the CPMP are then selected as rapporteurs; usually the manufacturer and the CPMP chairman suggest one rapporteur each. Rapporteurs are responsible for coordinating the assessment report on the application dossier, liasing with the applicant company on any questions or further information required during the assessment process and presenting the assessment report to the full membership of the CPMP before the latter determines a final opinion on authorization. Once an opinion has been delivered, the European Commission (EC) has another three months to make a decision on whether to adopt it or not. Overall, a marketing authorization is granted within 300 days and companies have the right to withdraw a dossier at any time before an opinion is reached. Table 4.2 presents a summary of the CPMP's opinions between January 1995 and December 2002.

The results of the dossier evaluation are summarized in the summary of product characteristics (SPC) (see Table 4.3 for the information that must be included in a SPC) and in a European public assessment report,[3] which reviews the documentation upon which the CPMP opinion is based. Opinions are adopted by consensus or by an absolute majority of members (16 votes). In the case of a negative opinion the company can make an appeal, which is discussed by the CPMP after having appointed two different rapporteurs.

Table 4.2 The EMEA's activities in its first 8 years, 1995–2002

Procedures	1995–2001	2002	Total
Applications submitted	335	31	366
Withdrawals	60	13	73
Positive CPMP opinions	208	39	247
Negative CPMP opinions	5	0	5
Marketing authorizations granted by the Commission	194	40	234
Type I variations	1254	463	1717
Type II variations, positive opinions	647	269	916
Type II variations, negative opinions	7	0	7
Extensions	74	14	88
Scientific advice	252	50	302
Follow-up to scientific advice	35	15	50

Source: CPMP Press Release, December 2002 (available from http://www.emea.eu.int/pdfs/human/press/pr/624802en.pdf).

Table 4.3 Outline of the summary of product characteristics (SPC)

1 Name of the medicinal product
2 Qualitative and quantitative composition
3 Pharmaceutical form
4 Clinical particulars
    4.1 Therapeutic indications
    4.2 Posology and method of administration
    4.3 Contraindications
    4.4 Special warnings and special precautions for use
    4.5 Interactions with other medicinal products and other forms of interaction
    4.6 Pregnancy and lactation
    4.7 Effects on ability to drive and use machines
    4.8 Undesirable effects
    4.9 Overdose
5 Pharmacological properties
    5.1 Pharmacodynamic properties
    5.2 Pharmacokinetic properties
    5.3 Preclinical safety data
6 Pharmaceutical particulars
    6.1 List of excipients
    6.2 Incompatibilities
    6.3 Shelf life
    6.4 Special precautions for storage
    6.5 Nature and contents of container
    6.6 Instructions for use and handling
7 Marketing authorization holder
8 Marketing authorization number(s)
9 Date of first authorization/renewal of the authorization
10 Date of revision of the text

An authorization can sometimes be granted 'under exceptional circumstances', when the applicant is unable to provide comprehensive data because the indications for the new product are too rare, or the scientific knowledge insufficient, or further research would be contrary to generally accepted principles of medical ethics. In such cases, a temporary approval is granted that requires post-authorization commitments in order to obtain permanent approval.

The CPMP also undertakes a number of other tasks. It is responsible for the pharmacovigilance of centrally licensed products until they are available on the market; that is, it evaluates the periodic safety update reports, which provide information on reported adverse events and reactions. It also renews marketing authorizations after five years, and accepts any changes to be inserted into the SPC. In cases of severe adverse reactions, the CPMP may call for an urgent safety restriction, requiring the distribution of a 'Dear doctor letter', and may suspend the drug in question or take it off the market. Moreover, in recent years the CPMP has set up the Scientific Advice Section, intended to help pharmaceutical companies prepare dossiers and, in particular, to design pivotal clinical trials for the approval of new products. Finally, the CPMP deals with referrals from member states in a number of circumstances, including:

- when there is disagreement in or among the member states about the SPC of a drug (Article 28 of Directive 2001/83/EC) (European Parliament and Council 2001);
- in the course of a mutual recognition procedure, when a member state believes that the medicinal product in question might pose a risk to public health (Article 29);
- in cases of divergent decisions by member states concerning the authorization of a drug (a different indication, for instance) or its suspension or withdrawal from the market (Article 30);
- when a suspension, withdrawal or change of marketing authorization is deemed to be necessary in the interests of the community because of a risk to public health (Article 31);
- and when a member state considers that a variation, suspension or withdrawal of a community-authorized product is necessary for the protection of public health (Articles 35, 36, 37).

A critique of the system

Although the EMEA lacks the tradition and size of the US Food and Drug Administration (FDA), its merits are undisputed and its effects on the European pharmaceutical sector should be acknowledged (see Table 4.4 for a comparison of the FDA and the EMEA). However, a number of issues relating to the EMEA's legislative provisions and internal rules now need to be revised to ensure that patients derive maximum benefit (Garattini and Bertele' 2001). The European Commission is currently reviewing the EMEA's functions and procedures (Commission of the European Communities 2001a,b), offering a good opportunity to improve the system (Garattini and Bertele' 2002; Garattini *et al.* 2003). The following considerations should be taken into account in the review process.

Institutional location

The EMEA is regulated by the European Commission's General Directorate of Enterprises even though its mission is 'to promote the protection of human health . . . and of consumers of medicinal products' (Council of the European Communities 1993). However, in all 15 member states the pharmaceutical sector is linked directly or indirectly to a ministry of health or social affairs, and never to ministries of trade and industry. Shifting the institutional location of the EMEA to the European Commission's Public Health Directorate would serve as a useful political indicator that the Agency is primarily patient-focused while still acknowledging the interests attached to the production and distribution of medicinal products. However, the Commission's current revision of the pharmaceutical legislation does not seem to take this point into consideration.

Table 4.4 Comparison of the FDA and the EMEA

	EMEA	FDA
Established in:	1995	1931
Dependent on:	European Commission Directorate-General for Enterprise	Department of Health and Human Services
Budget for 2001	€62 million (70 per cent as fees from the companies)	€1,450 million (10 per cent as fees from the companies)
Permanent staff	250	9000
Evaluation of drug documentation by:	External experts (two appointed by each member state included in the scientific committee – CPMP[a] – renewed every 3 years)	Internal (CDER[b] review team) and external (Advisory Committee) experts
Compulsory procedures	Biotechnology products	All drugs
Time of approval	7 months[c] to 15 months[d]	10 months[d] (standard medicines), 6 months (priority medicines)

Notes: [a]Committee for Proprietary Medicinal Products. [b]Centre for Drug Evaluation and Research. [c]Does not include 'clock stops' requested by companies. [d]Includes 'clock stops' requested by companies.

Financing the EMEA

The EMEA has two somewhat disproportional sources of finance: one part of its funding comes from a European Commission grant, while the remainder is collected through the fees charged to pharmaceutical companies for the evaluation of marketing authorization applications, variations to the conditions of the authorization, scientific advice, annual renewals and other services. In 2002, despite the dramatic decrease in marketing authorization applications for new products, 63.6 per cent of the EMEA's budget was made up of fees from industry and only 33.4 per cent was derived from EU financing. By way of comparison, since 1992 the Prescription Drug User Fee Act has authorized the US FDA to collect fees from the pharmaceutical industry. These additional resources are used to support additional staff for the review of human drug applications so that safe and effective drug products reach the public more quickly. However, these fees constitute only about 15 per cent of the FDA's overall budget (Food and Drug Administration Department of Health and Human Services 2003) and are less than the resources drawn from appropriated funds for the review of human drug applications. In collecting its own fees, the EMEA effectively has to compete with national agencies, since, with the exception of biotechnology products and orphan drugs, the pharmaceutical industry is free to follow the decentralized market authorization procedure through a member state national agency. Given this situation, the ideal would be to gradually eliminate the competition between centralized and decentralized procedures and have all applications for the European market made to a single agency, the EMEA. Moreover, any direct financial relationship between the EMEA and industry should be avoided. This could be achieved by industry paying the required fees to the European Commission, and by restructuring the budget formula so that fees make up a minority of the EMEA's total budget, thereby ensuring that the EMEA's financial sustainability is not adversely affected by fluctuations in fee revenues. In 2002, for example, the number of applications received was significantly lower than forecast, making it necessary to implement a contingency plan that cut all types of expenditure for internal and external activities (EMEA 2002). Again, the Commission's current review does not allow for such major changes (Garattini and Bertele' 2002; Garattini et al. 2003).

EMEA board membership

The EMEA management board includes two representatives from the European Parliament and two from the European Commission, in addition to representatives from the member states. It is our view that the new board structure currently being examined should not include representatives from the pharmaceutical industry as proposed by the Commission (2001a) and endorsed by the European Parliament (2002a). A management board without industry representation would avoid situations in which conflicts of interest could arise, especially given the fact that without this precaution the pharmaceutical industry would find itself in the dual position of exercising control over market authorizations while itself being the subject of such regulation.

CPMP membership

The present composition of the CPMP, though not homogeneous, allows for the inclusion of independent experts and representatives from national agencies. The former ensure critical analysis in evaluating new drugs, and the latter good relations with their organizations. However, the European Parliament has endorsed a proposal for member state representation on the CPMP to be cut from two members each to just one member.

Scientific advice

Scientific advice is fast becoming an important part of the CPMP's work. Accordingly, in 1999 a Scientific Advice Review Group was established as a permanent working group with the participation of several national delegations. This development is somewhat unusual in that it is uncommon for an organization, and in effect the same group of people (in this case the members of the CPMP), to be responsible for giving advice to industry about the best way to proceed with the development of a drug, and also to be responsible for approving drug authorizations and deciding on manufacturers' appeals in the event of initial rejections.

The impression is that today companies' requests for scientific advice are mostly a way of reaching agreement about how to prepare market authorization dossiers so as to avoid future objections. It is interesting to note that the Regulation concerned (Article 51 J) (Council of the European Communities 1993) lists among the tasks of the CPMP the following: 'where necessary, advising companies on the conduct of the various tests and trials necessary to demonstrate the quality, safety and efficacy of medicinal products'. This suggests that scientific advice should be given largely on the initiative of the CPMP rather than at the request of companies. In any case, the phrase 'where necessary' suggests that such advice need not be a systematic activity but undertaken on certain occasions. Therefore, it would be more appropriate for the tasks of providing scientific advice and presenting opinions on market authorizations to be undertaken by different groups working independently.

Objective assessment

For most diseases, physicians already have a range of different products available for prescription. Thus, public health needs would be better addressed by focusing on how new drugs compare with existing ones (in terms of efficacy, safety or both), on a sound scientific basis.

Despite the fact that the lack of adequate randomized controlled trials is a major cause of marketing authorization applications failing to obtain approval (Pignatti *et al.* 2002), currently new drugs can still be evaluated for their own quality, efficacy and safety with no comparison with alternative treatments. That is, such drugs can be proven to be effective and safe on their own, even though they may, in fact, be potentially less effective or less safe than other drugs currently in use. In those few cases where comparisons are made, the industry usually relies on demonstrating therapeutic 'equivalence' or 'non-inferiority', because this is enough to obtain a slice of the market. This results in a lot of uncertainty about the therapeutic role of new drugs (Bertele' *et al.* 1999). Therefore, new EMEA legislation could usefully include the requirement that, whenever feasible, clinical studies should be conducted in comparison with reference drugs, in accordance with the Declaration of Helsinki (World Medical Association 2000), so as to establish the relative benefit of a new drug. Assessment of relative benefit should then become an independent criterion for marketing authorization decisions.

In amending the European Commission's initial proposal, the European Parliament has suggested that: 'In the interest of public health, authorization decisions . . . should be taken on the basis of the objective scientific criteria of quality, safety, efficacy and added therapeutic value.' Drugs should be approved on the basis of data from comparative clinical trials aimed at demonstrating that 'the new medicinal product is more efficacious [than] . . . previously authorised medicinal products used to treat the same or a similar condition' (European Parliament 2002a). However, elsewhere in the revision document the risk/

benefit balance is regarded as a property that is intrinsic to each drug rather than related to other products (European Parliament 2002b). This inconsistency needs to be resolved in favour of stating that new drugs must offer some advantage over those already available in terms of efficacy, safety or ease of use, or at least in terms of cost. It is our view that the EMEA should adopt this criterion as a basis for marketing authorizations.

Moreover, among the several amendments aimed at improving clinical trial objectives and methods, and the transferability of their results to clinical practice, the Parliament also has presented a specific recommendation regarding ethics: 'Medicinal products should be approved only where the underlying clinical trials meet the ethical requirements' (European Parliament 2002b). This may be the basis for gradually phasing out or rejecting studies aimed at demonstrating the equivalent or non-inferior efficacy of new drugs as compared to available ones.

Summary of product characteristics

The increasing volume of biomedical knowledge poses problems for physicians who want to remain up to date on new developments and new products. Hundreds of new medicines are brought into the market every year and are often aggressively promoted by their manufacturers to bolster sales. A central feature of information geared towards marketing a new product is that its primary objective is to promote sales through advertising and not to act as an independent source of information. Currently, the large amounts of resources deployed by the pharmaceutical industry on advertising creates an imbalance in information sources available to the public. Fortunately, the European Parliament (2002b) rejected the Commission's proposal that information about prescription drugs (that is, direct-to-consumer advertising) should be made available to the public (Commission of the European Communities 2001b). The Commission had suggested that direct-to-consumer advertising on three chronic diseases – asthma, diabetes and AIDS – be allowed for a 5-year pilot period (see also Chapter 9). However, in our view, this proposal would have resulted in a proliferation of unmediated promotional information being disseminated through several routes, which would have confused patients and put undue pressure on physicians. Given the importance of providing rational and balanced pharmacological information, it is our recommendation that direct-to-consumer information should be supplied only by national regulatory authorities.

The best way for a physician to glean objective information about individual drugs is to read carefully the summary of product characteristics (SPC), a detailed description that, since 1995, has been prepared collaboratively by the manufacturer and the CPMP (see Table 4.3). In keeping with our recommendation that the efficacy of new drugs submitted for market authorization be compared with existing equivalent products, we also argue that the SPC should be reformulated from its current protocol of looking at each drug in isolation to a new format where comparisons are made with other drugs available for the same indications, with a similar mechanism of action. Moreover, it would be useful if doctors could obtain an idea of the characteristics of these active principles by reading just one SPC. This could be achieved by setting out in a table the therapeutic indications approved for each compound and the documented differences in the various sections of the SPC. This information would show whether the claimed differences in side-effects are real or just a matter of promotion, and whether the purported responses to one product by patients who are resistant to another are thoroughly documented. Finally, the SPC should also refer, albeit summarily, to any differences of opinion within the scientific community or among regulatory authorities. Awareness of the uncertainty surrounding some aspects of drugs' properties and use would make it easier for physicians to critically assess available data.

New drugs approved through the centralized EMEA procedure have now largely 'unified' the SPC format, but most drugs authorized by national agencies still circulate in Europe with different and often divergent SPCs. Therefore, much effort is required to iron out these discrepancies. A further concern is that frequently there are deficiencies in the documentation supporting the marketing authorization for the paediatric use of new drugs. Most drugs licensed for paediatric use have not actually been tested on children. The EMEA has published guidelines to promote clinical investigations in children (EMEA 1999), but unfortunately these have not yet increased the proportion of drugs with paediatric labelling in recent years ('t Jong *et al.* 2002).

Transparency

Over the years, the CPMP has certainly improved transparency by establishing rules to discipline any conflicts of interest of its members, assessors and experts, and making its decisions available through the EMEA website and press releases. However, there is still room for improvement (Abbasi and Herxheimer 1998; Abrahams and Lewis 1998). First, greater transparency in the approval process would be achieved if the appointment of rapporteurs were not influenced by the pharmaceutical industry; that is, the current practice of one rapporteur being nominated by the applicant manufacturer should be reviewed. Secondly, opinions – whether positive or negative – should be made public as soon as they are decided. The current practice is that opinions remain undisclosed for two weeks to allow companies to appeal. However, should a company wish to make an appeal, this could still be done publicly.

Thirdly, substantial improvements are needed in the stewardship of relations with the pharmaceutical industry in cases where negative opinions have been, or are about to be, issued. Currently, if a preliminary 'trend vote' by the CPMP tends towards a negative opinion, the rapporteur informs the company, giving it two options: either to let the full procedure take its course and accept a negative opinion (this usually occurs when the company plans to make an appeal) or to withdraw the dossier application. As of December 2002, only five negative opinions have been issued, whereas there have been 73 withdrawals. There were 247 positive opinions in the same period. It is important to point out that when an application is withdrawn, all the dossier information becomes confidential and is not publicly disclosed. However, it is in the interest of public health to know that a pending negative opinion has led to an application withdrawal, especially since public information on the reasons for withdrawal may also be very important for countries outside the EU, where a company may also be seeking market authorization approval.

Fourthly, another measure that would improve transparency concerns the explicit publication of the minority view. When a drug is not unanimously approved or rejected by the CPMP, we recommend that the minority divergent opinion should be reported and explained to the public. At present, minority views are attached to the opinion but there is a tendency for this document to be overlooked in the process of making the opinion public. In fact, no minority report has ever appeared on the EMEA website.

The European public assessment report does mention whether a product has been approved by consensus or by majority, but it does not present the minority's viewpoint. While it is acknowledged that the use of majority voting (16/30) is required when making decisions of a regulatory nature, when it comes to scientific matters, greater objectivity is best guaranteed through the presentation of all available information.

Pharmacovigilance

There is a growing need for the continuous monitoring of adverse effects, since unwanted effects can be expected to increase as drugs become more powerful. This should be a centralized task, although the participation of the member states will remain essential. One proposal is that the EMEA could set up a special body to collect information on all the drugs on the European market. Such a body would need adequate resources not only to store reports but also to support specific research to acquire information where necessary. In this respect, the European Parliament has proposed an improved pharma-covigilance system with an integrated network at EU level (European Parliament 2002a,b). In addition to making sure companies comply with their pharma-covigilance obligations (Arlett and Harrison 2001), under the Parliament's proposals, the EMEA and national public pharmacovigilance systems would operate interactively, with adverse reactions being monitored on a contin-uous basis by specialists in clinical pharmacology working for academia or qualified hospitals in collaboration with companies, pharmacists and patients' associations.

Mutual recognition

The current decentralized procedure for the approval of new drugs appears to conflict with the EMEA centralized procedure. Mutual recognition can some-times be perceived to be a less stringent form of evaluation, where the desire to obtain an extension of the marketing authorization throughout the 15 member states overrides the prerogative of a thorough-going critical evaluation of the drugs involved.

In the decentralized procedure, the member state that evaluates an applicant's dossier and whose assessment acts as a basis for marketing authorizations is called the 'reference member state'. Within 90 days of receipt of the assessment report, other member state(s) that have been requested to recognize the authorization – known as the 'concerned member state(s)' – should normally recognize the decision of the reference member state by granting a marketing authorization with an identical SPC.[4] While the CPMP is empowered to arbitrate in cases of disputes in the decentralized procedure, frequently recourse to such arbitration is avoided by withdrawing the application in the concerned member state that is withholding recognition. In fact, the CPMP has seldom been involved in arbitration. One of the problems with the alternative mutual recognition procedure is that it may lead to different outcomes in different member states, unlike the centralized EMEA procedure.

Market authorization renewal

Every five years, drugs have to be reviewed so that they can remain on the market. The pharmaceutical industry favours an evaluation that is essentially administrative: if a drug has no record of serious adverse effects, market authorization renewal should be automatic. In the interests of public health, however, an updated analysis of the benefit/risk profile would be preferable; 5 years of marketing could be an occasion to establish the record of side-effects, to determine whether the new drugs have made others obsolete or a second choice, to establish whether knowledge about the disease for which the drug is intended has substantially changed, and to clear the market of older drugs whose efficacy has never been proved. This could have been clearly spelled out in the new legislation, which, however, calls for a re-examination of the risk/benefit balance of new drugs only once, after the first 5 years a product has been on the market (European Parliament 2002b). In effect, this represents a compromise between the current five-year reviews and the Commission's proposal that the validity of an authorization should be perpetual (Commission of the European Communities 2001b). We recommend, instead, that a re-examination take place every five years.

Herbal and homoeopathic products

To protect consumers from harm and false expectations, the same standards of quality, safety, efficacy and added therapeutic value should be applied to herbal and homoeopathic products. The proposed introduction of the Committee on Herbal Medicinal Products only gives official status to products that are still assessed by standards that are far below those that are compulsory for pharmaceutical products (Commission of the European Communities 2001a).

Conclusion

The EMEA has brought advantages to patients, national health services and industry. Centralization could be gradually accentuated with the aim of concentrating and unifying all processes related to approval, monitoring and general policy making regarding medicinal products. The proposed revision of the EU's pharmaceutical legislation certainly aims to improve several aspects of the system, but it apparently will not tackle some major issues, including the political and financial independence of the EMEA. The criteria for approving new drugs should involve a comparative evaluation; it is no longer possible to consider quality, efficacy and safety as independent variables without any reference to an already crowded market.

If patients' interests are to be defended, then the drugs that are approved must be rigorously evaluated and demonstrate comparative benefit. For this to become reality, the EMEA must become a strong organization, with adequate resources to meet the challenges posed by the pharmaceutical industry.

Notes

1   We are indebted to Mrs Judy Baggott for helpful editorial assistance.
2   The content of SPCs is outlined in Table 4.3.
3   European public assessment reports can be found on the EMEA website (www.emea.eu.int).
4   The principle underlying the mutual recognition procedure is that the concerned member state should recognize the marketing authorization granted by the reference member state unless it feels that the medicinal product in question might present a public health risk.
5   All websites in the References last accessed on 10 January 2003.

References[5]

Abbasi, K. and Herxheimer, A. (1998) The European Medicines Evaluation Agency: open to criticism. Transparency must be coupled with greater rigour, *British Medical Journal*, 317: 898.

Abrahams, J. and Lewis, G. (1998) Secrecy and transparency of medicines licensing in the EU, *Lancet*, 352: 480–2.

Arlett, P.R. and Harrison, P. (2001) Compliance in European pharmacovigilance: a regulatory view, *Pharmacoepidemiology and Drug Safety*, 10: 301–2.

Bertele', V., Torri, V. and Garattini, S. (1999) Inconclusive messages from equivalence trials in thrombolysis, *Heart*, 81: 675–6.

Commission of the European Communities (2001a) Proposal for a Regulation of the European Parliament and of the Council laying down Community procedures for the authorization and supervision of medicinal products for human and veterinary use and establishing a European Agency for the Evaluation of Medicinal Products (available from http://pharmacos.eudra.org/F2/review/doc/finaltext/011126-COM_2001_404-EN.pdf).

Commission of the European Communities (2001b) Proposal for a Directive of the European Parliament and of the Council amending Directive 2001/83/EC on the Community code relating to medicinal products for human use (available from http://pharmacos.eudra.org/F2/review/doc/finaltext/011126-COM_2001_404-EN.pdf).

Council of the European Communities (1993) Council Regulation (EEC) No. 2309/93 of 22 July 1993 laying down Community procedures for the authorization and supervision of medicinal products for human and veterinary use and establishing a European Agency for the Evaluation of Medicinal Products, *Official Journal of the European Communities*, L214, 24.08.1993: 1.

European Medicines Evaluation Agency (1999) International Conference for Harmonisation Topic E11 (1999) Note for Guidance on clinical investigation of medicinal products in the paediatric population, CPMP/ICH/2711/99 (available from http://www.emea.eu.int/pdfs/human/ich/271199EN.pdf).

European Medicines Evaluation Agency (2002) Committee for Proprietary Medicinal Products 15–17 October 2002 plenary meeting: monthly report (available from http://www.emea.eu.int/pdfs/human/press/pr/497902en.pdf).

European Parliament (2002a) European Parliament legislative resolution on the proposal for a European Parliament and Council regulation laying down Community procedures for the authorization and supervision of medicinal products for human and veterinary use and establishing a European Agency for the Evaluation of Medicinal Products, p. 36 (available from http://www3.europarl.eu.int/omk/omnsapir.so/calendar?APP=PDF&TYPE=PV2&FILE=p0021023EN.pdf&LANGUE=EN).

European Parliament (2002b) European Parliament legislative resolution on the proposal for a European Parliament and Council directive amending Directive 2001/83/EC on the Community code relating to medicinal products for human use, p. 84 (available from http://www3.europarl.eu.int/omk/omnsapir.so/calendar?APP=PDF&TYPE=PV2&FILE=p0021023EN.pdf&LANGUE=EN).

European Parliament and Council of the European Communities (2000) Regulation (EC) No. 141/2000 of the European Parliament and of the Council of 16 December 1999 on orphan medicinal products, *Official Journal of the European Communities*, L018, 22.01.2000: 1–5.

European Parliament and Council of the European Communities (2001) Directive 2001/83/EC of the European Parliament and of the Council of 6 November 2001 on the Community Code Relating to Medicinal Products for Human Use, *Official Journal of the European Communities*, L311/67: 1–62.

Food and Drug Administration Department of Health and Human Services (2003) FY 2002 PDUFA Financial Report Required by the Prescription Drug User Fee Act of 1992 as Amended by the Food and Drug Administration Modernization Act of 1997 (available from http://www.fda.gov/oc/pdufa/finreport2002/executive).

Garattini, S. and Bertele', V. (2001) Adjusting Europe's drug regulation to public health needs, *Lancet*, 358: 64–7.

Garattini, S. and Bertele', V. (2002) Toward new legislation of drugs in Europe, *Expert Review of Pharmacoeconomics and Outcomes Research*, 2: 89–94.

Garattini, S., Bertele', V. and Li Bassi, L. (2003) Light and shade in proposed revision of EU drug-regulatory legislation, *Lancet*, 361: 635–6.

Pignatti, F., Aronsson, B., Gate, N. *et al.* (2002) The review of drug applications submitted to the European Medicines Evaluation Agency: frequently raised objections, and outcome, *European Journal of Clinical Pharmacology*, 58: 573–80.

't Jong, G.V., Stricker, B.H., Choonar, I. and van den Anker, J.N. (2002) Lack of effect of the European guidance on clinical investigation of medicines in children, *Acta Paediatrica*, 91: 1233–8.

US General Accounting Office (1996) *European Union Drug Approval: Overview of the New European Medicines Evaluation Agency and Approval Process*. Report to the Chairman, Committee on Labor and Human Resources, US Senate. Washington, DC: GAO (available from www.gao.gov/archive/1996/he96071.pdf).

World Medical Association (2000) The Declaration of Helsinki: ethical principles for medical research involving human subjects (available from www.wma.net).

chapter five

Measuring, monitoring and evaluating policy outcomes in the pharmaceutical sector

*Panos Kanavos, Dennis Ross-Degnan,
Eric Fortess, Julia Abelson and
Stephen Soumerai*

Introduction

The contribution of prescription drugs in improving health outcomes for many illnesses is indisputable. Yet some medications also present significant risks of iatrogenic injury, especially when misused (Leape *et al*. 1991). In addition, increasingly prohibitive costs of newly developed drugs, both marginally and highly effective, have caused concern among clinicians, policy makers and patients because of growing problems of access, and the economic, clinical and social impact of likely gaps in drug coverage in some health systems. Attempts to reduce the rate of growth of drug expenditure during the past three decades have seen the introduction of an array of drug cost-containment measures. In European countries, Australia and New Zealand, these have impacted on the entire pharmaceutical market, because of the universality of drug coverage schemes (Kanavos 2002; Rickard 2002; PHARMAC 2003). In the USA, they have predominantly affected low-income, elderly and disabled persons, through Medicaid coverage (Kaiser Commission 2002); in Canada, policies have been introduced by provincial governments to pay for prescription drug benefits for seniors.

Bearing in mind that about three out of four physician visits may result in at least one drug prescription (Cypress 1983), the intended effect of administrative interventions in pharmaceutical markets is to reduce drug overutilization, iatrogenic risks and contain expenditure growth. However, intervention may also produce unintended effects, including access restrictions, reduced use of cost-effective drug therapies, resulting declines in health status, substitution of less effective, more toxic or more expensive medications for non-reimbursed agents, and increased utilization of costly physician or institutional (inpatient or nursing) care. Among the hypothesized mechanisms for the increased medical and institutional care in low-income populations that has resulted from lack of access to effective drugs are objective declines in physical health status (Lurie *et al.* 1984), changes in patients' psychosocial health or perceptions of illness, increased ambulatory care visits to obtain medications, and the shifting of care to settings where reimbursement is available (Borus *et al.* 1985; Soumerai *et al.* 1991, 1994; Tamblyn *et al.* 2001).

Despite the proliferation of drug cost control policies in different settings – whether on the supply side or the demand side (Kanavos 2002; NPC 2002) – few investigations of the economic and health impact of these policies have been conducted, nor have recent studies been evaluated systematically and rigorously (Soumerai *et al.* 1993). The aim of this chapter is to critically appraise the methodological challenges present in research on the impact of educational and administrative interventions to improve drug use, and to identify and analyse the methodological flaws that are widespread in this literature, often casting doubt on many of the published conclusions. Methodological problems reviewed include threats to internal validity, regression towards the mean, incorrect unit of analysis, logistical issues, and the inability to detect effects on patient outcomes. We use carefully selected published and unpublished studies over the past three decades that evaluate the effects of administrative restrictions or measures (such as formularies, category exclusions, caps on the number of prescriptions, prior authorization requirements and reference pricing), applied on the demand side and limiting clinicians' ability to prescribe particular medications, as well as require patient cost-sharing to obtain medications. In addition, we demonstrate the nature and extent of likely design flaws that may lead to spurious policy conclusions. Whereas our focus is on studies that meet explicit research design criteria, we also discuss major sources of bias or imprecision in less well-controlled studies. In doing so, we hope to build on previous research on the subject, and portions of this chapter are based on a previous report (Soumerai *et al.* 1993). The selected literature in this chapter draws upon the US, European and Canadian experiences. Despite the majority of the reviewed published literature providing evidence of policies within the North American health care environment, the findings of the chapter are nevertheless also relevant for the system-wide policy context of European health care systems.

First, we provide a taxonomy of the methodological issues involved in assessing the impact of drug policy changes. We also describe the method used to select the studies to highlight the methodological challenges in evaluating policy outcomes, and then discuss these challenges. Finally, we summarize the findings, suggest methods to evaluate policy effects more reliably, and highlight important gaps in knowledge to be addressed in future research.

Key issues in evaluating policy interventions

Because policy interventions – so-called 'administrative restrictions' in the US context – may deny patients access to newer, more expensive and possibly more effective single-source agents, they have become increasingly controversial during the past 30 years. Proponents of administrative restrictions cite drug savings due to utilization of more established, cost-effective products. On the other hand, opponents argue that failure to reimburse effective drugs causes unintended reductions in quality of care and increased costs due to the use of sub-optimal substitute products, exacerbation of disease, or substitution of expensive physician and hospital services.

The potential for administrative controls on prescribing to produce unintended consequences depends on many factors, including their restrictiveness, the efficacy and substitutability of affected drugs, potential for irrational drug substitution effects, and the perceived need for a particular drug by a patient or physician. Clearly, restrictions on highly effective and non-substitutable agents could potentially result in increased physician visits or hospitalizations to gain access to treatment or to manage the sequelae of untreated disease (Fineberg and Pearlman 1981). On the other hand, withdrawing reimbursement for irrational drug combinations has been found to improve drug therapy for certain patients (Soumerai *et al.* 1991).

To understand the impact of administrative restrictions, one needs to study trade-offs between restricted drugs and (1) substituted drugs (first-order effects) and (2) substitution of other health services (second-order effects). For completeness, first-order effects should include changes in utilization of all plausible substitute therapies. Second-order effects include increased physician and emergency room visits, hospitalizations and nursing-home admissions that may result from changes in drug therapy. However, demonstrating a causal link between an administrative restriction and any second-order effect is more difficult for several reasons. Restrictions in access to individual drugs constitute only one of many factors that influence the likelihood of physician or hospital visits. For instance, countries or states with strict positive lists may simultaneously apply a variety of other cost controls on hospital or physician visits. Variations in recipient populations over time (e.g. through eligibility changes) may also seriously confound effects.

The presence of such known and unknown factors can lead to incorrect inferences about the cause of changes in drug and service utilization and emphasizes the importance of using strong research designs to evaluate the effects of policy changes. In light of this, the remainder of the chapter will address the methodological issues that arise in studies that evaluate the effect of restrictions on prescribing and whether such restrictions cause substitution of inappropriate drugs, increase utilization of more intensive medical services and increase total system costs.

Evidence of the impact of policy interventions

Published and widely referenced unpublished European and US reports evaluating the effects of specific drug cost-containment policies in national (in Europe) and state/provincial (through state Medicaid programmes in the USA and provincial schemes for seniors in Canada) pharmaceutical programmes were screened for inclusion in this chapter. The analysis was limited to administrative restrictions on prescribing, such as the imposition of a limited list of drugs eligible for reimbursement (formulary or positive list), the withdrawal of certain classes of drugs (a reduction in the scope of benefits), the requirement for prior authorization to receive specific drugs (a procedural regulation), and reference pricing (where a maximum reimbursement level is set requiring patients to pay the difference on their drugs of choice, if these are priced higher than the reference drug). We explicitly excluded studies on the impact of cost-sharing as well as those on financial prescribing incentives, which are analysed elsewhere in this book (see Chapters 10 and 13). We used the computerized Medline system and a manual search of citations to identify studies of target drug cost-containment policies published in the medical, pharmacy and social science literature between 1972 and 2002 in European countries, the US Medicaid programme and in Canada. The following keywords were used:

- drug/pharmaceutical cost containment
- drug formularies
- drug prior authorization
- drug/pharmaceutical reference pricing
- drug reimbursement limits
- drug reimbursement caps

On aggregate, the survey yielded 1110 titles. We excluded 121 titles focusing on the supply side, and a further 187 on strict medical content, 121 on aspects of cost-effectiveness, and 308 that addressed other aspects of the demand side or were altogether irrelevant to our broad study objectives. We focused on the remaining 373 studies. To be included in the discussion, studies were required to evaluate the impact of target national or state-level policies on one or more of the following processes or outcomes:

- overall or specific drug utilization/expenditures;
- frequency, cost or efficacy of drug substitutions in lieu of restricted drugs;
- under-use of effective medications;
- substitution of other health services for drugs;
- clinical outcomes.

Explicit criteria were developed to rate the adequacy of study methodologies in the following areas: overall research design; appropriateness of study population; data quality and availability; reliability of utilization measures; and adequacy of statistical analysis. The strength of overall research design is the most important criterion for evaluating a study's ability to suggest causal inferences. Studies with strong quasi-experimental designs, such as time-series with comparison series, are considered to be well-controlled, whereas studies utilizing time-series (without comparison series) or pre-post with comparison group

Table 5.1   Research designs in reviewed studies by type of cost-containment policy

Type of study	Administrative restrictions n=18 (%)
Time-series with CS[a,b]	2 (11.1%)
Pre–post with CG[a]	1 (5.5%)
Repeated measures[c]	1 (5.5%)
Pre-post	7 (38.8%)
Post only with CG[d]	4 (22.2%)
Post only	3 (16.7%)

Notes: [a] CS, CG indicate that design included an appropriate comparison series or comparison group. [b] Time-series are defined as analyses with six or more observations pre- and post-intervention. [c] Repeated measures designs include two to five observations pre- and post-intervention. [d] Category includes cross-sectional regression analyses.

designs are considered to be partially controlled. Studies with weak research designs, such as pre–post without a comparison group, or post-only observation (e.g. cross-sectional regressions), are considered likely to produce biased or unreliable assessments of the impact of target policies. We briefly discuss studies that were both adequately and inadequately controlled to describe their methodological shortcomings. These ratings indicate varying levels of control of potential bias in results, but do not consider limitations in resources or settings that may have precluded the use of stronger designs.

Several other methodological characteristics were also assessed. For example, we determined whether studies appropriately followed a specific sub-group at risk (i.e. target drug recipients) rather than the entire population of a drug benefit programme. Finally, we considered the adequacy of statistical analysis based on the presence of an appropriate denominator to calculate utilization rates, and calculation of appropriate error variances for estimated effects on utilization and expenditures.

On the basis of the above criteria, we identified a total of 18 studies that evaluated the effects of the target drug cost-containment policies. The distribution of the research designs employed in these studies is presented by type of policy in Table 5.1. Only four of the 18 studies even partially controlled for possible exogenous influences on study results; 10 had no comparison group; and four further studies with comparison groups only measured outcomes after changes had already been introduced. Descriptions of individual study findings that meet our minimum research design criteria, further reflections on their methodological adequacy, and solutions to the methodological problems that arise are discussed in the sections that follow.

Methodological challenges in evaluating policy outcomes

Internal validity

Poorly controlled studies produce misleading estimates of the effects of a variety of social programmes (Gilbert *et al.* 1975). Many non-intervention factors can affect drug utilization over time, such as marketing campaigns, mass media, regulatory policies, seasonal effects, changes in staffing of health care organizations, changes in eligibility for insurance programmes, and shifting demographics among others. Because randomized control trials are sometimes not feasible (e.g. contamination of controls within a single institution) or ethical (e.g. withholding quality assurance programmes from controls), other strong quasi-experimental designs should be used instead of weak one-group post-only or pre–post designs that do not generally permit causal inferences.

One such strong design is interrupted time-series that include multiple observations (often 10 or more) of study populations before and after interventions. Such designs permit investigators to control for pre-intervention secular changes in study outcomes and to estimate the size and statistical significance of sudden changes in the level or slope of the time-series occurring at initiation of the treatment. The availability of a comparison series collected from a similar, but unexposed, comparison group can further increase causal inferences if no simultaneous change in trend is observed for this group (Cook and Campbell 1979).

Our survey identified two studies with time-series designs, one on Medicaid patients and one on reference pricing in the Canadian province of British Columbia. Soumerai *et al.* (1991) used an interrupted time-series with comparison series design to evaluate the effect of withdrawing 12 categories of questionably effective or irrational drugs on the quality and cost of substitute agents among New Jersey Medicaid patients, using 42 months of claims data. Although withdrawn drugs accounted for 7 per cent of baseline utilization, the reimbursement restriction did not produce measurable reductions in overall medication use or expenditures. They found that eliminating reimbursement of even irrational agents does not address the perceived need for drugs by patients and physicians, and can result in both appropriate and inappropriate substitution effects.

Schneeweiss *et al.* (2002), in a carefully controlled study, analysed the impact of reference pricing in British Columbia and its impact on access to drugs as well as the impact on quality of care. They found that the probability of stopping antihypertensive therapy decreased when compared with that before the change in policy and 18 per cent of those prescribed with ACE inhibitors subject to cost-sharing switched to lower-priced alternatives. The switchers shared a moderate transitory increase in the rates of visits to physicians and hospital admissions through the emergency room during the two months after switching, but not subsequently. The study found that reference pricing for ACE inhibitors was not associated with changes in the rates of visits to physicians, hospitalizations, admissions to long-term care facilities or mortality.

Another popular design that can often lead to interpretable results is the pre–post with comparison group design. This design includes a single observation both before and after treatment in a non-randomly selected group exposed to a treatment (e.g. physicians receiving feedback on specific prescribing practices), as well as simultaneous before and after observations of a similar (comparison) group not receiving treatment. Although this design controls for many threats to the validity of causal inferences (e.g. due to the effects of testing or maturation), it cannot control for unknown factors (e.g. a regulatory policy) that might result in pre-intervention differences in trends between study and comparison groups.

Our review identified one such study by Hefner (1980). This study examined the effects of withdrawing reimbursement for cough and cold preparations, minor tranquillizers, combination anti-anaemia preparations, certain gastrointestinal remedies, vitamins, enzymes and anorexics in the Louisiana Medicaid programme and utilized a partially controlled pre–post comparison group design. Overall, prescription drug expenditures declined by 14 per cent, but this modest reduction in drug use was credited with a more than five-fold rise in hospitalization, an implausible finding given that the hospitalization effects were observed for the entire population, even those never affected by the drug payment restriction. These results suggest that important, unmeasured, non-formulary factors were responsible for the changes in hospitalization rates; therefore, such results ought to be interpreted with caution.

The weakest, and not uncommon, design is the one-group, post-only design, which consists of making only one observation on a single group which has already been exposed to a treatment. The one-group, pre–post design merely adds a single pre-intervention observation to the previous design. Such weak designs are unlikely to produce valid or reliable estimates of the effects of educational or managerial interventions. Nevertheless, 60 per cent of 76 studies designed to improve drug prescribing in primary care used the weakest non-experimental designs (Soumerai *et al.* 1989). The fact remains, however, that inadequately controlled studies may exaggerate the effectiveness of many interventions to improve prescribing.

The majority of our identified survey studies fall within this category and present a variety of methodological problems, which are outlined below. These include studies from the Medicaid context in the USA and some studies from Europe. Kozma *et al.* (1990) took advantage of a natural experiment in the South Carolina Medicaid programme, which switched from a 'restrictive' to a 'non-restrictive' formulary affecting a large number of therapeutic agents. Although this study used more reliable patient-level drug claims, a large and continuously enrolled population of non-elderly people, and a partially controlled repeated measures design, the lack of a sufficient pre-intervention period to model baseline utilization trends resulted in uninterpretable findings. For example, although the authors reported decreases in inpatient hospitalizations, no estimates were provided of either the magnitude of these decreases or of the reported 'increases' in outpatient hospital visits, physician visits and drugs.

Dranove (1988) evaluated the effects of adding several newer anti-infective agents to the Illinois Medicaid formulary. The study population included non-elderly patients with specific infectious disease diagnoses in the year before and after the policy change. Regression analyses comparing post-formulary and during-formulary periods suggested a light, non-significant decline in outpatient visits, which were attributed to 'faster cures'. However, a modest increase in ambulatory costs was also observed due to the added cost of the new medications. The absence of either adequate controls or pre-intervention trend data made it impossible to determine whether the modest changes were not simply the continuation of historical trends.

A pre–post study using three-month observation periods, one year apart, examined the effect of withdrawing reimbursement for propoxyphene napsylate, a marginally effective and abusable analgesic, from the Wisconsin Medicaid programme (Kreling *et al.* 1989). Prescribing of the alternative propoxyphene formulation on the formulary (propoxyphene hydrochloride) increased, as did use of NSAIDs, judged to be safer and more effective agents. The lack of control for prior trends is especially problematic given the rapid growth in NSAID use during the 1980s.

Smith and MacLayton (1977) used a pre–post design to examine the impact of withdrawing reimbursement for non-narcotic analgesics in the Mississippi Medicaid programme. They reported a 76 per cent increase in narcotic analgesic prescriptions, as well as increases in analgesic expenditures and pill supply per prescription after the policy change. However, the analysis did not control for the likelihood of differential prior trends in drug utilization across analgesic categories. Nevertheless, the large reported increase in use of narcotic analgesics suggests the possibility of inappropriate substitution for less toxic, non-reimbursed agents.

Bloom and Jacobs (1985) used a pre–post design to study the 'withdrawal' of cimetidine, an H2 blocker, due to the imposition of a closed formulary with prior authorization in the West Virginia Medicaid programme. Because of the established cost-effectiveness of this agent in preventing inpatient surgery for peptic ulcer, severe restrictions on access by low-income patients might have increased hospital service use, especially when no other H2 blocker existed at the time of the formulary change. The study contrasted a nine-month open formulary observation period with the same nine-month period a year later, during which West Virginia covered without prior authorization only a very restricted formulary of 66 products. Cimetidine use declined by 84 per cent among patients with peptic ulcer diagnosis at the same time that its use was increasing nationwide. Medicaid costs to treat peptic ulcer were 15 per cent lower during the closed formulary period. The percentage of patients hospitalized for ulcer disease did not vary significantly, although inpatient costs per patient-month rose somewhat. However, methodological problems made it difficult to be confident in the observed effects. No comparison group was available at a time when other cost-containment procedures (e.g. diagnostic related groups) were being implemented; the open formulary period excluded the medically needy for one-third of the period; and diagnostic ascertainment bias may have resulted in a comparatively sicker population during the closed formulary period because patients were likely to receive diagnosis later in their illness.

Moore and Newman (1993) also looked at the effects of restrictive formularies. Their study was based largely on a post-only, cross-sectional regression analysis of four years of aggregate Medicaid expenditure by state. No adjustments were made for pre-existing differences in Medicaid programme characteristics between formulary and non-formulary states (e.g. other drug cost control policies, differences in patient characteristics, other health care reimbursement policies). The analysis did not include sufficient time points to adjust for differential prior trends in expenditures among states with and without formularies. Although a second analysis purported to estimate changes associated with 'switches' between formulary and non-formulary status between 1985 and 1988 – a potentially adequate research design – the small number of observation periods and states affected precluded the use of more powerful time-series models. In addition, most states implemented changes in the first year of observation, resulting again in a weak post-only design.

Smith and Simmons (1982) examined the effect of reimbursement restrictions on 24 categories of medications in cross-sectional regression analysis, as well as two-group comparisons, using 8 years of aggregate Medicaid expenditure data obtained from the National Pharmaceutical Council. No consistent relationship was found between formulary controls and drug expenditures, and the validity of the reported findings is limited.

Several other cross-sectional regression analyses of the effects of formulary restrictions have also yielded uncertain results. In a study of 30 state Medicaid programmes, Schweitzer *et al.* (1985) constructed an index of formulary 'restrictiveness', which they found to be negatively associated with state-level aggregate Medicaid expenditures, but not associated with actual drug expenditures. The post-only design severely limits the scientific significance or policy relevance of these surprising findings. Hammel (1972) compared (without statistical analysis) four years of Medicaid expenditures in states with and without formularies and suggested that states with closed formularies had higher health care expenditures per recipient. However, trend data from the two states that shifted from open to closed formularies showed no change from preexisting expenditure trends. Smith and McKercher (1984) examined the effects of withdrawing reimbursement for laxatives, antacids, vitamins and nutritional supplements, cough and cold preparations, antivertigo medications and selected DESI[1] drugs in the Michigan Medicaid programme by conducting a post-only evaluation of 137 patients with prescriptions for one or more of the eliminated drugs. The small sample, the lack of a control group and danger of regression to the mean when following a cohort identified by previous use reduce confidence in the estimates of drug substitution effects.

Similar problems are inherent in the majority of studies from the broader European context, aiming to evaluate certain policy initiatives. Predominant among them are studies assessing the macroeconomic impact of reference pricing (Selke 1994; Zammit-Lucia and Dasgupta 1995; Schneeweiss *et al.* 1998). These studies are descriptive and do not rely on patient-related data or populations, but on aggregate expenditure data. Selke (1994) uses aggregate data from a sickness fund (AOK) to examine the net effect on prices of introducing reference pricing in Germany by taking into account the segment of the market subjected to reference pricing and the one that is not. He also describes the basic principles of the Dutch and Danish reference pricing systems and benchmarks these with the German system. The effect on quality is not examined and neither is the impact on hospitalizations. The study is exclusively concerned with the impact on prices, the extent of the coverage of the pharmaceutical market by the system, and whether reductions on prices have been observed in the segment of the market subjected to reference pricing. Zammit-Lucia and Dasgupta (1995) use aggregate data to examine the price, volume and substitution effects of reference pricing in several European countries, and conclude that modest price savings in all reference pricing systems are counterbalanced by strong switch effects. The contribution of these studies to our understanding of the operation and impact of reference pricing is undisputed, but the overall results may be subject to bias. The analysis recognizes but does not control for other cost-containment measures that were applied simultaneously to the reference pricing system and, in addition, aggregate data have unproven reliability.

The above findings provide further support for more widespread application of random controlled trials (RCTs) or, when RCTs are not feasible, time-series with comparison series designs to evaluate whether suddenly introduced interventions are associated with corresponding changes in the level or slope of the utilization series, after controlling for prior trends, as some studies indicate (Soumerai *et al.* 1987, 1991, 1994). If the collection of time-series data is not feasible, investigators may consider using pre–post with comparison group designs, which also control for most threats of history.

Regression towards the mean

Regression towards the mean – namely, the tendency of observations on populations, selected on the basis of exceeding a predetermined threshold level, to approach the mean on subsequent observations – is a common and insidious problem in much of the drug utilization literature. In Medicaid, for instance, the most common drug utilization programmes typically screen utilization data and eligibility files for possible co-occurrences of two interacting medications, or higher than recommended dosages for individual drugs. After case-by-case review by expert committees, letters are written to responsible physicians questioning the practice and asking for written responses. Unfortunately, however, the only published research evaluating this methodology utilized poorly controlled designs that are unable to control for regression to the mean. In one often cited drug utilization review (Groves 1985), 50 per cent of prescribing problems were absent several months after letters were sent, suggesting to the non-critical reader that the programme was effective. However, it is equally plausible that the offending medications were withdrawn because the patients' conditions improved or because the physicians detected the error on their own. If regression effects are unavoidable – for example, due to selection of at-risk (high-use) populations – investigators may consider including a 'wash-out' period after selection and before pre- and post-intervention observations (Soumerai *et al.* 1987).

Unit of analysis

A common methodological problem in physician behaviour studies is the incorrect use of the patient as the unit of analysis. Such a practice violates basic statistical assumptions of independence because prescribing behaviours for individual patients are likely to be correlated within each physician's practice. This often leads to exaggerated significance levels when the correct unit of analysis should be the physician or health care facility. As a result, interventions may appear to lead to 'statistically significant' improvements in prescribing practices when in fact no such claim is warranted. A review of articles on physicians' patient care behaviour found that 70 per cent of 54 articles incorrectly analysed the data using the patient as the unit of analysis (Divine *et al.* 1992). Similar errors can be made in drug policy studies, for instance, when using the number of drug packs consumed as opposed to defined daily doses.

The simplest, but conservative, solution to the problem of incorrect unit of analysis is to analyse data by facility or physician, or by using an internationally acknowledged measure of denomination, such as the defined daily dose, if the research question relates to drug consumption. Alternatively, new methods for analysing clustered data (Diggle *et al.* 1996) can control for clustering of observations at the level of patient, physician, facility as well as category of drug. Such models also allow aggregation at the patient level by controlling for correlation between patients cared for by the same provider or facility. The resulting significance levels for differences in prescribing rates between study and control groups are more conservative than assuming no intra-class correlation, but are greater than the most conservative methods of analysing at the provider or facility level.

Logistical issues

While continuity of care is a goal in most health care settings, many patients, particularly those treated within academic medical centres, see multiple primary providers over time. Although changing provider may or may not improve patient care, such changes almost always complicate and sometimes weaken research conducted in a clinical setting. Particularly in settings where providers may be assigned to both 'intervention' and 'control' patients, contamination problems are difficult to avoid. Even when interventions can be focused effectively on the intended patients or providers, informal communication among providers can lead to contaminated effects, thereby decreasing the likelihood of detecting significant changes.

To address these problems, investigators should identify through baseline interviews and organizational records the extent to which patients are cared for by multiple providers, and the patterns of consultations and referrals between caregivers within and between facilities. If randomization of clinicians is likely to lead to contamination of controls, or if patient–provider pairs are frequently broken, the entire facility or sub-unit should be assigned to the same study group (Soumerai *et al.* 1998). However, when this strategy is not feasible, because it results in a small sample of facilities and inadequate statistical power, investigators could collect data on drug use during multiple observation periods before and after the intervention, and to use time-series regression methods that can often detect modest changes in utilization after as few as 7–12 months (Soumerai *et al.* 1987, 1991; Avorn *et al.* 1988).

Detecting effects on patient outcomes

While a number of studies have demonstrated positive effects of various interventions on prescribing practices, almost no large well-controlled studies have linked such changes in prescribing to improved patient outcomes.

Available studies (Avorn *et al.* 1992; Marciniak *et al.* 1998; Schneeweiss *et al.* 2002) underline the difficulty of demonstrating statistically significant changes in patient outcomes in response to intervention. Explanations for the dissociation between improvements in prescribing and better patient outcomes include: (i) available clinical outcome measures may not be sensitive to the kinds of patient outcome that might be affected by the introduction or withdrawal of medications; (ii) changes in physician prescribing may lead to little or no change in patients' health status if patients do not adhere to the recommended regimens; and (iii) many medical therapies require months or years of continued compliance before clinical benefits become apparent. However, it has been demonstrated that drug reimbursement caps can increase nursing home admissions, emergency mental health utilization and partial hospitalizations, which are highly suggestive of adverse clinical outcomes (Soumerai *et al.* 1991, 1994).

Because of the above problems, sample sizes may need to be enormous to detect modest changes in patient outcomes. These problems are much less severe in standard drug trials because of experimenter control over the major independent variable – exposure to medications. However, process outcomes (e.g. use of recommended medications for acute myocardial infarction from EB practice guidelines) may often be sensitive and appropriate measures of quality of care (Brook *et al.* 1996a,b), and improvements in process should not be dismissed outright as surrogate outcomes. They may be important in and of themselves, as long as the processes are a measure of proven effective therapy.

Other threats to validity

Adequate research design is necessary but not sufficient to ensure validity. Other important characteristics to study design and analysis are essential. The first key issue is data availability. Reliable and complete data are necessary to estimate policy effects precisely. For instance, data on reimbursed claims provide reliable information on patient-level acquisitions of medications and other reimbursed health services, but no information on out-of-pocket purchases or co-payments. Aggregate data have unproved reliability for this purpose. They neither allow analysis of sub-populations at risk or monthly changes in utilization, nor do they control for patient-level differences. In addition, such key independent variables as formulary 'restrictiveness' are often measured imprecisely; therefore, studies relying on aggregate data may produce biased or unreliable results.

The second key issue is sub-groups at risk. A small proportion of chronically ill individuals consume disproportionate amounts of drugs. Such sub-groups are likely to be most sensitive to the impact of reimbursement decisions. Yet evidence suggests that only a small proportion of studies on cost containment follow high-risk sub-groups.

The third issue is the follow-up period. Reimbursement policy changes typically introduce a period of instability into established patterns of service utilization as providers and patients adjust their behaviour to the new context. Because patients and providers may learn to circumvent reimbursement regulations over time (e.g. by increasing quantity per prescription in the face of co-payments or caps), it is important to examine the 'durability' and long-term stability of changes in utilization. Ideally, follow-up observation periods should include two or more years of data. Realistically, however, 2 years of data may rarely become available and, in addition, many changes may occur in formulary or overall drugs policy in a two-year period. As a result, very few formulary studies have achieved a more modest criterion of six months follow-up.

Policy discussion

This review has so far suggested that great improvements in research methodology are needed before definitive recommendations are possible about how to implement cost control policies without compromising quality. In light of the existing studies' methodological failings, it is important for future research to take a number of steps as follows: first, to follow the basic principles of design needed to minimize internal and external threats to validity, including measurement before and after policy changes, and appropriate, well-chosen comparison populations. Second, incorporate multiple measurement points to better control for underlying trends in the use of drugs and other health services. Third, utilize patient-level data and appropriate denominators in outcome measures, so that changes in the size and mix of recipient populations do not bias the analysis. Fourth, investigate specific changes in health service use and clinical outcomes for well-defined populations at risk of these outcomes in order to build the chain of logic necessary to suggest causal relationships from non-experimental data. Fifth, measure the independent variables (e.g. formulary restrictiveness) more precisely. And sixth, apply appropriate statistical techniques to reduce the likelihood that observed differences are due to chance fluctuations, taking care to account for multiple comparisons and to aggregate data at the appropriate unit of analysis.

These methodological issues are of more than academic importance. Inadequate research methods reduce the scientific validity and reliability of study results and perpetuate the dissemination of inaccurate information about health care policies. If decision makers continue to base pharmaceutical policies on unproven assumptions about their economic and clinical impact, there will remain a disturbing potential not only to waste increasingly scarce health care resources, but also to further endanger the health of many of the most vulnerable members of society.

It is often argued that decision makers are not interested in the outcomes of academic research, or, indeed, in altogether evaluating policy measures introduced by themselves. This was certainly the case with the fundholding experiment in the UK (1991–1997). Despite the proliferation of studies on prescribing that fundholding led to, some of which were of good quality (see, for example, Bradlow and Coulter 1993; Glennerster *et al.* 1994), the policy was never properly evaluated[2] by the Conservative government that introduced it and was dismissed by the succeeding Labour government. However, there may be differences between Europe and North America in this matter, where adequate funding plays an important role in the capacity to measure outcomes of policy interventions.

Furthermore, despite the existence of a number of studies which approach methodological excellence, there are limitations to studying policy outcomes, which one needs to bear in mind. One such limitation is the nature of the health care system. Endogenous elements may affect the outcome of policy analysis, thus limiting its transferability across systems or settings. A second limitation is the questionable generalizability of results within a health system in that evaluating a policy intervention that applies to one drug or one drug class does not necessarily mean that the same result will be valid across all drug categories in the same system. A third limitation relates to data aggregation, which does not always lead to reliable estimates of policy outcomes. Finally, even with the best controlled studies, the effect of individual policies is very often difficult to isolate in the presence of other measures and this may lead to significant bias.

Notes

1 The Drugs Efficacy Study Implementation (DESI) programme was established to review the efficacy of a specified list of drugs already in the marketplace between 1934 and 1962, before the new FDA drug authorization process had been established legislatively in 1962. If a DESI review indicates a lack of substantial evidence of a drug's effectiveness for all of its labelled indications, the FDA will publish a Notice of Opportunity for a Hearing (NOOH) in the Federal Register concerning its proposal to withdraw approval of the drug for marketing. At that time, a manufacturer of that drug or identical, related or similar (IRS) drugs has the opportunity to request a hearing and provide the FDA with documentation of the effectiveness of the drug product before a final determination is made. Drugs for which a NOOH has been published are referred to as less-than-effective (LTE) drugs (see http://www.cms.gov/medicaid/drugs/drug11.asp).

2 In accordance with the criteria specified in this chapter. Clearly, there are studies (e.g. Audit Commission, 1994, 1996) which evaluate the performance of fundholding practices, but not that of non-fundholders.

References

Audit Commission (1994) *A Prescription for Improvement: Towards Rational Prescribing in General Practice*. London: HMSO.

Audit Commission (1996) *What the Doctor Ordered: A Study of GP Fundholders in England and Wales*. London: HMSO.

Avorn, J., Soumerai, S.B., Wessels, M. *et al*. (1988) Reduction of incorrect antibiotic dosing through a structured educational order form, *Archives of Internal Medicine*, 148: 1720–4.

Avorn, J., Soumerai, S.B., Everitt, D.E. *et al*. (1992) A randomised trial of a programme to reduce the use of psychoactive drugs in nursing homes, *New England Journal of Medicine*, 327: 168–73.

Bloom, B.S. and Jacobs, J. (1985) Cost effects of restricting cost-effective therapy, *Medical Care*, 23(7): 827–80.

Borus, J.F., Olendzki, M.C., Kessler, L. *et al.* (1985) The 'offset effect' of mental health treatment on ambulatory medical care utilisation and charges: month by month and grouped-month analyses of a five-year study, *Archives of General Psychiatry*, 42: 573–80.

Bradlow, J. and Coulter, A. (1993) The effect of NHS reforms on general practitioners' referral patterns, *British Medical Journal*, 306: 433–7.

Brook, R.H., McGlynn, E.A. and Cleary, P.D. (1996a) Quality of health care. Part 2: measuring quality of care, *New England Journal of Medicine*, 335(13): 966–70.

Brook, R.H., Kamberg, C.J. and McGlynn, E.A. (1996b) Health system reform and quality, *Journal of American Medical Association*, 276(6): 476–80.

Cook, T.D. and Campbell, D.T. (1979) *Quasi-Experimentation: Design and Analysis Issues for Field Settings*. Boston, MA: Houghton Mifflin.

Cypress, B.K. (1983) Drug utilisation in general and family practice by characteristics of physicians and office visits: National Ambulatory Medical Care Survey, *NCHS Advance Data*, 28 March, p. 87.

Diggle, P.J., Liang, K.Y. and Zeger, S.L. (1996) *Analysis of Longitudinal Data*. Oxford: Clarendon Press.

Divine, G.W., Brown, J.T. and Frazier, L.M. (1992) The unit of analysis error in studies about physicians' patient care behaviour, *Journal of General Internal Medicine*, 7: 623–9.

Dranove, D. (1988) Pricing by non-profit institutions: the case of hospital cost-shifting, *Journal of Health Economics*, 7(1): 47–57.

Fineberg, H.V. and Pearlman, L.A. (1981) Surgical treatment of peptic ulcer in the United States: trends before and after the introduction of cimetidine, *Lancet*, 1(8233): 1305–7.

Gilbert, J.R., Light, R.J. and Mosteller, F. (1975) Assessing social innovations: an empirical base for policy, in C.H. Bennett and A.A. Lumsdaine (eds) *Evaluation and Experiment: Some Critical Issues in Assessing Social Programmes*. New York: Academic Press.

Glennerster, H., Matsaganis, M., Owens, P. and Hancock, S. (1994) *Implementing GP Fundholding*. Buckingham: Open University Press.

Groves, R. (1985) Therapeutic drug-use review for the Florida Medicaid Programme, *American Journal of Hospital Pharmacy*, 42: 316–19.

Hammel, R.W. (1972) Insights into public assistance medical care expenditures, *Journal of the American Medical Association*, 219(13): 1740–4.

Hefner, D.L. (1980) *Cost-Effectiveness of a Restrictive Drug Formulary*: Louisiana *vs*. Texas. Washington, DC: National Pharmaceutical Council.

Kaiser Commission on Medicaid and the Uninsured (2002) *State Budgets Under Stress: How are States Planning to Reduce the Growth in Medicaid Costs?* Washington, DC: The Henry J. Kaiser Family Foundation.

Kanavos, P. (2002) *Pharmaceutical Pricing and Reimbursement in Europe*. Richmond, UK: PJB Publications.

Kozma, C.M., Reeder, C.E. and Lingle, E.W. (1990) Expanding Medicaid drug formulary coverage: effects on utilization of related services, *Medical Care*, 28(10): 963–77.

Kreling, D.H., Knocke, D.J. and Hammel, R.W. (1989) The effects of an internal analgesic formulary restriction on Medicaid drug expenditures in Wisconsin, *Medical Care*, 27(1): 34–44.

Leape, L.L., Brennan, T.A., Laird, N. *et al.* (1991) The nature of adverse events in hospitalised patients, *New England Journal of Medicine*, 324: 377–84.

Lurie, N., Ward, N.B., Shapiro, M.F. and Brook, R.H. (1984) Termination from Medi-Cal – does it affect health?, *New England Journal of Medicine*, 311(7): 480–4.

Marciniak, T.A., Ellerbeck, E.F., Radford, M.J. *et al.* (1998) Improving the quality of care for Medicare patients with acute myocardial infarction: results from the

Cooperative Cardiovascular Project, *Journal of the American Medical Association*, 279: 1351–7.

Moore, W.J. and Newman, R.J. (1993) Drug formulary restrictions as a cost-containment policy in Medicaid programs, *Journal of Law and Economics*, 36: 71–97.

National Pharmaceutical Council (NPC) (2002) *Pharmaceutical Benefits under State Medical Assistance Programmes*. Reston, VA: NPC.

PHARMAC (Pharmaceutical Management Agency of New Zealand) (2003) *Annual Review 2002* (available from www.pharmac.govt.nz/pdf/AR02.pdf) (accessed 20 March 2003).

Rickard, M. (2002) *The Pharmaceutical Benefits Scheme: Options for Cost Control*. Social Policy Group, Current Issues Brief No. 12 2001-02, 28 May 2002 (available from http://www.aph.gov.au/library/pubs/cib/2001-02/02cib12.htm) (accessed 22 March 2003).

Schneeweiss, S., Schoffski, O. and Selke, G.W. (1998) What is Germany's experience on reference based drug pricing and the aetiology of adverse health outcomes or substitution?, *Health Policy*, 44(3): 253–60.

Schneeweiss, S., Walker, A.M., Glynn, R.J. *et al.* (2002) Outcomes of reference pricing for angiotensin-converting-enzyme inhibitors, *New England Journal of Medicine*, 346(11): 822–9.

Schweitzer, S.O., Salehi, H. and Bolling, N. (1985) The social drug lag: an examination of pharmaceutical approval delays in Medicaid formularies, *Social Science and Medicine*, 21(10): 1077–82.

Selke, G. (1994) Reference price systems in the European Community, in E. Mossialos, C. Ranos and B. Abel-Smith (eds) *Cost Containment, Pricing and Financing of Pharmaceuticals in the European Community: The Policy Makers' View*. Athens: LSE Health and Pharmetrica SA.

Smith, D.M. and McKercher, P.L. (1984) The elimination of selected drug products from the Michigan Medicaid formulary: a case study, *Hospital Formulary*, 19(5): 366–72.

Smith, M.C. and MacLayton, D.W. (1977) The effect of closing a Medicaid formulary on the prescription of analgesic drugs, *Hospital Formulary*, 12(1): 36–8, 41.

Smith, M.C. and Simmons, S. (1982) *Proceedings: The effectiveness of medicines in containing health care costs*. Reston, VA: National Pharmaceutical Council.

Soumerai, S.B., Avorn, J., Ross-Degnan, D. and Gortmaker, S. (1987) Payment restrictions for prescription drugs under Medicaid: effects on therapy, cost, and equity, *New England Journal of Medicine* 317(9): 550–6.

Soumerai, S.B., McLaughlin, T.J. and Avorn, J. (1989) Improving drug prescribing in primary care: a critical analysis of the experimental literature, *Milbank Quarterly*, 67(2): 268–317.

Soumerai, S.B., Ross-Degnan, D., Avorn, J., McLaughlin, T. and Choodnovskiy, I. (1991) Effects of Medicaid drug-payment limits on admission to hospitals and nursing homes, *New England Journal of Medicine*, 325(15): 1072–7.

Soumerai, S.B., Ross-Degnan, D., Fortess, E.E. and Abelson, J. (1993) A critical analysis of studies of state drug reimbursement policies: research in need of discipline, *Milbank Quarterly*, 71(2): 217–52.

Soumerai, S.B., McLaughlin, T.J., Ross-Degnan, D., Casteris, C.S. and Bollini, P. (1994) Effects of limiting Medicaid drug reimbursement benefits on the use of psychotropic agents and acute mental health services by patients with schizophrenia, *New England Journal of Medicine*, 331: 650–6.

Soumerai, S.B., McLaughlin, T.J., Gurwitz, J.H. *et al.* (1998) Effect of local medical opinion leaders on quality of care for acute myocardial infarction: a randomised controlled trial, *Journal of the American Medical Association*, 279: 1358–63.

Tamblyn, R., Laprise, R., Hanley, J.A. *et al.* (2001) Adverse events associated with prescription drug cost-sharing among poor and elderly persons, *Journal of the American Medical Association*. 285(4): 421–9.

Zammit-Lucia, J. and Dasgupta, R. (1995) *Reference Pricing: The European Experience*. Health Policy Review Paper Series, No. 10. London: St Mary's Hospital Medical School, University of London.

chapter SiX

Regulating pharmaceutical prices in the European Union

Monique Mrazek and Elias Mossialos

Introduction

In the 1990s, pharmaceutical expenditures became a common target of health care cost-containment efforts. In general, such pharmaceutical policies are expected to yield lower costs in the subsequent year(s) while improving effi-ciency and equity. Policy makers in a number of countries see controlling drug prices as less politically sensitive than cutting the salaries of health professionals or rationing particular medicines or other health care services. The implications of doing so, at least on the incentives for innovation, are part of a wider debate that is beyond the scope of this chapter.

Total pharmaceutical expenditure is a function of the quantity of drugs dis-pensed, multiplied by price. Increases in total pharmaceutical expenditures are driven by many factors, including changing demographic patterns, changes in product mix, the introduction of new and often more expensive medicines, and an increasing number of 'me-too' drugs. Equally important are the imperfec-tions in the supply and demand of pharmaceuticals that lead to market failure (see Chapter 1). In an attempt to correct for market imperfections, and control other factors driving rising drug expenditures, most Western European govern-ments have aimed much of their cost-containment effort at the supply side of the market in the form of price controls, but demand-side measures such as financial incentives, quantity controls and educational initiatives for doctors have also been widely used with variable success (see Chapters 8 and 10).

Whether or how pharmaceutical prices are regulated varies among European Union (EU) countries, as shown in Table 6.1. The differing approaches reflect distinct national policy priorities: the need to contain pharmaceutical expend-itures; whether and how the demand for pharmaceuticals is regulated; and the relative weights of health policy and industrial policy objectives (for example, promotion of pharmaceutical research and development, employment, a

Table 6.1 Summary of approaches in the regulation of pharmaceutical prices in EU member states, 2003

	Market segment	Free pricing	Direct price controls	Use of international price comparisons	Profit controls	Reference pricing
Austria	In-patent		✔	✔		
	Off-patent		✔	✔		
Belgium	In-patent		✔	✔		
	Off-patent			✔		✔
Denmark	In-patent			✔		
	Off-patent			✔		✔
Finland	In-patent		✔	✔		
	Off-patent		✔	✔		
France	In-patent		✔	✔		
	Off-patent					✔
Germany	In-patent	✔				
	Off-patent					✔
Greece	In-patent		✔	✔		
	Off-patent		✔	✔		
Ireland	In-patent		✔	✔		
	Off-patent		✔	✔		
Italy	In-patent		✔	✔		
	Off-patent					✔
Luxembourg	In-patent		✔	✔		
	Off-patent		✔	✔		
Netherlands	In-patent		✔	✔		✔
	Off-patent		✔	✔		✔
Portugal	In-patent		✔	✔		
	Off-patent			✔		✔
Spain	In-patent		✔	✔		
	Off-patent			✔		✔
Sweden	In-patent		✔	✔		
	Off-patent		✔	✔		
UK	In-patent	✔			✔	
	Off-patent		✔			

Source: Updated from Mrazek (2002a).

positive balance of trade). Measures for directly controlling pharmaceutical prices have commonly included negotiated prices, maximum fixed price, international price comparisons and price cuts or freezes. These direct methods have been included here under the term 'direct price controls'. Alternative approaches include controlling reimbursement levels by trading-off price decreases against volume increases. Indirect approaches include regulating profits or setting reference prices (reimbursement limits).

The pricing of medicines in EU countries and their inclusion in national reimbursement systems has been loosely governed at the EU level since 1989 by what is known as the Transparency Directive (89/105/EEC; Council of the European Union 1989), which establishes that authorities must make price decisions within 90 days of receiving adequate information and indicate the manner in which any negative decisions are to be communicated. Furthermore, the Directive specifies that any price freezes be reviewed annually to determine whether macroeconomic conditions justify their continuance. It also stipulates that any direct or indirect mechanisms for controlling profits of those placing a medicine on the market need to be explicit, as must the reasons for inclusion of products on positive or negative lists for reimbursement (see Chapters 2 and 3).

The advent of parallel imports – legitimately produced goods imported legally into a country without the authorization of the trademark, copyright or patent holder (see Chapter 3) – suggests a way that the single European market is having an impact on pharmaceutical prices in national markets. Parallel imports are a growing component of pharmaceutical sales in the EU, with some estimates placing them between 2 and 4 per cent of total drug sales, but in some countries, such as Denmark (10 per cent), the Netherlands (15 per cent) and the UK (7 per cent), these numbers were much higher in 1999 (House of Commons 1999; Arfwedson 2003). Parallel imports are driven, in part, by single European market objectives stemming from principles of the free movement of goods and exhaustion of rights entrenched in the Treaty of Rome. Basically, the driving force behind parallel imports is cross-border price differences and the opportunity for arbitrage. They will likely represent a larger proportion of EU-wide pharmaceutical sales until prices level, through either changes in national price control mechanisms or the impact of EU-wide manufacturers' pricing strategies to launch products in countries with high prices so that these prices will be used as benchmark prices in low-price countries.

In this chapter, we examine the alternative approaches to regulating ex-manufacturers' prices in EU countries and the evidence of their impact. The intention is not to engage in a discussion of optimal pricing from a EU perspective – that is, concepts of Ramsey pricing (see Danzon 1998) – but rather to consider the impact of government pharmaceutical price controls on overall drug expenditures. In addition, we do not intend to present a price comparison between countries, as doing so alone will tell us little about the relative impact on drug expenditures of the particular measures used in a country. In fact, a number of studies have attempted to either directly compare drug prices between countries (Pharmig 2000; Productivity Commission Australia 2001; Department of Health 2002; LIF 2003), or to link price levels in different countries with the types of supply- and demand-side policies in place. However, it is difficult to compare the results between studies, as few adopted comparable methodologies. Common methodological differences include: the distribution chain point of comparison (ex-manufacturer, wholesale or retail price); the pricing unit (per unit, dose or package); the range of products compared; the units of currency conversion (exchange rates or purchasing power of parities); the use of weights to account for a product's market share; and the use of bilateral or multilateral comparisons. Unfortunately, many comparative studies have not provided a full and clear description of the methodology employed.

Studies that have attempted to link a price level in a given country and the regulatory framework adopted do provide some interesting insights. A study by the US General Accounting Office (1994) found that prescription drug spending controls in France, Germany, Sweden and the UK in the late 1980s and early 1990s were effective in keeping drug price increases lower than the overall inflation rate, but were unable to prevent the escalation of overall drug expenditures because of the volume effect. Similar evidence points to countries with strict price regulation (France, Italy and Spain) having systematically lower prices than countries with less stringent price regulation (Germany, Sweden and the UK) (Garattini *et al.* 1994; Jonsson 1994; Rovira and Darba 2001). Yet other studies that have analysed both on-patent and off-patent drugs suggest that in markets with less regulation, such as Germany and the UK, prices have tended to be kept lower through competition (Reekie 1998; Danzon and Chao 2000). The discrepancies in these studies' findings reflect their different methodological approaches, including the range of products considered (particularly whether off-patent generics were included), the period the data covered and the method of calculating the indices. Beyond the methodological difficulties that plague many international comparative pricing studies (Danzon and Kim 1998; Kanavos and Mossialos 1999), it is difficult to isolate causal effects in the cross-country comparisons because of the many factors influencing drug prices in a given market: differences in health system structure and financing, pharmaceutical subsidies, cost-containment policies, product mix and production costs (Productivity Commission Australia 2001).

Direct price controls

Direct price controls amount to the setting of fixed maximum pharmaceutical prices. The definition of what is a reasonable maximum price varies from one country to another and is dependent on a number of factors, including budget limits, prescribing behaviour, patterns of utilization and the importance of the pharmaceutical industry to the national economy. Direct price controls may apply broadly to all medicines whether or not they are reimbursed, or to specific groups of products (for example, reimbursed, inpatient/outpatient, on-patent/off-patent). In most EU countries, the regulated price is the market price, since legislation often stipulates that a medicine may only be sold at a single price. All EU countries apply direct price controls to on-patent drugs except Germany and the UK, where new patented drugs can be freely priced at launch; in the latter these prices are indirectly conditioned by profit controls. Since 2003, free pricing was also introduced in France, but only for products defined as innovative by the National Transparency Commission (accountable to the Ministries of

Health and Social Security); nevertheless, the French Economic Committee (in the same ministry, but includes representatives of the Ministry of Economics and Finance and the National Health Insurance Fund for Salaried Workers) can register its opposition to the proposed price within 15 days of receiving the proposal. Moreover, cuts and freezes to these maximum fixed prices have been common in many EU countries, often as regulators attempt to meet short-term budget constraints.

The various methods of directly controlling prices have as an objective to fix pharmaceutical prices at levels deemed 'reasonable' and affordable to the health care system; how a reasonable price is defined is highly dependent on the importance of the pharmaceutical industry to the national economy. Either prices are directly controlled through negotiations (Austria, France, Italy, Portugal, Spain) or are fixed by national authorities according to a list of factors, including discretionary criteria that are subjective, open to bias and result in a lack of transparency. What factors are considered depends on whether the primary objective of the regulator is to achieve the lowest possible price as part of a cost-containment strategy or whether it is to achieve a price level that balances industry incentives and profitability with cost-containment goals. Some countries reward companies that contribute to the national economy or invest in research and development, but determining what contributions should be rewarded and how much is not necessarily evident. For example, although Spain by law applied a cost-plus formula (manufacturer's costs plus a percentage margin) in the price control system, other factors such as therapeutic value and prices in other countries could be taken into account without being formally stated (Rovira and Darba 2001).

Price comparisons between similar products within a country, or comparisons with identical or comparable products in other countries, especially other EU countries, are also used in price fixing. Table 6.2 provides examples of some approaches to cross-country price comparisons. In some countries, comparisons are used only as one factor in price determination, while in other countries

Table 6.2 Examples of international price comparisons in price-setting schemes in EU member states, 2003

Country	Price comparison
Belgium	Ex-manufacturer's price in France, Germany, Luxembourg and the Netherlands
Denmark	Average European ex-manufacturer's price excluding Greece, Portugal, Spain and Luxembourg, but including Liechtenstein
Finland	Average EU wholesale price
Ireland	Average wholesale price of Denmark, France, Germany, the Netherlands and the UK
Italy	Weighted average ex-manufacturer's prices in EU (excluding Luxembourg and Denmark)
Netherlands	Average ex-manufacturer's price of Belgium, France, Germany and the UK
Portugal	Minimum ex-manufacturer's price of identical products in France, Italy and Spain

(Greece, for example) they are the main factor, and prices cannot exceed the average of the compared countries. Finland also includes the prices of comparable parallel imports in its system of average price comparisons (Sirkia and Rajaniemi 2001). Although price comparisons are meant to provide a basis to assess the fairness of the price-setting process, comparisons may suffer from methodological problems and is complicated by the fact that even if a product is available in a given market, there may be differences in the strength, formulation and package size of the product available across countries. Furthermore, these comparisons may potentially be circular in derivation: country A looks at an average of prices in countries B, C, D; country B looks at an average of A, C, D or perhaps A, C and E. The price comparison mechanism is based on the assumption that the prices in the country being considered have a sound basis and/or that the factors leading to those prices are appropriate for the country doing the pricing on the basis of such comparisons, none of which may be true.

Few countries now grant a reimbursement price 'for life'. Prices set at launch may be maintained for a period of time and then adjusted according to defined criteria. For example, in France, prices are set initially for a period of 5 years before being reassessed to take into account new indications, volume levels or any pharmacovigilance problems (Pelen 2000). In most countries, price cuts have been more common than granting a price increase for a particular drug.

While direct price controls may have gone some way to tackling the price side of the expenditure equation by slowing the rise in drug prices or in fact lowering the prices of at least some drugs, pharmaceutical expenditures in these same countries often continued to increase; this increase is best explained by a rise in the quantity of drugs used and/or a change in the mix of drugs as newer drugs were added to reimbursement lists. A study of the effects of price, volume and new product introductions in the Netherlands between 1990 and 2002 found that year-to-year growth in the quantity of drugs used was the primary contributor to total turnover; prices actually decreased in several years of the period examined (Nefarma 2002). In Sweden, real drug expenditures increased by 95 per cent between 1974 and 1993, due to a 22 per cent rise in the number of prescriptions – mainly due to newer, more expensive products – while relative prices decreased by 35 per cent (Jonsson 1994). In France, numerous supply-side policies aimed at controlling drug prices have been used since 1975, achieving some of the lowest prices in Europe. However, with volumes unconstrained, pharmaceutical expenditures increased with the number of prescriptions (Le Pen 1996; Lecompte and Paris 1998). In Spain, the relative price of drugs decreased by 39 per cent between 1980 and 1996, yet a 10 per cent increase in the number of items prescribed, mostly for new products (there was a 442 per cent increase in these) with little therapeutic gain, was associated with a 264 per cent increase in real drug expenditures over the same period (Lopez-Batisda and Mossialos 2000). A similar picture emerges from Greece, where from 1994 to 2000, despite a 17 per cent decrease in relative prices, the number of prescriptions increased by 16 per cent while drug expenditures grew by 204 per cent (Kontozamanis 2001). These examples serve only to emphasize that while direct price controls may be effective in lowering drug price, pharmaceutical expenditures may nevertheless increase. While the quantities of drugs used and mix of products may be necessary to meet patient need, and offset costs elsewhere in the system, it is nevertheless important that the use of medicines is rational (see Chapters 8 and 9).

Economic evaluations and drug pricing

Several EU countries are using economic evaluation data alongside other criteria for reimbursement decisions. As Chapter 7 discusses the rationale for using economic evaluations in drug reimbursement across the EU, the aim in this section is to discuss the role economic evaluation has actually played in determining drug prices. Finland is the only country to have officially adopted economic evaluation guidelines as part of the price-setting mechanism. In most other countries, economic evaluation informs the pricing decision only to the extent that it aids in forming a judgement as to the costs and benefits offered by a product relative to a comparator product(s); in this sense, it is a tool for price justification and potentially offers a margin for cost-effective innovation. Since the implementation of the Pharmaceutical Benefits Board in Sweden in 2003, evidence from comparative economic evaluations has been used to decide whether the price of the drug was too high and thus whether the drug should be excluded from reimbursement. The evidence of the effectiveness of using economic evaluation to secure 'value prices' is limited. Some evidence from Sweden suggests that higher margins are gained by drugs considered to be innovative (Lundkvist 2002), which may be a reflection of the use of economic evaluation. The case of the risk-sharing agreement for multiple sclerosis drugs in the UK (see Box 6.1) is a unique example of a price directly linked to a cost per quality-adjusted life year (QALY) ratio (see Chapter 7); however, the implementation of the scheme has faced multiple challenges.

Profit controls

The UK has had the Pharmaceutical Price Regulation Scheme (PPRS) in effect in various forms since 1957, indirectly regulating the prices of branded pharmaceuticals sold to the NHS by setting profit limits (Department of Health 1999). The PPRS is the result of periodical negotiations between the Association of the British Pharmaceutical Industry and the Department of Health and is reviewed every few years. Its objective is to achieve a balance between securing medicines for the NHS at reasonable prices and encouraging a profitable pharmaceutical industry capable of competitive development of innovative medicines. As a 'reasonably priced' medicine is not defined in the PPRS, it leaves room for differing interpretations on the part of industry, government and taxpayers.

Companies with NHS sales of £25 million are required to submit an annual financial return identifying those products with NHS sales above £500,000 and any details on the capital employed by each company in supplying these medicines. The data are used to assess a company's overall profitability on NHS sales and applications for price increases. New active substances may be priced at the discretion of the company on entering the market. Companies within the scheme have an allowable profit (or cap) of 21 per cent, measured as a return on

---

Box 6.1   The risk-sharing scheme for multiple sclerosis drugs in the UK

Thanks to the advocacy efforts of patient groups and the pharmaceutical industry, patients with multiple sclerosis in England and Wales who meet certain criteria have been eligible to receive prescriptions for four products (Avonex, Betaferon, Copaxone and Rebif) since May 2002, paid for under a risk-sharing scheme operated by the National Health Service (NHS). The scheme evolved despite a negative ruling by National Institute of Clinical Excellence in 2001 on the cost-effectiveness of these treatments. Under the scheme, the price for each product has been set according to evidence of its effectiveness derived from the outcomes obtained by patients participating in the scheme. If actual outcomes derived by a product fall short of targets within a margin of tolerance, the given company will have to make a repayment according to a sliding scale agreed in advance. There are many caveats to this approach, including the calculation and level of the cost per quality-adjusted life year threshold (see Chapter 7), patient selection and monitoring, and the implications for wider regulatory approaches of the NHS, such as the Pharmaceutical Price Regulation Scheme. Nevertheless, the risk-sharing scheme sets some precedence by linking price to volume to generate a performance-related price for reimbursement.

Source: Mrazek (2002b).

---

capital employed or return on sales for those companies that do not have major capital investments in the UK. If a company exceeds its target return, it can retain up to 40 per cent over the originally permitted return if it has not received a price increase for any product in the same year. If profits exceed the margin of tolerance, the company must reduce profits by cutting prices, repaying the excess profit to the Department of Health, or delaying or restricting previously agreed future price increases. The amount allowed for research and development can comprise up to 20 per cent of total NHS turnover and companies are permitted an additional 3 per cent, depending on the number of patented products sold in the UK. Companies are also allocated 6 per cent of their NHS turnover for promotional spending.

The success of the PPRS in securing low prices of medicines for the NHS is undetermined. Some authors have argued that the PPRS has done little to control the prices of medicines for the NHS, as the pharmaceutical budget has increased approximately 10 per cent per year from 1967 to 1997 (Maynard and Bloor 1997; Bloom and Van Reenen 1998). United Kingdom prices are among the highest in the EU (Department of Health 2002). This is despite one-off savings of £89.8 million resulting from 1993 price reductions (Borrell 1999). This partly reflects the fact that the UK is most often included as a reference country for international comparisons by other EU countries; its relatively free pricing means that companies are likely to establish their UK price first.

The PPRS is thought to have encouraged investment by maintaining a stable and predictable regulatory environment and allowing levels of research and development expenditures above the worldwide average (Mossialos 1997). The limitations of the PPRS are not uncommon to other rate-of-return-type regulatory schemes, which provide little incentive for efficiency, as increased costs can be recovered through allowable price increases. Moreover, to the extent that returns are calculated as a percentage allowance on the capital invested, the company may overinvest in capital equipment or artificially inflate its asset base. This is similar to the Averch-Johnson-Wellisz effect associated with rate-of-return regulation of public utilities (Baldwin 1995). Rate-of-return may also provide firms with incentives to shift production costs from an unregulated to a regulated division if they operate in several markets, as in the case of a firm manufacturing both PPRS-regulated patented medicines and generic medicines falling under another scheme. Finally, as target profits are negotiated and the process may not be transparent, there is the potential for 'regulatory capture'. The determination of the 'proper or fair' rate of return essentially requires insight into the structure, conduct and performance of the industry. The transparency of the PPRS is limited, and the recently produced annual reports based on aggregate data (Department of Health 2002) add limited additional understanding of this complex policy.

Other government–industry agreements

Government–industry agreements have commonly tried to make the industry responsible for overspending on public drug expenditure targets, resulting in price cuts and/or some repayment of the excess (Table 6.3). However, such agreements in Austria, Belgium, Denmark, Portugal and Spain have had a very limited impact in slowing the growth in public drug spending (OECD 2002). In

Table 6.3 Examples of government–industry agreements in EU member states

Country	Type of government–industry agreements
Austria	Agreement on drug expenditure targets for the Social Insurance Institution; growth to be slowed through price reductions
Denmark	Agreement on reduction in overall price level such that overall expenditure on subsidized pharmaceuticals is kept constant
France	Sector-based agreements on issues including exchange of information, promotion of compliance with national objectives, rational drug use, development of a generic drug market and others
Ireland	Agreement on supply terms, conditions and prices of medicines for the health service
Portugal	Agreement with industry to cap NHS drug expenditures and repay excess
Spain	Multiple agreements covering price cuts, expenditure targets and company repayment if spending targets are exceeded
UK	Pharmaceutical Price Regulation Scheme

addition, they have often been unpopular with industry, as their objectives are often short-term.

Some countries (Austria, France, Spain and Sweden) have negotiated price–volume trade-off agreements with individual companies. This mechanism works by setting prices according to expected or realized volume, such that if volume passes a threshold, the price level will decrease and/or companies have to repay the government or health insurance plan. It is not known whether these schemes have been successful or are respected by the industry. Furthermore, as summarized in Box 6.2, France has implemented both industry-wide and individual agreements with companies requiring repayments if government spending targets are exceeded. Such approaches are not uncontroversial. Belgium, for example, planned but never implemented price–volume contracts due to a debate between insurance funds and the pharmaceutical industry on how to classify products as innovative (Eggermont and Kanavos 2001). Another concern is how such an approach may effect an appropriate increase in volume and how this should be defined. Finally, Finland and Italy do not have formal

---

Box 6.2 Sector-wide agreements and agreements with individual pharmaceutical companies in France

France has implemented both industry-wide agreements and agreements with individual companies. Sector-wide agreements with the National Pharmaceutical Industry Union (LEEM, formerly SNIP) have been negotiated between the government and industry since 1994. These have generally defined common objectives, including meeting national health expenditure targets, promoting rational drug use, reduced company advertising and the development of a generic drug market. Within these agreements, if the health expenditure targets are exceeded, the pharmaceutical industry must make a repayment to the sickness funds through a sliding scale tax based on each company's turnover; this rule applied only to 15 companies in 2001, as the remainder were exonerated by having signed individual agreements with the government.

The individual agreements set price–volume conditions for individual products. The price of a drug is set with regard to the improvement it provides compared with other drugs in the same therapeutic class on the positive list; the exception is for drugs defined as innovative, which, since mid-2003, can be freely priced. The Improvement of the Medical Service Rendered (IMSR) is evaluated by the Transparency Commission. The price of a drug can only be higher than other drugs in its class if the IMSR is higher. The Economic Committee for Medical Products then uses the IMSR together with cost-effectiveness analysis and other factors, including the estimated sales volume as well as the expected and actual conditions of its use, in negotiations with individual companies.

price–volume agreements, yet both consider the forecasts of the number of users and sales level of a product in their direct price-setting systems.

Reference pricing schemes

Reference pricing schemes set fixed reimbursement limits for products assigned to the same group. Their purpose is to limit the rise in pharmaceutical expenditures by requiring patients to pay any excess of the price of the prescribed drug over the reference price. This additional cost is anticipated to increase patient and physician awareness of the prescribed drug's price and possibly result in the patient being switched to a drug listed at the reference price. If switching occurs, then a convergence of drugs in the same category to the reference price generally follows.

In the EU, reference pricing has gained popularity because it can be effective in reducing price differences among drugs defined as therapeutic substitutes by improving market transparency (Giuliani *et al.* 1998). Countries' schemes differ in coverage, pricing method and inclusion or exclusion of on-patent medicines. In general, reference pricing applies only to products that have been defined in the same category, having similar therapeutic mechanisms or clinical outcomes. However, if they are not generic equivalents, these classifications are often controversial (Rigter 1994). In Denmark, Germany and Spain (and Sweden until October 2002), the reference pricing schemes include only off-patent drugs. Almost uniquely in Europe, the Netherlands includes patented drugs in its reference price scheme. Germany, which included patented drugs in the early stages of its reference price scheme, may do so again should proposals for a reform of pharmaceutical legislation proceed (Busse and Wörz 2003).

Different mechanisms are used to calculate the reference price, as shown in Table 6.4. Evidence from studies in individual countries suggests that there is downward price convergence (Lopez-Casasnovas and Puig-Junoy 2000). In Sweden, the market share of reference price drugs decreased from 13 per cent by value at the start of the scheme in 1993 to 7.5 per cent by 1996 (Nilsson and Melander 2000); this was driven by a decrease in the price of both original brands and generic equivalents (Aronsson *et al.* 1998; Bergman and Rudholm 2001). Similar price decreases occurred in Germany after patients were switched to medicines at the reference price, sparing them the additional costs (Zweifel and Crivelli 1996; Pavcnik 2002). As a result, most companies in Germany reduced their prices and the label 'without co-payment' became one of the most important communication issues in physician-focused advertising campaigns (Vogelbruch 2000). There is evidence of switching in other reference price schemes such as that in British Columbia (Canada), where seniors were switched from angiotensin-converting-enzyme inhibitors listed above the reference price to cheaper alternatives (Schneeweiss *et al.* 2002).

Even where reference pricing resulted in some savings on pharmaceutical expenditures, the effect was generally only short-term in the Netherlands (Lopez-Casasnovas and Puig-Junoy 2000), Germany (Nink *et al.* 2001) and Italy (Donatini *et al.* 2001). One explanation is that an increase in the volume and

Table 6.4 Comparative definitions of reference price in selected EU schemes

Country	Year introduced	Definition of reference price
Germany	1989	Statistically derived median price for drugs containing the same active substance and having comparable efficacy
Netherlands	1991	Average price of drugs with similar pharmacotherapeutic effects
Denmark	1996	Lowest priced generic equivalent available on the market
Spain	2000	Arithmetic mean of the three lowest cost-per-treatment-day grouped by formulation and calculated by DDD
Belgium	2001	Equal to a price that is 26 per cent lower than the price of the original brand for generic equivalent products
Italy	2001	Lowest priced generic equivalent available on the market
Portugal	2003	Lowest priced generic equivalent available on the market

price of drugs outside the reference price system in general nullified any reductions in pharmaceutical expenditure from the scheme. Some German doctors, for example, preferred to prescribe products that were not included in the reference price scheme rather than sacrifice time to discuss co-payments with patients (Nink *et al.* 2001). In fact, the price of drugs outside the reference price system increased by over 20 per cent from the early stages of the German reference price system (Statistisches Bundesamt 1998). A similar outcome of reference pricing in New Zealand led the government to supplement it with cross-product agreements, where securing a particular price on a new drug required prices of drugs in unrelated markets to be reduced (Woodfeild 2001).

As reference pricing is often targeted at generic medicines where price competition should be possible (see Chapter 14), the challenge in many of these systems has been how to stimulate demand-side cost awareness, which is essential for competition and subsequently lowering the reference price. The lack of demand-side incentives in Norway was one reason given for the reference price scheme not achieving anticipated savings (ECON Centre for Economic Analysis 2000); in fact, a lack of satisfaction with reference pricing has resulted in both Norway and Sweden abandoning their schemes. Germany has supplemented the reference price scheme with what is referred to as the downward price coil in an attempt to move prices below the reimbursement limit (see Chapter 14); as pharmacists were paid such that the absolute margin increased with product price, they had little incentive to engage in discounting with wholesalers that would reduce a drug's market price. Despite the problems other countries have experienced with their reference pricing schemes, the practice continues to spread; France announced in 2003 that it would establish a reference pricing scheme for off-patent drugs.

There is a need for more thorough analysis of the impact of reference pricing systems, particularly in Europe. As mentioned in Chapter 5, the evidence on reference pricing is for the most part based on aggregate data, and while these studies do contribute to our understanding of how such schemes work, few have controlled for the impact of other cost-containment measures. It is also important that studies of reference pricing consider the impact on clinical outcomes, the health status of patients, total health system costs and drug innovation (Kanavos and Reinhardt 2003). Equity issues arising from the impact of reference pricing, particularly on the more vulnerable groups, needs also to be studied in more detail within a European context; several studies from British Columbia have shown that some of the province's cost-savings on reference pricing have resulted in higher costs for seniors (Grootendorst *et al.* 2001; Marshall *et al.* 2002).

Conclusions

Price controls certainly can have an impact on either slowing price increases or lowering drug prices. However, the impact of price controls on drug expenditures may be mitigated by growth in the quantity of drugs used or in the mix of products that includes more expensive medicines. Countries continue to face the challenge of determining what is a reasonable drug price and how to decide which drugs should be rewarded as being cost-effective innovations; the latter is important so that it acts as a signal to influence the innovative process.

One debatable issue is to what extent pharmaceutical prices can be deregulated. Certainly for competition to generate lower prices, there has to be cost-awareness on the demand side of the market for suitable alternative products. As discussed in Chapters 10, 11, 13 and 14, financial incentives targeting physicians, pharmacists and patients have led to greater cost-awareness for off-patent drugs. The extent to which these same incentives motivate the selection of comparable substitutes and competition for on-patent drugs is not clear, but is likely to be more limited than for generic drugs.

Another issue for debate is whether a single price control system for the EU would be a viable alternative to the multiplicity of national price control mechanisms. For the pharmaceutical industry it would mean a less complex European pharmaceutical market, but it could also mean a more restrictive market, as currently the number of products available differs across the national markets. From national perspectives, it is unlikely that a single EU price or reimbursement list would be acceptable, since willingness to pay for a drug may vary with national conditions such as relative price levels, epidemiology or patient valuations (Drummond 2003). It is therefore unlikely that there will be a single EU pharmaceutical price or reimbursement list in the near future.

References

Arfwedson, J. (2003) *Parallel Trade in Pharmaceuticals*. Brussels: Centre for New Europe Health (available from www.CNEhealth.org).

Aronsson, T., Bergman, M.A. and Rudholm, N. (1998) *The Impact of Generic Competition on Brand Name Market Shares: Evidence from Micro Data*. Umeå Economic Studies No. 462. Umeå: University of Umeå.

Baldwin, R. (1995) *Regulation in Question: The Growing Agenda 1995*. London: London School of Economics and Political Science.

Bergman, M.A. and Rudholm, N. (2001) *Potential Competition and Patent Expiration: Empirical Evidence from the Pharmaceutical Market*. Umeå: Research Institute of Industrial Economics, University of Umeå.

Bloom, N. and Van Reenen, J. (1998) Regulating drug prices: where do we go from here?, *Fiscal Studies*, 19(4): 347–74.

Borrell, J.R. (1999) Pharmaceutical price regulation: a study on the impact of the rate-of-return regulation in the UK, *Pharmacoeconomics*, 15(3): 291–303.

Busse, R. and Wörz, M. (2003) German plans for 'health care modernisation', *EuroHealth*, 9(1): 21–4.

Council of the European Union (1989) Council Directive 89/105/EEC of 21 December 1988 relating to the transparency of measures regulating the pricing of medicinal products for human use and their inclusion within the scope of national health insurance systems, *Official Journal of the European Communities*, L40, 11.02.1989.

Danzon, P.M. (1998) The economics of parallel trade, *Pharmacoeconomics*, 13(3): 293–304.

Danzon, P.M. and Chao, L.W. (2000) Does regulation drive out competition in pharmaceutical markets?, *Journal of Law and Economics*, 43(2): 311–57.

Danzon, P. and Kim, J. (1998) International price comparisons for pharmaceuticals: measurement and policy issues, *Pharmacoeconomics*, 14(suppl. 1): 115–28.

Department of Health UK (1999) *The Pharmaceutical Price Regulation Scheme*. London: Department of Health (available from http://www.doh.gov.uk/pprs.htm).

Department of Health UK (2002) *Pharmaceutical Price Regulation Scheme: Sixth Report to Parliament*, December. London: The Stationery Office (available from http://www.doh.gov.uk/pprs.htm).

Donatini, A., Rico, A., D'Ambrosio, M.G. *et al.* (2001) *Health Care Systems in Transition: Italy*. Copenhagen: European Observatory on Health Care Systems.

Drummond, M.F. (2003) Will there ever be a European drug pricing and reimbursement agency?, *European Journal of Health Economics*, 4: 67–9.

ECON Centre for Economic Analysis (2000) *Evaluation of the Reference Pricing System for Medicines*. Report 44/2000. Oslo: Centre for Economic Analysis.

Eggermont, M. and Kanavos, P. (2001) *Pricing and Reimbursement in Belgium*. London: London School of Economics and Political Science (available from http://pharmacos. eudra.org/F3/g10/p6.htm) (accessed 4 April 2002).

Garattini, L., Salvioni, F., Scopelliti, D. and Garattini, S. (1994) A comparative analysis of the pharmaceutical market in four European countries, *Pharmacoeconomics*, 6(5): 417–23.

Giuliani, G., Selke, G. and Garattini, L. (1998) The German experience in reference pricing, *Health Policy*, 44(1): 73–85.

Grootendorst, P.V., Dolovich, L.R., O'Brien, B.J., Holbrook, A.M. and Levy, A.R. (2001) Impact of reference-based pricing of nitrates on the use and costs of anti-anginal drugs, *Canadian Medical Association Journal*, 165(8): 1011–19.

House of Commons UK (1999) *Trade and Industry, 8th Report*. Trade and Industry Committee. London: The Stationery Office.

Jonsson, B. (1994) Pricing and reimbursement of pharmaceuticals in Sweden, *Pharmacoeconomics*, 6(suppl. 1): 51–60.

Kanavos, P. and Mossialos, E. (1999) International comparisons of health care expenditures: what we know and what we do not know, *Journal of Health Services Research and Policy*, 4(2): 122–6.

Kanavos, P. and Reinhardt, U. (2003) Reference pricing for drugs: is it compatible with US health care?, *Health Affairs*, 22(3): 16–30.

Kontozamanis, V. (2001) *The Greek Pharmaceutical Market*. Athens: Institute for Industrial and Economics Studies.

Lecompte, T. and Paris, V. (1998) Le controle des depenses en medicament en Allemagne, en France et au Royaume-Uni [Controlling drug expenditure in Germany, France and the UK], *Economie et statistique*, 312(13): 109–24.

Le Pen, C. (1996) Drug pricing and reimbursement in France, *Pharmacoeconomics*, 10(suppl. 2): 26–36.

(LIF) Lægemiddelindustriforeningen (2003) *Tal & Data 2002*. Copenhagen: LIF (available from http://lif.albatros.dk/sw231.asp) (accessed 9 July 2003).

Lopez-Bastida, J. and Mossialos, E. (2000) Pharmaceutical expenditure in Spain: cost and control, *International Journal of Health Services*, 30(3): 597–616.

Lopez-Casasnovas, G. and Puig-Junoy, J. (2000) Review of the literature on reference pricing, *Health Policy*, 54(2): 87–123.

Lundkvist, J. (2002) Pricing and reimbursement of drugs in Sweden, *European Journal of Health Economics*, 3: 66–70.

Marshall, J.K., Grootendorst, P.V., O'Brien, B.J. *et al.* (2002) Impact of reference-based pricing for histamine-2 receptor antagonists and restricted access for proton pump inhibitors in British Columbia, *Canadian Medical Association Journal*, 166(13): 1655–62.

Maynard, A. and Bloor, K. (1997) Regulating the pharmaceutical industry, *British Medical Journal*, 315: 200–1.

Mossialos, E. (1997) An evaluation of the PPRS: is there a need for reform?, in D. Green (ed.) *Should Pharmaceutical Prices be Regulated?* London: Institute of Economic Affairs.

Mrazek, M. (2002a) Comparative approaches to pharmaceutical price regulation in the European Union, *Croatian Medical Journal*, 43(4): 453–61.

Mrazek, M. (2002b) Risk-sharing scheme for the provision of MS drugs, *Hospital Pharmacy Europe*, Autumn, pp. 40–4.

Nefarma (2002) *Jaarverslag 2002* [Annual Report 2002]. The Hague: Nefarma.

Nilsson, J.L.G. and Melander, A. (2000) Use of generic drugs and effects of the reference price system in Sweden, *Drug Information Journal*, 34: 1195–200.

Nink, K., Schroder, H. and Selke, G.W. (2001) Der Arzneimittelmarkt in der BDR [The pharmaceuticals market in the Federal Republic of Germany], in U. Schwabe and D. Paffrath (eds) *Arzneiverordnungs-Report 2001*. Berlin: Springer.

OECD (2002) *Health Data 2002*. Paris: OECD.

Pavcnik, N. (2002) Do pharmaceutical prices respond to potential patient out-of-pocket expenses?, *RAND Journal of Economics*, 33(3): 469–87.

Pelen, F. (2000) Reimbursement and pricing of drugs in France: an increasingly complex system, *Health Economics in Prevention and Care*, Trial issue 0: S24–S27.

Pharmig (2000) *Facts & Figures 1999/00*. Vienna: Pharmig.

Productivity Commission Australia (2001) *International Pharmaceutical Price Differences*. Canberra, ACT: AusInfo.

Reekie, W.D. (1998) How competition lowers the costs of medicines, *Pharmacoeconomics*, 14(suppl. 1): 107–13.

Rigter, H. (1994) Recent public policies in the Netherlands to control pharmaceutical pricing and reimbursement, *Pharmacoeconomics*, 6(suppl. 1): 15–21.

Rovira, J. and Darba, J. (2001) Pharmaceutical pricing and reimbursement in Spain, *European Journal of Health Economics*, 2(1): 39–43.

Schneeweiss, S., Walker, A.M., Glynn, R.J. *et al.* (2002) Outcomes of reference pricing for angiotensin-converting-enzyme inhibitors, *New England Journal of Medicine*, 346(11): 822–9.

Sirkia, T. and Rajaniemi, S. (2001) *Pricing and Reimbursement in Finland*. LSE Study on Healthcare in Individual Countries. London: London School of Economics and Political Science (available from http://pharmacos.eudra.org/F3/g10/p6.htm) (accessed 4 April 2002).

Statistisches Bundesamt Gesundheitsbericht für Deutschland (1998) *Pharmazeutische und medizinische Industrie* [*The Pharmaceuticals and Medicinal Products Industry*], Teil 2, Kapitel 6.14. Wiesbaden: Statistisches Bundesamt.

US General Accounting Office (1994) *Prescription Drugs: Spending Controls in Four European Countries*. GAO/HEHS-94-30. Washington, DC: GAO.

Vogelbruch, B. (2000) *Festbetrage fur arzneimittel: ein neues instrument zur kostendampfung im Gesundheitswesen und sein einfluss auf das wettbewerbsverhalten auf dem arzneimittelmarkt* [*Fixed Prices for Medicines: A New Cost-Containment Measure for the Health Care System and Its Influence on Competitive Behaviour in the Pharmaceutical Market*]. Hamburg: Duisburger Economic Papers.

Woodfeild, A. (2001) Augmenting reference pricing of pharmaceuticals in New Zealand with strategic cross-product agreements, *Pharmacoeconomics*, 19(4): 365–77.

Zweifel, P. and Crivelli, L. (1996) Price regulation of drugs: lessons from Germany, *Journal of Regulatory Economics*, 10: 257–73.

seven

Reimbursement of pharmaceuticals in the European Union

Alistair McGuire, Michael Drummond and Frans Rutten

Introduction

In this chapter, we outline the impact that the imposition of additional regulatory instruments will have on the reimbursement (i.e. public subsidy) of pharmaceutical products. The general argument proposed is that all reimbursement affects the research and development (R&D) base of the pharmaceutical sector through its sales revenue. There is a concern that the increasing implementation of cost-effectiveness analysis, as part of the reimbursement environment, will dampen innovative activity considerably. While it is certain to have an impact, it is argued here that it is uncertain what the aggregate impact will be. The other major regulatory mechanisms relating to reimbursement, co-payment structures and selected lists have been implemented with little consistency across Europe. The criteria underlying cost-effectiveness analysis could be argued to have more consistency and this particular mechanism may, in any case, eventually replace the selected list approach to determining the reimbursement status of pharmaceuticals.

Theoretical impact of reimbursement rules

It is generally acknowledged that the free market allocation of pharmaceutical products would be prone to inefficiency. Patients do not have adequate knowledge about treatment options and in any case do not bear the full cost of purchase. The clinician, acting as the agent for the patient, does not bear full, if any, financial responsibility for the purchase and may be affected by promotional activities of the companies. Indeed, the main interaction in this market is between the health care funder and the pharmaceutical industry. While a major objective of pharmaceutical reimbursement is undoubtedly the capping of expenditure on an easily identifiable component of the health care budget, funders are aware that reimbursement mechanisms have an impact on research and development and, ultimately, on the treatment choices faced by individual patients.

The pharmaceutical industry is characterized by an oligopoly structure, with monopoly power in particular markets at particular times. The monopoly power is both a reflection of the tendency towards potential scale and scope effects in R&D and a result of patent protection of innovation. The length of this protection varies depending on the length of time devoted to the discovery and development phases of the new product and the maximum time limit of the patent period. The diversity of regulation in the pharmaceutical market is aimed at dampening the economic rents enjoyed by such monopoly. The regulation, however, must not be too severe so as to add to the already substantial costs involved in bringing new products into this market. Cockburn and Henderson (2001) report that for 10 major international pharmaceutical firms, average expenditure on product development has increased from US$40 million in the mid-1960s to over US$200 million by 1990. The average duration of both successful and unsuccessful projects was just under five years, with less than one in five compounds that moved into substantial clinical testing being approved for use in the market.

The costs of developing new products are therefore substantial. A rationally planned inventive effort will be undertaken only if the expected revenue of the innovative product, or portfolio of products, is likely to exceed the expected cost. The aim of optimal reimbursement policies is to provide adequate reward to invention to stimulate future investments in research, while at the same time to depress economic rent to ensure that those purchasing the new technologies – whether these are individuals or governmental payers – are not being overly exploited. Figure 7.1, taken from Vernon (2001), gives the individual pharmaceutical firms' perspective.

Rational inventive effort is undertaken to the point where the marginal cost of capital (mcc) used to fund the process is equal to the marginal rate of discounted return (mrr) on the inventive effort. The inventive effort is correlated with the level of R&D expenditures as given on the horizontal axis. To finance new innovation, the individual firm has to raise capital. It can do so in three broad ways. First, it can raise internal funds through sales revenue. Even for large firms this will normally be inadequate to cover the broad scope of R&D required to develop a successful product. Secondly, it can debt finance. This is shown by the sloped section of the mrr curves, with the slope reflecting increasing leverage of debt (the more debt incurred, the higher the price). Finally, the firm can issue new equity.

Clearly, if reimbursement is curtailed, this will have an impact on the firm's marginal rate of return (mrr) on innovation. As shown in Figure 7.1, the mrr curve shifts inward (from mrr_1 to mrr_2) as the expected marginal rate of return on all R&D projects falls. This reduces R&D expenditure (from $R\&D_1$ to $R\&D_2$)

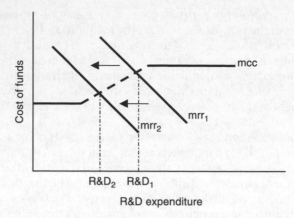

Figure 7.1 Rational inventive effort from the pharmaceutical firm perspective.

on all future projects and, given the high failure rate in developing new projects, the impact of decreases in reimbursement could have a significantly greater impact on those innovations that are of market potential.

Reimbursement levels reflect the outcome of negotiation between the pharmaceutical company and the purchaser. Prices are regulated in a number of ways, including the direct means of reference pricing, formulary pricing, capping or item-by-item price negotiation, as well as indirectly through rate-of-return regulation. However established, the resultant price is the outturn of a negotiated process between a monopolist (the firm with the innovative product) and a monopsonist (the purchaser who is normally a regulatory body). The objective pursued by the monopolist can be characterized as profit maximization, while the objectives of the purchasing body are more complex. They can generally be thought of as pursuing the maximization of social welfare. Welfare, however, may relate to a number of arguments. These are normally characterized as the pursuit of consumers' welfare, in this case by ensuring monopoly rent is not excessive and that the new technology diffuses in an optimal manner, as well as maintaining adequate return to the pharmaceutical sector to ensure continued innovative activity, or even employment levels. These goals may, however, be conflicting. In several regulated industries, notably the utilities sector, the consumer faces a price per unit that is equal to the marginal cost of producing that output (that is, the addition to total cost of producing this unit of output). It is well established in economic theory that if this is not the case, then both the firm and the consumer can be made better off by appropriately changing the quantity produced in return for a transfer of money.

Given the R&D base at the root of the pharmaceutical industry, it can be characterized as a sector that has increasing returns to scale and scope such that average cost decreases with output levels. If this is the case, average cost will be higher than the marginal cost of production. If the regulator desires that an incentive be retained for further innovative activity, then the suitable product price will be pitched higher than average cost (and therefore marginal cost). In other words, to create an incentive for innovative behaviour, the regulator will allow some monopoly profit to be retained by the industry. This moves the pricing of any pharmaceutical product away from the regulatory norm of marginal cost (or even average cost) pricing. With asymmetry of information over the costs of production, such that the regulator cannot fully observe R&D costs, further complexities ensue. Given the uncertainties that prevail regarding the basic innovative process within the pharmaceutical industry, and the cross-subsidy that exists between successful marketable products and unsuccessful product development, it is difficult for the regulator to observe the firm's cost-reducing effort. Appropriate price-setting becomes extremely difficult.

What can be said of reimbursement mechanisms under such circumstances? Essentially there is a bilateral monopoly. A single seller faces a single buyer. The pricing outcome under such circumstances is indeterminate. The actual reimbursement price established will be determined by the bargaining skills, and the political and economic power of the two monopolies. The monopoly will attempt to attain as high a price as possible, the monopsonist will attempt to push the price as low as possible.

Regulation has traditionally dealt with safety, efficacy and quality, with reimbursement negotiations following these concerns. Increasingly, however, a number of countries are considering what has been referred to as the 'fourth hurdle' of regulation, which, notwithstanding the conceptual problems outlined above, attempts to set pharmaceutical product prices.

The regulation of prices is seen, by some, to be an extension of the existing regulations aimed at curtailing pharmaceutical expenditure. Selected lists are the most obvious example of this regulatory instrument. We suggest that this is a blunt regulatory reimbursement instrument, which, additionally, has at least a perceived detrimental impact on pharmaceutical companies' R&D return through inhibiting the development of new products in the therapeutic areas listed. This was an argument put to the UK Parliamentary Committee on Health Affairs, for example. Particularly if companies are risk-averse, they may weight the impact of a blunt regulatory tool more highly than an instrument that is more flexible in its implementation. On the other hand, flexibility places greater discretion in the hands of the reimbursing agency. If flexibility is also coupled with transparency, however, this may temper any abuse of discretion. In this chapter, we argue that the emerging use of economic evaluation as a reimbursement instrument in several countries could be useful in replacing blunter instruments, especially listing of pharmaceuticals, as it is a more flexible and transparent instrument, but that a number of problems are faced in implementation.

Reimbursement background

Chapter 6 covers the area of pricing and the reader is referred to that chapter for further detail. Here, discussion will centre on listing and economic evaluation as regulatory instruments. However, to the extent that these instruments are complementary to pricing controls, a few points relating to pricing are highlighted. Health care funders design reimbursement criteria to affect the price and utilization of pharmaceuticals. While there are a broad range of criteria embedded within any reimbursement regime, here we merely highlight that, on the pricing side, reference pricing is common, while on the utilization side, selected lists are prevalent. Neither instrument, unlike economic evaluation, draws information on cost and health outcome together.

There is extensive use of reference-pricing schemes where the health care funder sets the level of public payment for a pre-defined group or cluster of drugs. Manufacturers are free to set the price of their product above the reference price but the patient has to pay the difference (the impact of co-payments are dealt with in Chapter 14). Generally, the introduction of reference price systems has led to a one-off reduction in the prices of referred drugs, but firms have raised the prices of non-referred drugs. On the other hand, the attractiveness of generics was argued to have decreased as branded product prices have fallen. This general trend with regards to reference pricing has been witnessed in a number of countries, including Germany, the Netherlands and Sweden (Drummond *et al.* 1997). In each of these countries, substantial once-and-for-all budget savings have been witnessed on the introduction of the reference price savings. Arguably, such a system may continue to see savings on the budget as the non-referred products fail to increase prices to an extent that offsets the regulated effect of the reference prices. Whether this is a continuing process, however, depends on the manner in which reimbursement limits are set. In most countries, these limits are rather fixed over time. Since introduction in the Netherlands, for example, they have been changed only once yet prices have risen sharply since 1992. Indeed, it was observed that the prices of several generic drugs were raised towards the maximum reimbursement level or were maintained at the same level when products went out of patent in the Netherlands. Competition between manufacturers and wholesale companies resulted in pharmacists being provided with bonuses and discounts in an attempt to persuade them to prescribe specific pharmaceutical products. So the potential gains to society arising from the erosion of the protection of branded products was not realized and was transformed into large gains for pharmacists.

As a result, the failure of the reference price system has been widely acknowledged in the Netherlands and the new policy is to gradually abandon this system and make way for a more active role of the monopsony power of the insurance companies. The cholesterol-lowering drugs and gastrointestinal drugs will be the first drugs to exit the reference price system in 2003. Health care insurers may purchase these drugs directly from pharmaceutical companies or contract for large bulks with wholesale companies. As patents expire for some of the products in these two areas, there is potential for large price reductions. Strangely enough, other countries like France are just about to introduce reference pricing, without the accompanying controls on other parts of the health care system that the Dutch experience indicates is necessary. It seems that countries do not learn from experiences elsewhere, although there is a general recognition that reference pricing does not display any information relating price to treatment efficacy. The proponents of economic evaluation argue that one strength of this instrument is the explicit linkage of treatment cost to health benefit.

Utilization may be regulated through the establishment of national formularies, which may define positive or negative lists, the development of treatment guidelines, the encouragement of generic prescribing and the ongoing provision of information to prescribers on the cost and volume of their prescription patterns. Historically, the most common regulatory instrument in reimbursement has been the adoption of selected lists; that is, the explicit listing of a pharmaceutical product by the health care funder indicating whether or not a specific product may be adopted for reimbursement. Such lists are most common in Europe, where a positive list approach (the identification of products that may be reimbursed) is normally adopted. Germany is the major current exception to this rule, although it is proposed that the negative list in operation be abolished and a positive list be implemented within the next few years.[1] Although the precise criteria that will allow selection onto the list remain unclear, these are thought to relate to therapeutic benefit, quality and low-risk factors, and there is a possibility that cost-effectiveness analysis may also be invoked. The principle behind the adoption of such lists is that drugs which are ineffective or are more expensive than equally effective drugs should not be prescribed.

It is common for countries to classify pharmaceuticals within their lists. The use of such lists has spread over the past 20 years. In the USA, 12 states have recently adopted a positive list for their Medicaid pharmaceutical reimbursement. It is common to find different classifications within listings, although the more classifications there are tends to lead to more manipulation and discretion. Italy, for example, has recently reduced its three categories to two – essential and a catch-all category. The latter includes all drugs that have no efficacy information and are more costly than comparator drugs. Notes restricting use, that define the appropriate indication and the circumstances under which reimbursement will follow, accompany the list. Countries practising reference-based pricing tend to pursue a notion of additional therapeutic benefit for listing purposes.

All listing schemes suffer from similar disadvantages. Opponents of such schemes state that they are not open to adequate consultation, discussion and openness. They are seen to lack flexibility, such that once a decision has been reached it is difficult to reverse even if new information is disclosed. This latter criticism could be overcome through a prescribed period being defined, after which a drug could be reviewed. It has been argued that by their nature, selective lists discourage R&D as they are a blunt regulatory instrument that may result in no reimbursement if products do not make the list or dampen the incentive to innovate in areas already covered by existing drugs. The argument here is that as new drugs have to prove additional therapeutic benefit over and above pre-existing drugs, there is an incentive to move on to virgin areas. This seems a weak argument not least on the grounds that, with or without the existence of lists, marginal benefit in areas with existing competitor products would always be more difficult to maintain than in areas with weak competition.

Economic evaluation

Against this general background, the approach of reimbursing with recourse to the cost-effectiveness of a specific health care technology has recently been advocated in a number of countries. Dickson *et al.* (2003) note that, in general, pharmacoeconomic assessment is diffusing quickly across the OECD countries. They suggest that an increasing emphasis on value-for-money, particularly for new drugs and related reimbursement and pricing issues, lies behind this spread of use. While their survey of the use of such assessment across 11 OECD countries suggested marked differences in application, they did note an improvement in informational exchanges across national assessment agencies.

Why has this increased use of economic evaluation occurred? There appears to be a number of contributory factors. First, there is a growing awareness of escalating health care costs in a number of countries with the implicit argument that existing regulation is failing to contain costs. In most OECD countries, the rate of growth in health care costs is higher, sometimes substantially higher, than that in gross domestic product (GDP). While pharmaceutical prices are generally not increasing markedly, the number of prescribed items continues to grow apace. More significantly, there is a propensity towards prescribing newly introduced drugs. It is generally recognized that these new products tend to have higher average prices than existing products. The market share of newly introduced drugs does vary across countries. In the UK in 2001, 16 per cent of market share by value went to new drugs launched in the five years prior to this date. In the larger US and German markets, the respective comparable figures were 32 and 25 per cent (UK Pharmaceutical Industry Competitiveness Task Force 2002). The pharmaceutical market is therefore seen to be one of high activity with regards to new products. Given the tendency to pursue high prices for new products, as linked to the justification to cover innovative activity, there is increasing concern over the growth in the pharmaceutical budget in most countries. Moreover, in most countries pharmaceutical budgets can be easily identified, making them a clear target for specific constraint.

As noted above, setting a price makes it possible to explicitly judge the economic efficiency of a new product. While price regulations attempt to set a price compatible with incentives to innovate while ensuring adequate diffusion of the pharmaceutical product, it may be argued that cost-effectiveness attempts to evaluate the relative value-for-money provided by a new health care technology through explicitly linking treatment costs to health outcomes. The implication is that formal adoption of cost-effectiveness evidence ties reimbursement to a consideration of the cost of acquiring a new product, which increases health status. Cost-effectiveness analysis establishes the comparative costs and health outcomes under review. Used in conjunction with reimbursement regulation, this amalgamates information on treatment costs with relative effectiveness. This relates reimbursement to comparative effectiveness in a manner that is explicit. Moreover, in highlighting effectiveness, this regulatory instrument also aids the definition of the indications or patient groups where the new therapy will be of greatest value.

Table 7.1 highlights the general regulatory background with respect to pharmaceutical reimbursement for a number of countries. As can be seen from this table, there is no general consensus on the use of cost-effectiveness as part of reimbursement across the countries indicated. However, as well as those indicated in Table 7.1, a number of EU member states have imposed or have signalled an intent to impose some requirement for cost-effectiveness data as a

Table 7.1 Reimbursement and related features affecting the pharmaceutical market in selected countries

	France	Germany	Italy	Netherlands	Spain	Sweden	Switzerland	UK	Australia	Canada	NZ	USA
Conditional/limited reimbursement exists	Yes	Yes	Yes	Yes	Yes	Yes	No	Yes	Yes	Yes	No	Yes
National guidelines on pharmacoeconmics	Planned	No	No	Yes	No	No	No	Yes	No	No	No	No
Pharmacoeconomics used in pricing decisions	Possible	No	Some products	Some products	No	Yes	Sometimes	Not directly	Yes	Some provinces	Yes	Sometimes, locally
Drugs budget funded by	National	National	Regional	National	Regional	Local	Local	National	National	Provincial	National	Mix
Co-payment culture exists	Yes	Yes	Yes	No	Yes	Yes	Yes	Yes	Yes	Yes	Yes	Yes
Capped profits/ sales rebates	Yes	No	Yes	No	Yes	No	No	Yes	No	No	Yes	No
Company free to set launch price	No	Yes	No	No	No	No	Yes	Yes	No	No	No	Yes

Source: UK Pharmaceutical Industry Competitiveness Task Force (2002).

condition for full adoption for some, if not all, pharmaceutical products. These countries include Belgium, Portugal, Italy, the UK, Sweden, Spain and the Netherlands. Indeed, formal requirement of cost-effectiveness also exists in Australia, certain provinces of Canada and for a major health insurer in the USA (Blue Shield Blue Cross). Moreover, other countries, such as France, Finland, Norway and Denmark, include cost-effectiveness as supporting evidence for reimbursement or pricing.

While Table 7.1 represents the current situation, the near future beckons even greater changes. For example, while in the Netherlands economic evaluation has been used to aid pricing decisions in certain therapeutic areas, it has not been used systematically to date. At the time of writing, a voluntary scheme is being introduced whereby pharmaceutical firms are being encouraged to submit cost-effectiveness studies with their pricing dossier when innovative products are being submitted to the Health Insurance Advisory Board for 'premium' pricing. Innovative products are defined as those outside the reference-based pricing scheme, where products are clustered and one level of reimbursement is given to the cluster. This scheme will become compulsory in 2005. In Spain, regional health technology assessment centres are being implemented with a remit to consider cost-effectiveness of new technologies. A recent announcement from the Spanish government signalled an intention to adopt cost-effectiveness as a formal requirement in the reimbursement process. In Italy, new innovative products must include economic evaluation as part of their reimbursement submission. In Germany, the Health Insurance Funds (*Kranenkassen*) will be actively encouraged to review pharmaceutical products on the basis of their cost-effectiveness. The German government is currently reviewing the introduction of cost-effectiveness as a requirement for pharmaceutical registration and pricing decisions within the establishment of a new health technology assessment structure. Perhaps the most surprising development is the initiation of discussions between the Centres for Medicare and Medicaid Services (CMS)[2] and the Food and Drug Administration (FDA) in the USA aimed at the establishment of a joint office to evaluate the cost-effectiveness of pharmaceutical products, although this is on hold with economic analysis currently relegated to a bit part in the setting of reimbursement by the CMS.

An obvious question is whether there is broad agreement on the guidance on the implementation of cost-effectiveness across the countries that have begun to implement this instrument. A recent analysis of 25 published sets of guidelines found that, other than slight methodological differences, broad general principles were maintained (Hjelmgren *et al.* 2001). All countries generally adopt the most commonly used therapy as their comparator within their evaluation guidelines. Two European countries, the Netherlands and Portugal, specify the comparator to be chosen, while the majority of other European countries leave some discretion to the product sponsor to define the appropriate comparator. Generally, cost–benefit analysis is discouraged, but only the Netherlands specifies that cost-effectiveness must be undertaken. In most countries, effectiveness evidence is sought from clinical trials where available, with conversion to quality-adjusted life years (QALYs) gained being encouraged. The main areas of disagreement in implementation were, according to these authors, concerned with the choice of perspective, which ranged from a societal to a health purchaser viewpoint, and consequently which costs were to be included in any analysis. The choice of time horizon is also in the main left to the discretion of the submitting party, although the Netherlands asks that this be the period most valid to the decision maker. Interestingly, some countries, for example the Netherlands and Portugal, which have introduced economic evaluation into the regulatory process, do not allow appeal against official decisions.

Undoubtedly, there is increasing awareness and utilization of economic evaluation within the regulatory context. While this is to be encouraged as a move which links price, cost and outcome data explicitly, there are a number of concerns. Such concerns arise over the conceptual basis for introducing economic evaluation, practical issues of implementation and methodological issues. Each is now addressed in turn.

While the theory of economic evaluation has a long history, there is a weak link between the use of cost-effectiveness as a regulatory tool and as a concept for pursuing traditional notions of economic efficiency. There have been a number of attempts recently to reconcile the conceptual framework with the application of cost-effectiveness (Garber 2000). Essentially, these rely on relating cost-effectiveness to cost–benefit analysis and, in particular, the defence of QALYs as a measure of individual preferences defined over health states. This is only possible through imposing severe restrictions both on the perspective of the analysis and on the underlying (mathematical) properties that support the measurement of QALYs. For cost-effectiveness to be related to cost–benefit analysis, the investigators have to believe that decision makers are concerned with conventional, academic notions of economic efficiency. This is unlikely. Indeed, given that cost-effectiveness feeds into a more general regulatory framework, it is much more plausible to think of cost-effectiveness as playing the more limited role of providing information on the opportunity cost of various treatments. In other words, cost-effectiveness should be seen to be aiding decisions rather than being the basis for making decisions.

That said, it is likely that if cost per QALY becomes the standard measure sought, then there will be increasing pressure for decision makers to identify the target threshold value of cost per QALY associated with the willingness to pay for a new treatment. The Canadian guidelines have recognized this and set an explicit threshold value level. In some other countries, including the UK, it would appear that the threshold may be inferred from the general trend in adoption of treatments below a set level of cost per QALY. The adoption of explicit or implicit threshold values would seem to imply that efficiency criteria are being given greater weight currently by decision makers than equity or distributive criteria more generally.

Quality-adjusted life years are commonly used to support the notion of opportunity cost, as they are a commensurate measure that allows comparison across treatment areas. However, there is a growing concern that QALYs are really a measure of health benefit that is not related to individual preferences over health states (Broome 1993). In accepting this limited definition of the QALY, the notion of efficiency becomes one of merely maximizing health, as defined by QALYs. This has very restrictive properties. For example, if QALYs are generally gained more by the young than the elderly, merely because they have more life to gain than the elderly, an efficiency criterion that maximizes QALYs will redistribute health resources from the elderly to the young. This raises redistributional concerns. A different approach would retain the QALY as a measure of health benefit but incorporate explicit weights to reflect distributional concerns. In either case, the health decision maker is using some distributional judgement to alter the efficiency outcome. It is rare for these distributional weights to become explicit. In other words, while cost-effectiveness can aid transparency in the allocation of resources, this transparency can become lost when distributional concerns are introduced.

Several practical issues have arisen in the application of cost-effectiveness as a regulatory instrument. The first practical issue relates to the selection of drugs for appraisal. In the UK, the National Institute for Clinical Excellence (NICE) selects, for appraisal, 'technologies that are likely to have a major impact on the NHS'. To date, around two-thirds of the technologies appraised have been pharmaceuticals. The authorities in the Netherlands and Portugal have been similarly selective.

The second practical issue concerns whether drugs should be appraised individually, as in Australia and Ontario, or whether groups or classes of drugs should be appraised together. If several drugs can be assessed as a group, this has the advantage that comparisons can be made among them, so as to guide choice of drug. However, a major difficulty exists in that, for new drugs, it is unlikely that head-to-head clinical trials will have been conducted. This leads to methodological difficulties (see below). In the UK, NICE has undertaken several appraisals of groups of drugs (e.g. proton pump inhibitors, atypical antipsychotics, Cox-II inhibitors) but rarely distinguishes among them unless there is compelling evidence of differences in cost-effectiveness.

A third practical issue concerns transparency in the appraisal process. In most jurisdictions, the economic dossiers submitted by drug manufacturers are regarded as commercial-in-confidence. In the UK, NICE has sought to increase transparency by publishing its technology assessment reports. However, these have to be stripped of any commercial-in-confidence material. This means that the evidence base, on which the authorities make decisions, may not be in the public domain. This can make the decisions hard to explain, which is problematic at a time when several parties, including drug manufacturers, are demanding more transparency in public decision making (Drummond 2002).

Turning to the methodological issues, the first relates to the lack of head-to-head clinical studies comparing the drug of interest with the relevant alternative. This issue was alluded to above in the context of comparisons of new drugs, but could also arise if current care differs among European countries. Therefore, if the drug of interest had been compared, in a trial, with current care in one country, this may not be relevant in other settings. Indeed, selecting the appropriate comparator may not be straightforward generally. If when the alternative to which the new drug is to be compared is standard therapy, this may be difficult to identify as medical practice varies substantially even within countries. When head-to-head comparisons are not available, it may be possible to synthesize these (indirectly) if both therapies have been compared, in separate clinical studies, to a third therapy. Such indirect comparisons are open to bias, but a recent study by Song *et al.* (2003) showed that, among 46 comparisons, the indirect (synthesized) comparisons only differed substantially from the head-to-head studies in three cases.

Moreover, even where evidence is available it must relate to the appropriate patient population. Cost-effectiveness relies on data being available for the patient group for which the drug is being licensed. It is rare that such data exist; for example, there are few clinical studies relating to the elderly. The cost-effectiveness of any individual therapy is also, of course, likely to change over time. This raises the issue of whether reimbursement should be given for an initial phase and then reconsidered after the drug has been on the market for some time. An additional advantage of such a strategy would be that additional data on effectiveness could be gathered after the launch of the drug.

Another methodological issue relates to the need, in economic evaluations, to extrapolate beyond the follow-up period of the clinical trial. Of course, a 'within-trial' analysis could be conducted but this would probably be overly conservative and may not incorporate relevant endpoints such as QALYs. The problem is that, for new drugs, there is often no clear basis on which to make such projections. It may be possible to use the open-label extensions of clinical trials to assess compliance and long-term clinical benefit for those who were originally randomized to the study drug. However, ideally one would require long-term observational studies of the drug as used in regular clinical practice. These uncertainties have led some authorities to propose risk-sharing deals, whereby the final level of payment for the drug is dependent on long-term outcomes. An example of such an arrangement is that developed for the beta interferons (for multiple sclerosis) in the UK.

There exists little agreement over the best method to extrapolate outcomes. A number of studies have proposed extrapolation of hazard rates as based on survival techniques, but there is no guarantee that, even if available, the hazard rates experienced within a trial period will be give rise to adequate forecasts of future outcomes. That said, at least a range of methods does exist for extrapolating outcomes. There is no agreement over the appropriate manner in which to extrapolate treatment costs. In fact, there is little agreement over how best to analyse within-trial costs, again even where this information is available, when problems relating to censoring, missing data and skew exist (Heyse *et al.* 2001).

More generally, there may only be evidence on intermediate outcome measures, for example on changes in blood pressure rather than changes in coronary heart disease morbidity or mortality. If this is the case, this will require a model to extrapolate the intermediate outcome through disease progression into the final outcome.

Finally, a further methodological issue concerns problems regarding the lack of generalizability, from setting to setting, of economic evaluations (Drummond and Pang 2001). This means that decision makers in one European country may not be able to use cost-effectiveness results from elsewhere. None of the European jurisdictions requiring economic evidence insist on all the data coming from their own country. However, they do generally require that the data are relevant to their setting. This issue arose in the NICE appraisal of glycoprotein 3b/2a inhibitors in the treatment of heart disease. All of the clinical data came from trials in the USA, where the patient population and cardiology practice were thought to differ from those in the UK. Therefore, Palmer *et al.* (2002)

estimated the pooled relative risk reduction (comparing drug with placebo) from the American clinical trials through meta-analysis and then applied this to the levels of risk that exist among the patient population in the UK.

As economic evaluation is applied, as part of the drug pricing and reimbursement process, in more European countries, other practical and methodological issues are likely to arise. However, in drawing together information on both treatment costs and health benefits, economic evaluation remains a powerful tool for regulating pharmaceutical reimbursement.

Conclusions

Following price setting, the reimbursement policies operating within Europe vary markedly. At least three distinct mechanisms appear relevant in the reimbursement process: co-payments and deductibles, selected listing and, most recently, cost-effectiveness. Co-payments and deductibles have been dealt with elsewhere in this book and are not considered here. The selected listing of pharmaceutical products appears to be common but is applied inconsistently across individual countries. Most countries appear to operate, or are moving towards, a positive list. That apart, the criteria used for selection are often vague or not open to discussion. Although selected lists clearly address issues of relative effectiveness, they are a blunt regulatory instrument and do not tie cost to health benefit.

The requirement to undertake cost-effectiveness analyses also considers relative effectiveness, but within the context of value for money. Therefore, to an extent, this instrument competes with the notion of a selected list. Indeed, it is of interest that since the implementation of cost-effectiveness criteria through NICE in the UK, the NHS selected list, which formally still exists as a negative list, has not been added to. Moreover, the Netherlands appears to be moving away from reference pricing towards the implementation of cost-effectiveness as a regulatory requirement. In other words, it could be suggested that the cost-effectiveness criteria are replacing the effectiveness control exercised through the selected list in the UK and the use of reference pricing in the Netherlands. Whether this will happen elsewhere is an open question, given the increased application of cost-effectiveness within Europe. Moreover, there has been little consistency in reimbursement regulation across Europe to date. However, it could also be argued that, although no common criteria are invoked in all countries, there is greater consistency in the application of cost-effectiveness across various regulatory regimes than is seen with the other two reimbursement mechanisms considered above.

In returning to the theoretical argument posed at the beginning of this chapter, clearly reimbursement rules will reduce the marginal rate of return on innovative behaviour. It is likely that, in a risky business, increasing the risk will, all other things being equal, dampen R&D. If the reimbursement criteria are clear and new instruments of regulation replace older, blunter instruments, there is an argument that the detrimental impact on R&D will be reduced. That is, the consideration of value for money in cost-effectiveness studies means that the added value (in increased cost-effectiveness) achieved through innovation can be rewarded. While it remains to be proven, it might be argued that the increased use of cost-effectiveness, if this replaces selected lists, will do just that.

Notes

1   However, given the history of several failed attempts in Germany to introduce positive lists, it is unclear whether the current proposal will be successful.
2   The Centers for Medicare and Medicaid Services (CMS) is a Federal agency within the US Department of Health and Human Services. The agency administers Medicare, Medicaid and the Child Health insurance programmes. Formerly called the Health Care Financing Administration (HCFA) (see http://cms.hhs.gov/)

References

Broome, J. (1993) QALYs, *Journal of Public Economics*, 50: 149–67.

Cockburn, I.M. and Henderson, R.M. (2001) Scale and scope of drug development: unpacking the advantages of size in pharmaceutical research, *Journal of Health Economics*, 20: 1033–57.

Dickson, M., Hurst, J. and Jacobzone, S. (2003) *Survey of Pharmaceutical Assessment Activity in Eleven Countries*. Paris: OECD.

Drummond, M. (2002) Should commercial-in-confidence data be used by decision makers when making assessments of cost-effectiveness?, *Applied Health Economics and Health Policy*, 1(2): 53–4.

Drummond, M.F. and Pang, F. (2001) Transferability of economic evaluation results, in M.F. Drummond and A.J. McGuire (eds) *Economic Evaluation of Health Care: Merging Theory with Practice*. Oxford: Oxford University Press.

Drummond, M., Jonsson, B. and Rutten, F. (1997) The role of economic evaluation in the pricing and reimbursement of medicines, *Health Policy*, 40: 199–211.

Garber, A. (2000) Advances in CE analysis, in A.J. Culyer and J.P. Newhouse (eds) *Handbook of Health Economics*. Amsterdam: North-Holland.

Heyse, J., Cook, J. and Carrides, G. (2001) Statistical considerations in analysing health care resources, in M.F. Drummond and A.J. McGuire (eds) *Economic Evaluation in Health Care: Merging Theory with Practice*. Oxford: Oxford University Press.

Hjelmgren, J., Berggren, F. and Anderseeon, F. (2001) Health economic guidelines – similarities, differences and some implications, *Value in Health*, 4: 225–50.

Palmer, S., Sculpher, M., Philips, Z. *et al.* (2002) *A Cost-Effectiveness Model Comparing Alternative Management Strategies for the Use of Glycoprotein IIb/IIIa Antagonists in Non-ST-Elevation Acute Coronary Syndrome*. Technology Assessment Report. London: National Institute for Clinical Excellence (available from http://www.nice.org.uk).

Song, F., Altman, D.G., Glenny A.-M. and Deeks, J. (2003) Validity of indirect comparison for estimating efficacy of competing interventions: empirical evidence from published meta-analyses, *British Medical Journal*, 326: 472.

UK Pharmaceutical Industry Competitiveness Task Force (2002) *Competitiveness and Performance Indicators*. London: Department of Health and the Association of British Pharmaceutical Industry.

Vernon, J. (2001) The economics of pharmaceutical research and development: investment models, capital market imperfections and policy considerations. Unpublished PhD thesis, City University, London.

chapter eight

Good prescribing practice

Steve Chapman, Pierre Durieux and
Tom Walley

Introduction

The aim of this chapter is to examine and evaluate some aspects of prescribing practice. The key questions we address are: What is good prescribing and how can we define and measure it? How can we measure how much prescribing is necessary and in what areas? And, where prescribing is deficient in quality or quantity, then how can current prescribing be improved?

What is good prescribing?

The term 'good prescribing' is widely used by health care policy makers, politicians and practitioners alike, yet a clear definition is elusive. There are a range of stakeholders in prescribing and each might define good prescribing differently. Governments, or third-party payers with a responsible view, might define it as the lowest cost prescribing that meets public health needs. They may be keen to monitor prescribing and may measure good prescribing according to the available data. Since their data often relate to drug costs, their definitions of good prescribing emphasize this. The pharmaceutical industry might describe good prescribing as prescribing of the latest (and by implication the most effective) drug, to all patients who meet the diagnostic criteria. Evidence-based practitioners might define it as the use of therapies proven to be most effective in randomized controlled trials (RCTs), or perhaps in accordance with an evidence-based guideline.

Although each of these definitions has some validity, they can at best tell only part of the story. They are based on a biomedical model of prescribing: disease ⇒ diagnosis ⇒ treatment. In reality, the general practitioner (GP), who is the most common prescriber, is faced with uncertainty: about diagnosis, since he is often seeing early disease with limited access to diagnostic facilities; about the best treatment for this particular patient, who would probably never have fitted the criteria for a trial anyway, for instance because of co-morbidities; and evidence of what the best treatment might be but which is often less clear than some would have us believe. A decision to prescribe a drug without a clear diagnosis may be a means of reducing the uncertainty inherent in general practice (Weiss 1997). So the GP often has to work with a 'best formulation' of the patient's problem rather than a firm diagnosis in the RCT style, and GPs might therefore define good prescribing differently. Parish (1973) defined good prescribing as 'appropriate (for the condition), safe, effective and economic', in that order. Bradley (1991) noted a lack of empirical evidence on how best to judge quality in prescribing, but favoured a definition that balanced the evidence of the most effective way to treat conditions with the associated costs. Marinker and Reilly (1994) went further in stressing the pivotal role of doctors as the arbiters of good prescribing by defining it as whatever doctors could justify to their peers. They further describe GPs as satisfiers, rather than optimizers – that is, their response has to be 'good enough' to meet the formulation of a patient's problem rather than be perfect enough to meet a clear diagnosis.

Barber (1995) criticizes the definitions of both Bradley and Parish, as they only consider appropriateness from the perspective of the prescriber. This took no account of the view of the patient. He illustrates this with an example from his own experience as a pharmacist: a dying man came into hospital during the last few days of his life having been on a particular brand of sleeping tablet that had been blacklisted by the UK National Health Service, and would not normally have been supplied within the hospital. The evidence for the equal or better efficacy of the alternative that was available in the hospital was sound, and as Barber states, would easily meet Parish's definition of being appropriate, safe, effective and economic. However, it took no account of the needs of the patient or the particular circumstances.

Barber (1995) suggests that rather than define what good prescribing is, we should define what the prescriber is trying to achieve. He used the model illustrated in Figure 8.1 to demonstrate the dynamic tension between the four key aims: maximizing effectiveness, minimizing risk, minimizing cost and respecting the patient's choice. There are clear parallels to beneficence, non-malfeasance, distributive justice and autonomy, the cornerstones of medical ethics (see Chapter 21). Good prescribing, then, is a balance between these.

This model is very close to Marinker and Reilly's vision of quality in prescribing, but it has flaws. For instance, for an external assessor to judge the appropriateness of the prescribing would be almost impossible without extensive detailed knowledge of the case. Another potential flaw is that not only is patient preference difficult to assess (Protheroe et al. 2000), but it may change according to the financial contribution patients have to make to their own health care. If the patient has to pay extra – as, for example, in a reference pricing system – they may choose to endure a 'minor' side-effect in return for a lower acquisition cost. Involving the patient in this way may be a luxury that neither the patient nor the health service can afford in health systems in transitional countries, or those with a low gross domestic product, which do not generate sufficient income from taxation to generate a fully state-funded system for medicines. But a failure to consider the patient's perspective may be a cause

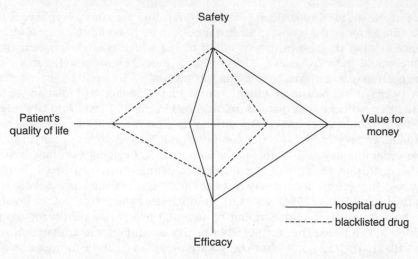

Figure 8.1 Barber's prescribing model (reproduced with permission from Barber 1995).

of poor patient adherence to prescribed medicines; this is discussed further in Chapter 9.

Finally, good prescribing from everyone's perspective should perhaps be measured by its outcomes – that is, does the patient get better? However, our data sources – usually administrative in origin – record the process of prescribing rather than its outcomes. Good prescribing is therefore sometimes defined as the lack of irrational prescribing – irrational in its choice of drug, or polypharmacy, or the co-prescribing of interacting drugs. This is an unsatisfactory compromise forced on us by the availability of data, which is discussed in more detail below.

Prescribing needs assessment

Understanding the clinical needs of an individual in order to inform Barber's model of good prescribing is a matter of good interview skills, taking a comprehensive clinical history, then applying one's knowledge, supported by an evidence base. Trying to assess the need for prescribing in a population is another matter entirely. There are many possible definitions of 'need' that could be based on evidence-based medicine, epidemiology, the quality of the service and by affordability within the service. Where 'need' shades onto 'demand' is discussed in Chapter 17.

From a governmental perspective, the most useful way of assessing the public health need for drugs may be to estimate the level of morbidity that can be treated by medicines. Assessing morbidity is not easy. The World Health Organization has performed a large exercise to assess burden of illness in terms of numbers of disability-adjusted life years (DALY) (Murray and Lopez 1996), but this is of less relevance to most developed countries. The problem is that there is no single comprehensive and universally valid measure that takes into account all the diverse aspects of health. In many countries, the absence of a sufficiently detailed database on morbidity leads to the use of surrogate measures such as standardized mortality rates, which at least allows some measure of the importance of different diseases. The problems of mortality data are well known. Some GP computer systems, such as the General Practice Research Database in the UK (used also for drug safety monitoring), or Mediplus in the UK and Germany (used for market assessment by the pharmaceutical industry), might be used to evaluate levels of diagnosis of different conditions in some GP practices, and by extrapolation of the whole country. These data are dependent on the recorded diagnosis and are vulnerable to cultural influences.

Other possible data sources are hospital data on morbidity, but these do not identify the bulk of chronic illness managed in the community or never diagnosed at all. Specific cohort studies for disease prevalence can be useful but differing definitions undermine their value. For instance, the prevalence of insomnia ranges across Europe from 4 to 38 per cent depending on the study and the definitions it used. Even when standard definitions are used, cultural factors still result in variation in the apparent prevalence of insomnia from 4 per cent in Germany to 22 per cent in the UK (Chevalier *et al.* 1999).

A simpler alternative is to use prescribing data as a proxy. In countries such as the UK, France, Italy, Germany and Spain, the government has access to nationwide prescribing data (Cosentino *et al.* 2000). This may seem like a tautology, to evaluate need for prescribing by measuring prescribing, but in fact it can produce useful results. For instance, the prevalence of angina can be gauged by measuring the use of glyceryl trinitrate (Clarke *et al.* 1994) and this can be extrapolated to identifying the appropriate extent of statin use in secondary prevention. The advantage of these data is that they are comprehensive; the disadvantage is they provide no information about the diagnosis for which prescriptions were used (Chapman 2001). They are therefore often too insensitive to determine disease prevalence.

Prescribing quality

Quality in prescribing at a population level is the sum of quality of the individual prescriptions. Buetow *et al.* (1997) define appropriateness as the outcome of a process of decision-making that maximizes net individual health gains, within society's available resources. This balance is along the lines proposed by Barber, but again may be difficult to judge in any given case. Buetow advocates combining explicit criteria, as in the Medical Appropriateness Index (MAI), with independent review in cases of uncertainty and disagreement. The MAI is the most widely used instrument to estimate appropriateness at the level of the individual prescription and patient. Although it has been found to be reliable and valid in a number of settings, it is yet to be validated in general practice (Samsa *et al.* 1994) and is not useful for health care planning or monitoring in populations. The MAI assesses each prescription on 10 dimensions: (1) indication, (2) effectiveness, (3) dosage, (4) directions, (5) drug interactions, (6) drug–disease interactions, (7) expense, (8) practicality, (9) duplication and (10) duration.

At a population level, health care providers and payers are keen to have a benchmark of some kind to be able to assess quality, however defined. There has, therefore, been a growth in performance indicators in prescribing and elsewhere. As performance indicators of quality should generally relate to the aspects of care that are controlled by the health care provider being measured (i.e. the prescriber; Giuffrida *et al.* 1999), the most accurate measurement of performance comes from MAI-type assessment, including the diagnosis, full clinical history and treatment of individual patients. This is excessively data-intensive and expensive for routine use, and therefore not an option for third-party payers. Alternative proxy measures are therefore needed (Veninga 1990), such as evidence of wide variances in practice (Melnychuk *et al.* 1993; Delesie and Croes 2002), the occurrence of polypharmacy, or the use of medicines 'of limited clinical value' (Audit Commission 1994).

For example, in the UK, very high-quality data on what drugs are prescribed, by which practice and at what cost are available to both prescribers and health authorities (Prescribing Analysis and CosT, or PACT, data) (Chapman 2001). Care must be taken with interpretation, as there are no data on the underlying morbidity or burden of disease. A survey of the measures used to judge 'good prescribing' by prescribing advisers in the UK (see Chapter 10) demonstrated that over half were cost-driven (e.g. generic prescribing rate, or potential generic savings as a percentage of total drug expenditure). Others were weak 'quality' indicators (e.g. number of prescriptions for antibiotics per head, volume of use of benzodiazepines per head – a smaller number being 'good prescribing') (Campbell *et al.* 2000). These markers lacked any clear scientific basis, although the principles behind some of them (e.g. discouraging use of benzodiazepines) seem sound. The benchmarks for such performance indicators (i.e. what constitutes good or bad prescribing) are sometimes an arbitrary target or sometimes a comparison with other GPs in a given locality. These performance markers, although unsatisfactory, can turn into targets and may be used to define who receives incentive payments (see Chapter 10).

A key issue with these measures is what they are for: information and education or performance management, which most doctors would find threatening. It may be better to use these figures to highlight a possible problem, and then to seek to understand it with further investigation (Pryce *et al.* 1996). In practice, creating simple prescribing indicators from prescribing cost and volume data alone has very low validity with prescribers and those who advise them (Campbell *et al.* 2000). Similar disadvantages to using indicators based just on individualized prescribing data were reported by researchers in the Netherlands (Veninga *et al.* 2001). They found that using rankings of performance based on such analyses is only likely to alienate prescribers and make them more obdurate to change. Linking prescribing to diagnosis would be better; such techniques applied in France showed ineffective drugs were prescribed in 32–88 per cent of orders according to the target disease (Coste and Venot 1999). So the ideal markers of good prescribing would tell us about both diagnosis and outcomes (McGavock 2001), but our data systems cannot achieve this at present.

Influencing prescribers

Prescribers are subject to many influences: patient pressure, financial incentives and government directives are discussed elsewhere in this book. Here we will consider how a government or third-party payer can persuade prescribers to change their practice and improve prescribing. A bureaucrat might ask why doctors have to be persuaded, rather than just told what to do: the answer lies in the strength of professional autonomy, which allows the doctor to consider the patient ahead of the payer. A corollary of this is that any attempt to change behaviour by persuasion must focus on creating a gain for the patient, as well as the doctor and of course the payer. A problem in evaluating the effectiveness of these interventions (see Chapter 5) is that they are rarely applied singly and, if they are, the situation may be so artificial as to have little meaning in reality. In general, persuading prescribers to change their habits can be laborious (Lohr *et al.* 1998) and expensive. By comparison, the pharmaceutical industry in the UK is usually quoted to spend at least £10,000 (€14,000) on each general practitioner per year on promoting their products, and given the constraints of the Pharmaceutical Price Regulation Scheme (PPRS) described in Chapter 6, this is probably one of the lowest in Europe. Government agencies, on the other hand, spend far less time and resources on these efforts.

In any prescribing, the doctor is faced with two decisions: first, whether or not to prescribe a drug at all and second, the selection of drugs. The first is far more difficult to change than the second. The doctor's knowledge of a condition and its preferred treatment does not necessarily predict appropriate treatment (e.g. antibiotic prescribing for non-bacterial upper respiratory tract infections is common). The issuing of a prescription reinforces the professional and expert role of the doctor, and provides both the patient and doctor with the perception of an unambiguous diagnosis and a course of treatment to validate the patient's illness (Comaroff 1976). This is often the case in antibiotic prescribing. In one Scandinavian study (Cars and Hakansson 1995), the prescription of antibiotics varied between general practitioners in the same practice, from 76 per cent of patients for the most generous doctor to 21 per cent by the most restrictive doctor. Although during the study period (four years) there were continuous discussions within the practice regarding principles of antibiotic prescribing, the doctors were found to be extremely reluctant to change their prescribing habits. The authors concluded that doctors have an individual and very constant pattern of prescribing antibiotics. This indicates that not only are doctors' beliefs about prescribing stable and consistent over time (Taylor and Bond 1991), but so may their behaviour be too. Strategies to implement guidelines and change prescribing choice for the long term will need to tackle these beliefs and habits.

Formularies

Formularies are restricted lists of medicines, to which prescribers are encouraged or required to adhere. This helps consistency of prescribing, ensures that doctors are familiar with a range of medicines, and may be a useful cost-containment measure by encouraging generic prescribing and restricting the use of more expensive medicines (Pearce and Begg 1992). In practice, almost all doctors work to a formulary, whether it is written down or not (i.e. a list of favoured medicines, perhaps developed as a matter of habit without clear rational thought). In the UK, local and practice level formularies are encouraged by government and local primary care organizations, but these never try to impose a restricted formulary, except where this is agreed by the local consensus of doctors.

There is some limited evidence that formularies improve the quality of prescribing and constrain costs (Beardon 1987; Avery *et al.* 1997), at least in the short term. A danger of formularies is that they may allow the definition of good prescribing to be based simply on adherence to its recommendations. Marinker and Reilly (1994) reject this on the grounds that prescribing can only be good or bad in the light of the management of the condition that prompts it, and not solely on the choice of drug.

Guidelines

Guidelines address some of these issues by considering the overall management of a condition. They also allow the application of the best evidence to a clinical situation. In a landmark paper, Grimshaw and Russell (1993) undertook a systematic review of rigorous evaluations of the effect of clinical guidelines on medical practice and found that in all but four of 59 studies, significant improvements in care outcomes were detected. The size of the effect was very variable; the most effective strategies involved *local* rather than national guideline development and dissemination, and near-patient reminders to apply the guideline. The least effective methods were national guideline development combined with unrequested mailshots (Grimshaw and Russell 1993).

Despite goodwill towards guidelines among practitioners, there is a growing consistent story of difficulty in their implementation. Grol *et al.* (1998) indicate that the following attributes are necessary for acceptance and effective guideline implementation. They must:

- be compatible with doctors' existing values;
- not be too controversial;
- not demand too much change to existing routines;
- be defined precisely with specific advice on actions and decisions in different cases;
- be supported by an explicit description of the scientific evidence; and
- be straightforward and consistent.

In addition, Langley *et al.* (1998) suggested that guidelines were more acceptable and used by GPs if they were:

- brief, clear and simple;
- locally relevant;
- produced by people who are known and trusted;
- include GP input; and
- had a 'common ownership'.

A further factor that reduces the likelihood of uptake of guidelines is that of 'guideline fatigue' – a sense of demoralization when faced with mounting evidence of the inadequacies of one's practice and a mountain of paper to help one improve it (if only one could find the right guideline when one needed it).

Within the UK, the responsibility for centrally generated guidelines has been adopted by the National Institute for Clinical Excellence (NICE). The openness and transparency of the process should help generate credibility, but there remain problems of dissemination and implementation – for guidelines to be successful, they have to be either mandatory and closely monitored, or prescribers have to be persuaded and educated to comply with them. The former can generate cynicism and suspicion such as with health maintenance organizations in the USA, while the latter is resource-intensive. Other professional bodies also produce guidelines as well as sources sponsored by pharmaceutical companies; little wonder, then, that fatigue can set in with so many different voices. Issues regarding mandatory guidelines in France are discussed in Chapter 10.

Computerized decision support systems

Combining these problems with the difficulties and expense of keeping such guidelines up to date and disseminating them and promoting their use, a solution might be to make such guidelines available in GP computer systems. Computer-based clinical decision support systems (CDSS) are defined as 'any software designed to directly aid in clinical decision making in which characteristics of individual patients are matched to a computerized knowledge base for the purpose of generating patient-specific assessments or recommendations that are then presented to clinicians for consideration'. Simple systems covering one or two areas work well (Durieux *et al.* 2000), but real value would lie in the development of a more comprehensive system for primary care. The development of such a system (PRODIGY: www.prodigy.nhs.uk; Purves 1996) funded by the UK government seemed particularly appropriate given the already high levels of GP computerization funded by the state (over 90 per cent of GPs use computerized records in varying ways). PRODIGY provides a comprehensive series of guidelines, triggered by the entry of a diagnosis. These are evidence-based where possible, otherwise consensus-driven, and are now available on almost all GP computer systems. It includes a choice of prescriptions where appropriate, but the GP can change these at will.

It is less clear how valuable this system is. It is not widely used, as many doctors and patients find the use of a computer during the consultation to be intrusive. A recent UK trial of a system related to PRODIGY found no significant effect on consultation rates, process of care measures (including prescribing) or reported patient outcomes (Eccles *et al.* 2002). By contrast, researchers in the Netherlands have found the decision support tool to be effective, but in these studies the GPs had financial incentives to use it. If a CDSS is removed, physicians revert to their previous practice, so for a sustained effect the CDSS should be maintained (Durieux *et al.* 2000).

Feedback and education

A theme of those who wish to improve prescribing has been that if only doctors were convinced of the right thing to do, then they would immediately implement it. This is simplistic and ignores all the baggage that comes with a consultation and the difficulties of actually changing practice. Informing the doctor is not, therefore, just a matter of education, by written material or other format.

One traditional method is to provide postgraduate education for prescribers through postgraduate medical centres or universities. These, however, only attract those who are motivated and so, unsurprisingly, generally produce no change and can even have negative effects (Oxman *et al.* 1995; Grimshaw *et al.* 2001). However, more interactive sessions can be effective at bringing about at least temporary change. Mailings of information are also ineffective. The pharmaceutical industry equivalents of these are advertising and mailshots: the comment usually is that industry has no proof that advertising works but feel obliged to carry on just in case it does! Although none of these alone seems to alter what doctors do, they have been shown to change levels of knowledge and so prepare the ground for more focused means of changing practice.

One problem faced by prescribers who wish to modify their prescribing is actually knowing what they have prescribed. Feeding back prescribing data in a constructive way to prescribers, alongside the evidence for the required change, should help to change attitudes if managed appropriately. Again experience has shown that after an initial change, fatigue sets in and doctors need to be motivated to keep examining their prescribing in this way.

Academic detailing or educational outreach visits

Direct visits from pharmaceutical company detailers or 'academic' detailers employed by government agency seem to be far more effective. They have several roles: they allow exchange of information, but also a degree of negotiation and persuasion so as to win the prescriber around to the detailer's point of view. Pharmaceutical detailers usually offer small gifts, the influence of which is thought to be out of all proportion to their value (Dana and Loewenstein 2003). Company detailers are extensively trained for this task; in general, academic detailers have had far less training but may carry more personal credibility when they visit prescribers.

The seminal study on academic detailing was undertaken by Avorn and Soumerai (1983). In this study, pharmacists were trained in communication and influencing skills as well as clinical knowledge, and then made visits to physicians using specially designed support materials to reinforce the key points. This approach was adapted in the UK as the IMPACT model (Chapman 1998) and EBOR (Freemantle *et al.* 2002); the latter was a rigorous study, in which a definite but limited effect was seen. A similar programme in the Netherlands showed that messages about acute situations that were clear and easy for GPs to implement were most successful (Veninga 1990). This approach has also been followed in German studies and seems to have produced the most change among those doctors who previously had prescribed with minimum quality and cost-consciousness (though this may have been regression to the mean).

The effects of pharmaceutical industry detailing are never published but, for instance, companies can use returns from local pharmacies to wholesalers to pay their detailers productivity bonuses, suggesting that in their view at least, the benefits of detailing can be measured. These detailing visits, however, do not occur in a vacuum but against a background of a carefully built-up relationship between doctor and detailer over many years with a history of reciprocal favours. In contrast, the academic detailer will be in a position to audit the response of the GP to the suggestions made, and can invoke local peer opinion to help change the practice of the recalcitrant GP. However, the academic detailers need to be careful in the messages they deliver: they must be credible, well communicated and brief, and repeated, as the effects of a single detailing visit are usually limited. These visits can be especially effective when tied into incentives of some kind (see Chapter 10), but then the effects of each are difficult to distinguish.

The key lessons to take away from this review of how practice may be changed are that single interventions have demonstrated limited effectiveness; a more sophisticated multifaceted approach is required, which can be adapted to the needs of the individual practitioner or the situation. Administrative interventions such as financial incentives or those that involve other changes must be supportive of these. Finally, any such interventions must be sustained, so as the effects of any intervention are usually short term. If sustained for a prolonged period, they become habit and more engrained and then acquire the status of established practice and themselves become difficult to alter.

New drugs

New drugs pose a particular challenge to good prescribing practice. Producing new and more effective drugs is difficult and expensive, but essential for treating existing disease in a more effective way. But the reality is that most new drugs are not innovative: many are often copies of existing drugs, produced to capture a share of a very lucrative market, such as hypertension. Thus in Europe we have 11 ACE inhibitors and 10 dihydropyridine calcium channel blockers, none of which is of proven superiority to any other.

New drugs are a major driver of the rise in prescribing costs (see Chapter 1), and usually they are displacing existing therapies, rather than extending therapeutics into new areas. New drugs are supported with intensive marketing. Within countries, companies will be aware of which doctors are the 'early adapters' to be targeted for promotional activities, and which the 'laggards' to be ignored.

For the prescriber, the marketing obscures any difference between the 'me too' drugs and the useful advances. The rate of uptake of new drugs across Europe differs: in the past, the highest users of new drugs were the Germans and the lowest users were the British (Griffin 1995). The British way of prescribing has been attributed to spending constraints or to quality of undergraduate education in prescribing, and has been both praised and criticized. Interestingly, the one-year snapshot of causes of the rising drug bill in Chapter 1 (Table 1.2) suggests that the UK now spends proportionately more on new drugs than most other countries, so this innate therapeutic conservatism may have been eroded over the years. Over the period 1992–2000, most (over 85 per cent) of this increase in cost was not due to new drugs treating patients where previously there was no treatment, but displacing older, less expensive drugs with more expensive, newer drugs, in areas where treatment was already established (Department of Health and ABPI 2002).

Concerns about new drugs include: their uncertain safety profile, with several well-publicized withdrawals of drugs recently come to market (e.g. mibefradil, cerivastatin); lack of firm evidence of their superiority over existing drugs (see Chapter 4), especially in long-term use (some of the benefits of a new therapy may not be obvious when first launched and its proper place in therapeutics may only become apparent with time); their usually high cost compared with existing therapy and possibly poor value by comparison; and constraints on their use as a result of non-reimbursement. There are therefore clinical and financial uncertainties.

National bodies such as the UK's NICE will increasingly provide economic and clinical evaluations of these drugs. Some countries control this by refusing reimbursement to new therapies until some of these issues have been resolved. The UK has adopted a novel risk-sharing approach in funding the use of beta-interferon for multiple sclerosis, defining expected improvements and the costs to be paid on the basis of an economic evaluation, and agreeing reimbursement by the manufacturer if pre-set targets of long-term effectiveness are not met (Mrazek 2002).

The best advice to a prescriber, therefore, is to prescribe new drugs only with caution, and when convinced of their superiority to report all suspected adverse reactions, and neither be the first to embrace the new nor the last to abandon the old!

Conclusions

Good prescribing is a Holy Grail: ever elusive and usually only imperfectly seen or defined. Good prescribing must be considered to start with the patient and prescribing most appropriately for that individual, but must at the same time consider the wider context of the health of the whole population. An ideal way of evaluating quality of prescribing would be to move away from measurements of the process of prescribing, to looking at the outcomes of prescribing; realistically, however, this is some way off. Clearly, as with any goal, if it is to be achieved it has to be defined and so we may identify elements of good prescribing along the way to the holy grail, even if we cannot see the grail itself.

A range of interventions to try to achieve these elements can be applied but individually seem to have little or uncertain effect. Combined and repeated, however, their success is more convincing. Continuing to generate centrally endorsed guidelines will not by itself change practice, and equal emphasis needs to be given to strategies for implementing such guidance. Academic detailing has had some success with this. Computer-based clinical decision support systems may also be useful, but need more thought on their implementation. Time spent in helping doctors to manage new drugs may be well rewarded, and is certainly more acceptable than blanket proscription of their use.

References

Audit Commission (1994) *A Prescription for Improvement: Towards More Rational Prescribing in General Practice*. London: HMSO.

Avery, A.J., Walker, B., Heron, T. and Teasdale, S.J. (1997) Do prescribing formularies help GPs prescribe from a narrower range of drugs? A controlled trial of the introduction of prescribing formularies for NSAIDs, *British Journal of General Practice*, 47: 810–14.

Avorn, J. and Soumerai, S.B. (1983) Improving drug-therapy decisions through educational outreach: a randomized controlled trial of academically based 'detailing', *New England Journal of Medicine*, 308: 1457–63.

Barber, N. (1995) What constitutes good prescribing?, *British Medical Journal*, 310: 923–5.

Beardon, P.H.G. (1987) Introducing a drug formulary to general practice: effects on practice prescribing costs, *Journal of the Royal College of General Practitioners*, 37: 305–7.

Bradley, C. (1991) Decision making and prescribing patterns – a literature review, *Family Practice*, 8: 276–96.

Buetow, S.A., Sibbald, B., Cantrill, J.A. and Halliwell, S. (1997) Appropriateness in health care: application to prescribing, *Social Science and Medicine*, 45: 261–71.

Campbell, S.M., Cantrill, J.A. and Roberts, D. (2000) Prescribing indicators for UK general practice: Delphi consultation study, *British Medical Journal*, 321: 425–8.

Cars, H. and Hakansson, A. (1995) To prescribe – or not to prescribe – antibiotics: district physicians' habits vary greatly, and are difficult to change, *Scandinavian Journal of Primary Health Care*, 13: 3–7.

Chapman, S. (1998) Educational outreach in medicines management, in R. Panton and S. Chapman (eds) *Medicines Management*. London: BMJ Books.

Chapman, S. (2001) Prescribing information systems: making sense of primary care data, *Journal of Clinical Pharmacy and Therapeutics*, 26: 235–9.

Chevalier, H., Los, F., Boichut, D. *et al.* (1999) Evaluation of severe insomnia in the general population: results of a European multinational survey, *Journal of Psychopharmacology*, 13: S21–S24.

Clarke, K., Gray, D. and Hampton, J. (1994) Defined daily doses: insensitive in determining disease prevalence, *Pharmaceutical Journal*, 252: 334–5.

Comaroff, J. (1976) A bitter pill to swallow: placebo therapy in general practice, *Sociological Review*, 24: 79–96.

Cosentino, M., Leoni, O., Banfi, F., Lecchini, S. and Frigo, G. (2000) An approach for the estimation of drug prescribing using the defined daily dose methodology and drug dispensation data: theoretical considerations and practical applications, *European Journal of Clinical Pharmacology*, 56: 513–17.

Coste, J. and Venot, A. (1999) An epidemiologic approach to drug prescribing quality assessment: a study in primary care practice in France, *Medical Care*, 37: 1294–307.

Dana, J. and Loewenstein, G. (2003) A social science perspective on gifts to physicians from industry, *Journal of the American Medical Association*, 290: 252–5.

Delesie, L. and Croes, L. (2002) Monitoring the variability in drug prescribing patterns: benchmarking and feedback in Belgium, *European Journal of Clinical Pharmacology*, 58: 215–21.

Department of Health and ABPI (2002) *PPRS: The Study into the Extent of Competition in the Supply of Branded Medicines to the NHS*. London: Department of Health.

Durieux, P., Nizard, R., Ravaud, P., Mounier, N. and Lepage, E. (2000) A clinical decision support system for prevention of venous thromboembolism: effect on physician behavior, *Journal of the American Medical Association*, 283: 2816–21.

Eccles, M., McColl, E., Steen, N. *et al.* (2002) Effect of computerised evidence based guidelines on management of asthma and angina in adults in primary care: cluster randomised controlled trial, *British Medical Journal*, 325: 941.

Freemantle, N., Nazareth, I., Eccles, M. *et al.* (2002) A randomised controlled trial of the effect of educational outreach by community pharmacists on prescribing in UK general practice, *British Journal of General Practice*, 52: 290–5.

Giuffrida, A., Gravelle, H. and Rowland, M. (1999) Measuring quality of care with routine data: avoiding confusion between performance indicators and health outcomes, *British Medical Journal*, 319: 94–8.

Griffin, J.P. (1995) Therapeutic conservatism: more costly in the long term? A UK perspective, *Pharmacoeconomics*, 7(5): 378–87.

Grimshaw, J.M. and Russell, I.T. (1993) Effect of clinical guidelines on medical practice: a systematic review of rigorous evaluations, *Lancet*, 342: 1317–22.

Grimshaw, J., Shirran, L., Thomas, R. *et al.* (2001) Changing provider behavior: an overview of systematic reviews of interventions, *Medical Care*, 39: II2–II45.

Grol, R., Dalhuijsen, J., Thomas, S. *et al.* (1998) Attributes of clinical guidelines that influence use of guidelines in general practice: observational study, *British Medical Journal*, 317: 858–61.

Langley, C., Faulkner, A., Watkins, C., Gray, S. and Harvey, I. (1998) Use of guidelines in primary care: practitioners' perspectives, *Family Practice*, 15: 105–11.

Lohr, K.N., Eleazer, K. and Mauskopf, J. (1998) Health policy issues and applications for evidence-based medicine and clinical practice guidelines, *Health Policy*, 46: 1–19.

Marinker, M. and Reilly, P. (1994) Rational prescribing: how can it be judged?, in *Controversies in Health Care Policies: Challenges to Practice*. London: BMJ Books.

McGavock, H. (2001) Prescription pricing databases should include more details to assess prescribing rationality, *British Medical Journal*, 322: 173–4.

Melnychuk, D., Moride, Y. and Abenhaim, L. (1993) Monitoring of drug utilization in public health surveillance activities: a conceptual framework, *Canadian Journal of Public Health*, 84: 45–9.

Mrazek, M. (2002) Risk sharing scheme for the provision of MS drugs, *Hospital Pharmacy Europe*, Autumn, pp. 40–4.

Murray, C.J.L. and Lopez, A.D. (eds) (1996) *The Global Burden of Diseases: A Comprehensive Assessment of Mortality and Disability from Diseases, Injuries and Risk Factors in 1990 and Projected to 2000*. Cambridge, MA: Harvard University Press.

Oxman, A., Thomson, M., Davis, D. and Haynes, R. (1995) No magic bullets: a systematic review of 102 trials of interventions to improve professional practice, *Canadian Medical Association Journal*, 153: 1423–31.

Parish, P. (1973) Drug prescribing – the concern of all, *Journal of the Royal Society of Health*, 4: 213–17.

Pearce, M.J. and Begg, E. (1992) A review of limited lists and formularies: are they cost-effective?, *Pharmacoeconomics*, 1: 191–202.

Protheroe, J., Fahey, T., Montgomery, A.A., Peters, T.J. and Smeeth, L. (2000) The impact of patients' preferences on the treatment of atrial fibrillation: observational study of patient based decision analysis. Commentary: patients, preferences, and evidence, *British Medical Journal*, 320: 1380–4.

Pryce, A.J., Heatlie, H.F. and Chapman, S.R. (1996) Buccaling under the pressure: influence of secondary care establishments on the prescribing of glyceryl trinitrate buccal tablets in primary care, *British Medical Journal*, 313: 1621–4.

Purves, I. (1996) Prodigy, a computer assisted prescribing scheme: interim data show that it is worth taking the scheme further, *British Medical Journal*, 313: 1549.

Samsa, G.P., Hanlon, J.T., Schmader, K.E. *et al.* (1994) A summated score for the medication appropriateness index: development and assessment of clinimetric properties including content validity, *Journal of Clinical Epidemiology*, 47: 891–6.

Taylor, R.J. and Bond, C.M. (1991) Change in the established prescribing habits of general practitioners: an analysis of initial prescriptions in general practice, *British Journal of General Practice*, 41: 244–8.

Veninga, C. (1990) *Improving Prescribing in General Practice*. Groningen: University of Groningen.

Veninga, C.C.M., Denig, P., Pont, L.G. and Haaijer-Ruskamp, F.M. (2001) Comparisons of indicators assessing the quality of drug prescribing for asthma, *Health Services Research*, 36: 143–61.

Weiss, M. (1997) Whose rationality? A qualitative analysis of general practitioners prescribing, *Pharmaceutical Journal*, 259: 339–41.

chapter nine

Patients and their medicines

Colin Bradley, Ebba Holme Hansen and Sjoerd Kooiker

Introduction

Regulation of the supply and distribution of medicines is one of a range of factors acting on patients and influencing their consumption of medicines. The consumption of medicines is strongly influenced by cultural factors that affect patients and health care professionals alike. These cultural factors are themselves mediated and developed through the interactions between patients or medicine users and health care professionals, particularly doctors. The traditional information and power imbalance between patients and doctors is beginning to shift, with patients gaining greater access to information about diseases and medicines and indeed to the medicines themselves. The extent of these shifts is still limited and variable but future pharmaceuticals policy needs to be framed in a manner that anticipates and, where appropriate, encourages these trends.

Culture and prescribing

The consumption of pharmaceuticals varies widely across geographic boundaries. Variations are found at the sales level (Cars *et al.* 2001), the prescriber level (Mölstad *et al.* 2002) and the population level (Hansen *et al.* 2003). In spite of attempts to harmonize the regulation of pharmaceuticals across the European Union (EU), wide variations in the use of pharmaceuticals persist over time (Holme Hansen *et al.* 2003). A Norwegian analysis of the associations between medicine consumption and health care system characteristics had the expressive conclusion 'wide variations, little explanations', stating that explanations should be found in local traditions and preferences (Haugen *et al.* 1978).

That such variations occur should not surprise us, as many aspects of medicines use are deeply embedded in the culture of the prescriber and the patient.

Responses to symptoms are culturally determined. This has been studied in particular with respect to pain. Bates (1996), for example, found marked differences in pain behaviour between Latinos and Italians on the one hand, who were very expressive about their pain, and Poles, the Irish and Anglo-Americans on the other, who were more restrained. The definition of illness differs from culture to culture and even from country to country within Europe. Payer (1988) observed that in France (vague) symptoms are often attributed to the malfunction of the liver, whereas in Germany (vague) symptoms are often attributed to malfunction of the heart. In the USA and the UK illness is often believed to be caused from external sources (germs), whereas in continental Europe illness is often seen as disturbance of the balance within the body. Helman (1990) has noted that the total drug effect on the individual is determined by:

1 the attributes of the drug itself, like taste, shape, colour and name;
2 the attributes of the patient receiving the drug;
3 the attributes of the person prescribing or dispensing the drug (personality, sense of authority); and
4 the setting in which the drug is administered (the doctor's office, a laboratory).

All of these aspects of drug effect are at least modulated by patient beliefs, which, as already noted, vary from culture to culture.

These differences are easily observed in comparisons of how patients in different countries respond to similar symptoms. In a cross-cultural study on health care utilization, a sub-sample of people in the Belgian, Dutch and German part of the Rhine-Maas area were shown a list of both serious and minor symptoms and asked if they would seek help for these symptoms (Lüschen *et al.* 1995). While the scores for serious symptoms did not differ much, the Dutch had by far the lowest inclination to seek medical treatment for minor symptoms and the Belgians the highest. The Germans were somewhere in between but in the larger sample of the same study were the most likely to worry about their health and also reported more illnesses than respondents from other nations.

In a comparison of antibiotics sales among the 15 member states of the EU in 1999, the Dutch had the lowest sales (8.96 DDD per 1000 inhabitants per day where DDD = defined daily dose), whereas neighbouring Belgium was among the countries with the highest sales (26.72 DDD per 1000 inhabitants per day) (Cars *et al.* 2001). The mechanisms leading to these differences were explored in a qualitative study on the management of upper respiratory symptoms conducted in 1997–1998 in both the Netherlands and in Flanders (Deschepper *et al.* 2002). Belgians worried more about disease and were more used to leaving the consulting room with a medicine. The Belgians rated their upper respiratory tract diseases often as bronchitis and the Dutch mostly as cold or flu and never as bronchitis. Moreover, Belgians more often consulted their doctor when ill (obtaining a sick leave notification from a doctor is obligatory in Belgium but not in the Netherlands) and the episodes of bronchitis almost always led to a prescription of antibiotics. The predominant coping strategy in the Netherlands

Table 9.1 Patients' responses to minor respiratory illnesses in France, Germany, Sweden and the USA,[a] as a percentage of families[b]

Behaviour	Countries (% of families)			
	France	Germany	Sweden	USA
See doctor or nurse	21	37	1	10
See alternative practitioner	2	3	0	1
Take OTC medicine	62	46	56	88
Use home remedies	18	46	15	31
Stay at home	14	27	40	62
Do nothing	27	19	55	34
Don't know	1	1	1	0

[a] The question asked was 'What do you normally do when you have a cold or a fever?'
[b] Totals may exceed 100 per cent as more than one response was allowed.
Source: Procordia and Trygg Hansa SPP (1992), Alsterlind (1993).

was to nurse one's illness, sometimes in combination with over-the-counter (OTC) medicines and home remedies; Dutch patients did not want to trouble their general practitioner (GP) with their symptoms as they were aware of busy GP waiting rooms. However, in Belgium there are three times as many GPs as in the Netherlands (13.7 in Belgium versus 4.9 in the Netherlands per 10,000 inhabitants in 2000).

With regard to how people tend to deal with minor ailments, there are also quite marked variations. Table 9.1 illustrates the findings of another study on how patients in different countries tend to respond to minor respiratory illnesses. The Germans are much more likely to seek formal care, while the Swedes are more likely to 'do nothing' and use OTC medicine only. Using OTC medicine is the predominant response to illness among the Americans and the French, but the French are also somewhat more inclined to seek help from a health care professional.

Cultural factors, it should be noted, do not operate in isolation. They exert their influence in combination with other factors related to economic development, geography and so on, and are, in turn, themselves determined by these factors.

Ethnic minorities and pharmaceuticals

Ethnicity is a complex concept that can be defined by objective criteria (immigrant status, citizenship, nationality, country of birth, parents' country of birth, language, religion) or by subjective criteria (the feeling of or the perception of belonging to a culturally different population group). When we talk about ethnicity, we usually mean culturally distinct minority groups in a given country. Studies often show that ethnic groups' attitudes to medicines and medicine-taking behaviours differ from those of indigenous populations. For example, surveys of the illness behaviour of Turkish immigrants in the Netherlands based on interviews with GPs in Rotterdam with a high number of Turkish immigrants in their practice lists revealed that:

- Turkish immigrants have more health complaints than the Dutch and present their health complaints more expressively. They have less knowledge than the Dutch about the functioning of the body.
- Turkish immigrants are more likely to seek care for common symptoms than the Dutch, a finding in both the patient surveys and interviews with GPs.
- Because Turkish immigrants are more likely to seek a medical solution for their symptoms, they are less likely than the Dutch to apply self-care or adopt a 'wait and see' policy.
- Turkish immigrants are more likely than the Dutch to expect a medical intervention (physical examination, prescription) from their GP, which is, presumably, based on their experiences with Turkish doctors. These expectations are difficult to change once in the Netherlands (Leeflang 1994; Denktas *et al.* 1999).

However, from an international perspective (see above), the Dutch are reluctant users of medicines, so it understandable that Dutch GPs have difficulties with the expectations of their Turkish patients.

A Swedish study, comparing the coping behaviour of immigrant and Swedish female patients with diabetes mellitus, reached similar conclusions. The study reported that most of the female refugees from Arab nations like Iraq 'had a lower threshold for health care seeking, were more reliant on professional care even in the case of insignificant symptoms. In activity level they fell in between the majority of Yugoslavians, who showed a passive self-care attitude, and Swedes, who, in general showed an active self-care behaviour, being more technically oriented and knowledgeable' (Hjelm *et al.* 2003).

In a Danish study, ethnicity was defined by the language spoken in the household (Hansen *et al.* 2003). This study deals with children's and adolescents' medicine use for headache, stomach-ache, difficulties in getting to sleep and nervousness. The authors found that non-Danish-speaking children reported higher prevalence of the four symptoms than Danish children. Boys and girls from both Western and non-Western minorities used medicine for each of the four symptoms more often than Danish children and adolescents.

Mediation of cultural influences through interpersonal interactions

These cultural influences are expressed through decisions made by people to take medicines. Although in the case of home remedies, the decision to take a medicine may be made by the person themselves, many (probably most) decisions about medicines use are influenced by others. In the case of self-treatment with either folk remedies or over-the-counter medicines, the decision will be influenced by other family members and sometimes by health professionals, particularly pharmacists. In the case of prescription medicines, the key influence will usually be the doctor (in most cases a family doctor), although other community-based health professionals, especially nurses and pharmacists, have an increasing role. Central to the decision-making process is the kind of interaction that occurs between the patient and the health professional. These interactions have been studied most intensively in the case of doctor–patient interactions.

Doctor–patient communication

Studies of doctor–patient communication from the 1970s onwards have highlighted the tendency for consultations between doctors and their patients to be controlled almost exclusively by the doctor in a manner that was dubbed 'doctor-centred' (Byrne and Long 1976). The drawbacks of this style of communication were identified even in these early studies and, from the outset, researchers in this area have promoted the use of a more 'patient-centred' style of communication. What constitutes a patient-centred style has in recent times been more clearly articulated by Stewart and colleagues from London, Ontario (Stewart *et al.* 1995). They stress the need for doctors to explore the illness experience of the patient, which means striving to obtain the patient's point of view of what the illness means in terms of what the patient has experienced and not just a list of his or her signs and symptoms. They also stress the need to 'understand the whole person', which is about getting a much deeper level of connection with the patient such that an understanding of who the patient is (what sort of person the patient is, their lifestyle, concerns and so on) is achieved. This involves a level of interpersonal engagement that goes beyond taking the usual social history. This approach also recognizes that the ultimate action plan, including decisions about taking any medicines prescribed, must be implemented by the patient. The patient ultimately calls the shots and, therefore, the doctor and patient need to negotiate a plan of management that is acceptable to both, though especially the patient. This sort of negotiation of a mutually agreed plan is also resonant with the concept of concordance (see next section).

In a review of the impact of 21 high-quality studies of doctor–patient communication, Stewart (1995) found that in 16 studies more patient-centred styles that included one or more components of Stewart and colleagues' (1995) definition of patient-centredness were associated with positive effects on health outcomes, including improved patient adherence to their medication regimen.

Doctor–patient communication, while having broadly similar characteristics everywhere, does vary in certain respects from country to country. Two major studies of communications between GPs and their patients have detected differences in the balance of different styles of communication in ten different European countries (van den Brink-Muinen *et al.* 1999, 2003). By detailed examination of a sample of videotaped consultations and questionnaires to doctors and patients, these authors were able to characterize the prevalent styles of communication in each country and the attitudes of doctors and patients to various issues in doctor communication. While these differences are almost certainly related to cultural differences between countries, the researchers also found that certain differences could be associated with features of the health care system (itself, of course, a product of national culture, among other factors). They found that in countries in which GPs have a major gatekeeping role – that is, where patients have to be referred by a GP to access other secondary care resources – that both doctors and patients tended to display more of certain affective behaviours in their consultations. Thus, there tended to be more paraphrasing of the patient by the doctor and checking of understanding. However, other affective behaviours such as showing empathy and social talk showed no difference. With regard to what the researchers termed 'instrumental behaviour' (i.e. mainly questioning and sharing information), there were even fewer differences between different countries, with GPs in gatekeeping countries perhaps asking fewer questions. The addition of three central European countries to the study (namely Estonia, Romania and Poland) showed similar inter-country differences depending on whether or not GPs had a gatekeeping role. No East/West differences were observed and the payment system for GPs (whether self-employed or employed) did not appear to exert any consistent effect on communication. All inter-country differences were less pronounced than the differences in communication observed between patients based on age and sex, but differences in the particular nature of the patient's problem seemed to exert the largest influence.

Recent work by Britten and colleagues (2000) has examined communication between doctors and patients specifically in relation to medicines and medicine taking. They found that while patients attending GPs often have an expectation to receive a medication, they also have more complex agendas (Barry *et al.* 2000). They often hold quite ambivalent attitudes to medicines and medicine taking with aversion to taking a medicine being quite common, although rarely explored in the consultation. Thus, misunderstandings between doctors and their patients arise quite frequently and these can contribute to the incorrect use of medicine or non-adherence to doctor's advice or to treatment regimens prescribed (Britten *et al.* 2000). The miscommunication identified in this study can also be described in terms of Mischler's concepts of the 'voice of medicine' and the 'voice of the lifeworld' and the variable extent to which these two voices are heard in consultations (Barry *et al.* 2001). The 'voice of medicine' is the name Mischler applies to the use of language that focuses on technical aspects of medicine, scientific rationality and abstract concepts such as disease, while the 'voice of the lifeworld' refers to talk about contextually grounded experiences of events and the challenges of everyday life, including the patient's lived experience of their illness (Mischler 1984).

For patients with complex and chronic health problems, having their 'voice of the lifeworld' either ignored or blocked by their doctor was found to be a possible contribution to non-adherence in medicine taking and to poorer consultation outcomes. It was also noted that the conditions for 'shared decision making', which has been advocated as a way of improving concordance between doctor and patient about treatment, were generally not fulfilled (Stevenson *et al.* 2000).

Many researchers in the field of doctor–patient communication are advocating more involvement of patients in decisions about their health care, particularly treatment decisions. However, there can sometimes be a conflict between the treatment the patient wants or thinks they need and the treatment that is identified on the basis of best evidence as optimal. This has led to the articulation of the concept of 'evidence-based patient choice' (Edwards and Elwyn 2001), which seeks to negotiate treatment plans for patients that incorporate the best treatment for the patient's condition on the basis of an effective review of the best evidence available as well as the patient's wishes, beliefs and values. The implementation of this rather idealistic model requires the doctor to possess highly developed skills in both the acquisition and evaluation of relevant evidence from biomedical literature with effective techniques and skills for eliciting and incorporating the patient's perspective. As sources of high-quality evidence-based treatment recommendations become more readily available and as techniques for presenting treatment choices in ways that are utilizable by patients improve, this ideal may become more achievable; and the costs and benefits of this approach to patient care can then be evaluated.

Patient non-adherence

A crucial influence on medicines consumption is the decision made by the patient after a prescription has been written on whether or not to take the medicine recommended by the doctor. It has long been recognized that patients sometimes do not take their medicines as prescribed and sometimes not at all. This phenomenon, traditionally referred to as 'non-compliance' but much more recently has been termed 'non-adherence' on the grounds that this term is less pejorative of patients who behave in this way, has both clinical and economic consequences. Medicines prescribed and dispensed, but not taken, cost the health system in both pharmaceutical expenditure and in continuing and, possibly worsening, of the conditions for which the medicines were prescribed. Medicines prescribed but not dispensed or discontinued at the patient's discretion may, however, sometimes save health care expenditure, especially if the anticipated clinical consequences of non-adherence do not occur.

The extent of the non-adherence problem is difficult to ascertain precisely because what constitutes adherence is not that straightforward and all the techniques for measuring adherence are limited in some way. Simply classifying patient behaviour as either 'adherent' or 'non-adherent' fails to allow for the extent to which different medicines are 'forgiving' of strict adherence to dosing regimens. Arguably, it is more relevant to base the measurement of adherence on the level required for the desired therapeutic response. Therefore, to expect that medicine users should comply with standard dosage regimens – as expressed by, for example, formularies – is to overlook the difference in needs due to inter-individual variations in the metabolism of medicines. Thousands of studies using, for instance, electronic devices to monitor when medicines have been opened or used have, over three decades, suggested that adherence often follows a Gaussian distribution such that about one-quarter of patients are between 75 and 100 per cent adherent, a half of patients are between 25 and 75 per cent adherent, and one-quarter are less than 25 per cent adherent; however, in other studies, the distribution may be skewed towards non-adherence and/or higher degrees of adherence (Gordis *et al.* 1969; Roth *et al.* 1970). More recent longer-term studies suggest that medicine taking declines the longer the patient is on a medicine, especially for preventive therapies and in patients who have not had symptoms (Monane *et al.* 1994; Benner *et al.* 2002; Jackevicius *et al.* 2002). Overall, it has been concluded that about half of all medicines prescribed are taken sufficiently well for their main therapeutic benefit to be accrued and in about half of all cases, this is not the case; however, this varies, sometimes quite critically, depending on the therapeutic profile of the medicine and the condition being treated (McGavock *et al.* 1998). Non-adherence with therapeutic regimens is especially common when:

- more medicines are used concurrently;
- the illness is without noticeable symptoms or is a psychiatric illness;
- the medication has troublesome side-effects; and
- the illness is chronic (Christensen 1978; Haynes *et al.* 1979; Hingson *et al.* 1981).

Early studies of non-adherence identified the problem as mainly one of a failure of communication on the part of the doctor, or a lack of understanding or incapacity to remember on the part of the patient. Other possible reasons for non-adherence include the occurrence of adverse effects, a patient's failure to appreciate the purported benefits of the medicine, or the patient not placing as high a value on the benefits as the prescriber. The failure to appreciate benefits or to value them as highly as doctors is a particular problem with preventive medicines, where the patient may receive deferred or, indeed, no benefit. However, several studies of medicine taking over the past decades have identified that, in addition to this so-called 'unintentional non-adherence', medicine users frequently regulate their medicine use as a result of a conscious and deliberate choice. Arluke (1980) demonstrated how arthritis patients test and evaluate their medicine use according to their own experience. Since then, studies on epilepsy (Conrad 1985), asthma (Harding and Modell 1985; Larsen and Hansen 1985) and other patient groups (Hansen and Launsø 1988) have confirmed Arluke's findings. Across studies it can be summarized that:

- people use medicines in accordance with their own experience, including their previous medications;
- people experiment with the effects and side-effects of medicines by increasing and decreasing the dose;
- not taking a medicine is another way to test both effects and side- effects; and
- taking some additional medicine, like anti-asthma remedies or analgesics, can be a tool to allow participation in social events.

These factors can arise from: a general mistrust of medicines or pharmaceuticals in particular; a mistrust of the doctor or doctors in general; or a desire to deny the fact of having an illness or the need to take medicines to control it. The strategies and techniques required to deal with these two forms of non-adherence are quite different.

Thus, unintentional non-adherence can be improved by techniques that make it easier to remember to take the medicine, easier to actually take the medicine and which make the benefits of medicine taking clearer. The provision of written, in addition to verbal, instructions about the medication regimen and the use of various prompts and reminders also can assist. It also helps if medication regimens can be kept simple with once or twice daily regimens being much easier to comply with than ones which require more than twice daily dosing. The clarity of instructions, the simplicity of instructions and the repetition of instructions all help to promote adherence, especially where non-adherence is accidental (or unintentional). Generally speaking, the more information the user has about the medicine and the rationale for its use, the more likely he or she is to adhere to the treatment. However, sometimes it is the case that facets of the medication might be inappropriate for the patient. Health professionals should be aware that non-adherence may have both undesirable and desirable effects.

It was mainly through a recognition of the reality of intentional non-adherence that the concept of concordance was devised. This concept, developed and promoted by the Royal Pharmaceutical Society of Great Britain, specifies that medicine taking should be the result of a mutually arrived at agreement between doctor and patient and not, as was traditionally the case, the result of the patient's more or less reluctant compliance with orders issued by their doctor (Royal Pharmaceutical Society of Great Britain 1997).

The informed patient

The advocacy of both patient-centred medicine and concordance are expressions of the newly emerging dominance of patient autonomy as a consideration in medical ethics. Another expression of this ethical principle is the belief that for patients to be fully able to express their autonomy, they need to be able to provide informed consent to treatment and this, in turn, is dependent on the patient having access to adequate, reliable and comprehensible information relevant to their needs. Happily, there are developments afoot that do increase patients' access to appropriate information, although in this information age not all the information available to, or accessed by, patients is of assistance to them in making the best choices regarding their health care.

Recent studies on consumers' expectations and demands have documented a wide discrepancy between older and younger population groups. Young people and families with children, much more than older population groups, not only demand access to medicines from a wide range of retail outlets, but they also want to receive information from many different professional and other sources. For the youngest groups, this includes access to information from the internet. These tendencies reflect a development towards what has been termed 'the new consumer' (Schytte-Hansen 2003).

One indication of the trend towards an expectation that patients be provided with fuller information on their prescription medicines is EU Directive 2001/83 (European Commission 2001), which requires that all pharmaceutical products are packaged with an approved patient information leaflet. The directive stipulates what must be included in the patient information leaflet, although this deals mainly with the possible adverse effects of the medicine and how the medicine is to be taken. Consumer groups have been critical of the content of leaflets, alleging them to be often so detailed as to be confusing; sometimes unnecessarily alarming for patients and written in language and in a size of print that can be difficult to read or understand (Anonymous 2000). Other important developments that increase patients' access to information, albeit of variable quality, include the growth of the media in general and the amount of attention given, in the media, to health and health-related matters; the emergence of the internet; the revival of public health medicine now encompassing a major emphasis on health education and health promotion; the emergence of patient support and advocacy groups; and the increasing involvement of the pharmaceutical industry in conveying information to patients and potential patients by all possible means.

Educating the patient

Providing information to patients is not sufficient of itself to ensure safe and effective use of medicines by patients. Patients require to be educated in a more general sense about medicines and their benefits and limitations, and information needs to be presented at a time and in a way that facilitates the patient's assimilation and understanding. Patients tend to hold quite black-and-white views of medicines as either things to be avoided at all costs or panaceas to be used to sort out all of life's ills. There is a need for a wider understanding of medicines as commodities that are neither intrinsically good nor bad but rather as substances with potential for both good and harm. Usually there is a trade-off between these properties, with the medicines that are most potent in relieving suffering being those with the greatest propensity for harm if used excessively or inappropriately. More recently developed medicines do seem to escape this trade-off to some extent, with medicines that are very powerful sometimes being relatively free of adverse effects in ordinary usage. An example might be proton pump inhibitors for the relief of acid-related diseases of the gastrointestinal tract. However, sometimes there are more subtle trade-offs – with the limitations of medicines use being related more to opportunity costs of resources going to where benefits are small relative to cost, or the continuing of a medicine allowing the continuation of an unhealthy lifestyle, which, if amended, would lead to a more sustained and cost-effective improvement in health.

When it comes to education of patients about the use of specific medicines, there is a need for clarity of information and skill in its delivery. Thus, for example, it has been shown that patients retain information better when it is provided in simple, clear, jargon-free language, when the key message is given early in the consultation, is repeated and is reinforced by written information (Ley 1988). This is facilitated by the use of peer-reviewed patient information leaflets on diseases and their treatment, such as those available in certain GP computer systems (e.g. EMIS and PRODIGY in the UK).

A minimum data set of the type of information patients should be given before commencing treatment has also been proposed (Bradley 1999). It is proposed that this should include:

- the name of the drug or drugs – this should, ideally, be both the brand name and the generic name but one of these as a minimum;
- what the drug is supposed to do;
- how and when they are to be taken;
- how long they are to be taken for;
- common adverse effects and interactions the patient should look out for;
- the extent to which the medicines are thought, by the doctor, to be essential to health.

The role of the media

As well as education directed at individual patients, there is a need for education directed at the general public to make them more aware of issues in medicines use. The evidence suggests that using the public media for health education is effective in raising public awareness of health issues, but is less effective in conveying more complex information or in promoting behavioural change. There is a need for a multifaceted approach, with coordination of public health education across different media and individualized approaches.

As well as being consciously exploited as part of a deliberate public health education endeavour, the media has a very important role in influencing public knowledge, attitudes and behaviour in relation to health issues. The influence of the media can be both positive and negative in terms of information (or sometimes misinformation) conveyed to the public and the influence can occur both deliberately and inadvertently. Health information is conveyed in all sorts of media. Not only is it conveyed in obviously health-related news and features, but it is also conveyed in correspondence sections, dramas (such as soap operas) and so on. In relation to many health issues, including developments in pharmaceuticals, there is a tendency for media coverage to oscillate between hyping new advances as 'breakthroughs' and being scandalized by the revelation of adverse effects or limitations of medical technologies.

The role of the internet and eHealth care

There is, as yet, no agreed definition of eHealth. The term is used to refer to a great variety of methods of health care provision delivered using information technology, particularly the internet (Anonymous 2001). Thus it encompasses the provisions of health information and health advice (both general and specific) over the internet. It is also taken by some to encompass other aspects of the impact of information and communication technology on health care, such as telemedicine, electronic storage and retrieval of patient records and the sale of pharmaceuticals via the internet.

Seeking information on health is said to be the fourth most common use of the World Wide Web. However, a major problem with the internet is its unregulated nature, so that there is a danger of misinformation as much as reliable information being acquired from this source (Consumers International 2002). There are many sites with health-related information that are regulated and quality assured but it can be difficult, particularly for the general public, to distinguish reliable from unreliable sources. Most of the information provided on the internet is of a general or non-specific nature for the information of anyone who seeks it out. However, there are an increasing number of sites, many of them accessible from more general advice sites, that offer more detailed and specific advice in response to a user's specific questions. This advice is usually claimed to be provided by a doctor but it is difficult to know how this can be assured. Thus, there is even more concern about these sites as they are much more likely to influence the behaviour of patients. There is a worry that patients may act in an ill-advised fashion on the basis of information from such a site or may try to use it as a substitute for obtaining medical advice from a face-to-face consultation with a health professional. Another concern is the inherent risks that follow from consumers' direct access to prescription-only medicines that some internet sites provide.

Direct-to-consumer advertising

Traditionally, access to many medicines has been tightly controlled, with a patient usually only able to obtain medicine using a prescription from a doctor. In this environment, advertising of medicines was also tightly regulated and a major feature of such regulation was that prescription-only medicines could only be advertised to doctors. Direct advertising to patients was forbidden. However, in 1997, the US Federal Drugs Administration (FDA) relaxed regulations governing the advertising of prescription medicines directly to the public. This highly controversial move has resulted in a substantial increase in expenditure by pharmaceutical companies on advertising to the public, particularly on television. Although such advertising has been restricted to a relatively narrow range of products, for those products heavily advertised in this way there have been substantial gains in market share. Direct-to-consumer advertising is also allowed in New Zealand, but this has arisen not so much from a relaxation of regulation as through an absence of regulation. This position, too, is under review, with a recent comprehensive review of the issue concluding, on the basis of both local and international experience, that 'the net effect on the public health of direct to consumer advertising of prescription medicines is adverse' (Toop *et al.* 2003).

The purported benefits of direct-to-consumer advertising are that it raises awareness in the general public of the availability of medicines they might not have been aware of and, presuming these medicines are more effective than their current treatment, accessing these medicines should improve their health. Of course, the benefit to the advertisers will be increased sales of their pharmaceutical product. These benefits need not necessarily be in conflict, but there are concerns that direct-to-consumer advertising leads to inappropriate demands for medicine by patients for whom they are not the optimal treatment. There are also more general risks to the quality and content of doctor–patient interaction that might be initiated in response to advertising rather than real medical need and that might be dominated by consideration of the particular advertised product rather than other wider issues related to the patient's more general health. The New Zealand review concluded that the information provided to patients through direct-to-consumer advertising was neither appropriate nor adequately balanced to provide proper guidance to patients, and they have proposed a ban on such advertising as well as the development of an independent medicine and health information service free from commercial interests.

Direct-to-consumer advertising is still prohibited in the EU, although in July 2001 a change in European law was proposed that would allow such advertising in three specific disease areas – AIDS/HIV, diabetes and asthma – for a 5-year period to be followed by a review. On 2 June 2003, EU health ministers rejected a proposal by the European Commission to relax the EU ban on advertising prescription-only medicines to the public. The EU Health Council decision was part of the review of the European legislation on medicines. However, the emergence of this proposal from the Directorate General for Enterprise is an indication of the pressure that is building from industry and the supporters of free trade to have all restrictions on the advertising of pharmaceuticals lifted.

A recent comparison of attitudes towards direct-to-consumer advertising among interested parties in the USA and Denmark found a remarkable difference. In the USA, all groups but some consumer leagues supported the right of companies to have 'free speech' in relation to their products. However, everybody thought that such advertising should be regulated by the FDA. The Danish parties were much more reluctant and in general against such advertising. Although most parties found that the manufacturers had some right to inform the public about their prescription-only medicines, this should be passed by health professionals or patients' organizations, depending on who was asked (Bacher 2003).

The European regulation of advertisements for over-the-counter medicines follows the licensing regulations in the EU and in the respective countries. The licensing of such medicines generally requires that the medicine exerts low toxicity, is not to be injected, has no risk of dependence, is indicated for minor health problems only and that long-term experience exists (Fallsberg and Hansen 1995).

Access to medicines and the changing agency relationship

Medicines, unlike most other goods and services, are typically purchased on the advice or prescription of a doctor rather than being selected by the patient or consumer on the basis of his or her own determination of the costs and merits of competing products. Furthermore, in many health care systems, medicines are paid for in whole or in part by a third-party payer, such as an insurance provider or by the state. This has been likened to a scenario in which a diner goes to a restaurant but another party comes and orders her meal for her and yet another party pays the bill. However, this situation is changing. Patients are increasingly well informed about their medicines (see above) and more often have quite clearly formulated ideas on what medicine or medicines they see as necessary or appropriate for their condition. Regardless of how informed they are, there is also an emerging tendency for patients to be less willing to trust professionals without question. There is also an increasing expectation that health professionals will inform patients about decisions affecting their health (including treatment decisions) and involve them actively in those decisions. Furthermore, pressures to contain health care costs have led to the development of schemes that oblige patients to pay part or all of the cost of their medicine. In many health care systems, there are also efforts to encourage patients to treat their own minor ailments using an ever-widening range of over-the-counter medicines (which, of course, will also be paid for by the patient). Thus, the previously outlined scenario is not as widespread as it once was.

The traditional agency relationship in which the doctor selects the medicine for the patient is changing in other ways too. Pharmacists have long been involved as an intermediary between the doctor who prescribes the medicine and the patient who takes it, but their role was historically as a manufacturer or compounder of the medicine. As modern pharmaceutical technology has rendered this role redundant, their role has evolved (see also Chapter 11). They have developed roles in acting as a safety net for prescribing errors (by the doctor) and as an information source for patients. The concept of 'pharmaceutical care' encompasses the pharmacists' obligations to identify and deal with patients' medicine-related problems (Hepler and Strand 1990). Pharmaceutical care has been officially recognized by the World Health Organization as an element of the role of the pharmacist (WHO 1996). Pharmacists are also beginning to develop more independent professional relationships with patients – that is, independent of doctors. They have become more active in providing advice and treatment on minor ailments without reference to doctors and have also begun to provide preventive care with in-store blood pressure measurement, cholesterol testing and so on. They are also becoming actively involved in the provision of care management packages for patients with specific long-term illnesses such as asthma, ischaemic heart disease and diabetes. They are also developing a more active advisory/drug information role for doctors and other primary care workers, especially in the context of managing drug budgets where these apply. These developments are being actively encouraged and extended in some health care systems, partly as a way of increasing the accessibility and availability of primary care services, but also as part of cost-containment endeavours (as pharmacists' salaries are less than those of doctors).

Although the precise role of pharmacists varies between countries, they have always had, in addition to the role of dispensing medicines prescribed by doctors, the capacity to advise patients on the use of other non-prescription medicines. As the range of drugs available over the counter has expanded, so too has the scope for the pharmacist in respect of recommending and advising on the use of these drugs. The pressure to allow patients greater access to medicines, where safety considerations do not preclude their having unimpeded access, is manifest most clearly in the shift in pharmaceuticals licensing policy promoted by the EU (Directive 2001/86/EC), which clarifies that the default position should be that a medicine for which there in no strong reason as to why it should be prescription-only should be licensed as available over the counter. More detailed discussion of over-the-counter medicines is provided in Chapter 15.

Nurses, too, who traditionally worked almost exclusively under the direction of doctors and had very little role in medicines management, are beginning to become more actively involved in the prescribing process. They have, in reality, often provided patients with information about their medicines and have advised on the management of minor ailments but their roles, until recently, were not 'officially' recognized. These roles are now being recognized and some nurses are being sanctioned to prescribe medicines. These prescribing responsibilities, though, are being restricted to more specialized or qualified nurses who have received additional pharmacology and therapeutics training and to a more limited formulary of medicines than doctors.

The role of patient groups

Another major development that is having an impact on the traditional relationship between doctors and patients is the growth of patient groups. Two types of patient groups can be recognized, although the functions of both can sometimes be subsumed within a single group. Support groups tend to focus mainly on providing information and support for patients with a particular ailment and their carers. Advocacy groups, on the other hand, aim to provide assistance to patients and carers in getting access to appropriate services on an individual or collective basis. Collective activity often includes lobbying for service improvements and/or access to new treatments. Both types of groups tend to raise charitable funds and both may also become involved in funding medical research in the disease area on which they are focused. Recent developments of patient groups with implications for medicines use have been: the growth of links between such groups and the pharmaceutical industry; their lobbying for earlier and insurance or state-funded access to newer medicines; and lobbying for the accelerated approval of new medicines.

Mail order and online pharmacies

Another important development that gives patients easier access to medicines is the development of mail order pharmacies and pharmacies on the internet. These developments are well advanced in the USA, where there is relatively easy access to medicines via the internet and/or by mail order. The current struggle in Europe between those favouring online and mail order pharmacies and those opposed is discussed in Chapter 11. It appears likely that online and mail order pharmacy will develop in Europe and other policies should be framed in the light of this.

Conclusions and recommendations

It is clear that the relationship between patients and their medicines is evolving. Although medicines and their use are moulded by history, culture-common trends are emerging across Europe. These trends are tending to put more information and more power in the hands of patients with regard to accessing and using medicines. Policies designed to maintain the control of information or medicines in the hands of professionals seem doomed to failure. However, there are dangers to patients in policies that are too liberal. Medicines used inappropriately are even more likely to do harm than they already can do even when used appropriately. Furthermore, inadequate regulation would allow the pharmaceutical industry a free hand to market medicines and create demand for pharmaceuticals even in the face of little or no health threat and leading to the consumption of health care resources that might be better deployed on other types of interventions for more significant health problems. Thus it is important that while educating the public and granting them greater access to information about medicines, that such information be placed in the context of a wider understanding of medicines and their benefits and drawbacks. The public also need more guidance on the quality and appropriateness of different information sources and help in accessing the more useful and relevant resources. In individual encounters, doctors and other health care professionals need to become more skilled in patient-centred medicine and in arriving at concordances with their patients on the medicine(s) to be used. However, changing the attitude and behaviour of doctors is not enough on its own. Patients will also have to become better informed and take more responsibility for their own medicines use, not least because they are being given increasing access to an ever widening range of drugs. Interventions to improve patients' use of their medicines will also have to be culturally appropriate. For example, prescribing guidelines for doctors are relatively firmly embedded in the Netherlands because they are part of the professionalization of general practice as a speciality within medicine, and not primarily motivated to save costs. Scientific guidelines fall on fertile soil in this country because they also appeal to the Dutch sense of frugality, rationality and to the Dutch tendency of lending authority to written rules (rather than to authoritarian rulers).

Policies on medicines need to take account of the cultural background and personalities of people (both patients and health care professionals) and of the realities of how policies will be implemented in the interactions between patients and their health care professionals.

References

Alsterlind, G. (1993) Health management – consumer perspectives, in *Proceedings of the Members' Meeting of the European Proprietary Medicines Manufacturers' Association: Pharmacy – Growing Self-Medication: The Marketing Challenge*, Paris, 24 January.

Anonymous (2000) Prescription for confusion, *Health Which?*, August, pp. 24–5.

Anonymous (2001) What is eHealth?, *Journal of Medical Internet Research*, 3(2): e20.

Arluke, A. (1980) Judging drugs: patients' conceptions of therapeutic efficacy in the treatment of arthritis, *Human Organization*, 39: 84–8.

Bacher, P. (2003) Direct-to-consumer advertising. Masters thesis, the Danish University of Pharmaceutical Sciences.

Barry, C.A., Bradley, C.P., Britten, N., Stevenson, F.A. and Barber, N. (2000) Patients' unvoiced agendas in general practice consultations: qualitative study, *British Medical Journal*, 320: 1246–50.

Barry, C.A., Stevenson, F.A., Britten, N., Barber, N. and Bradley, C.P. (2001) Giving voice to the lifeworld: more humane, more effective medical care? A qualitative study of doctor–patient communication in general practice, *Social Science and Medicine*, 53: 487–505.

Bates, M.S. (1996) *Biocultural Dimensions of Chronic Pain: Implications for Treatment of Mutli-Ethnic Populations*. Albany, NY: State University of New York Press.

Benner, J.S., Glynn, R.J., Mogun, H. *et al.* (2002) Long-term persistence in use of statin therapy in elderly patients, *Journal of the American Medical Association*, 284: 455–61.

Bradley, C. (1999) Ethics and prescribing, in C. Dowrick and L. Frith (eds) *General Practice and Ethics*. London: Routledge.

Britten, N., Stevenson, F.A., Barry, C.A., Barber, N. and Bradley, C.P. (2000) Misunderstandings in prescribing decisions in general practice: qualitative study, *British Medical Journal*, 320: 484–8.

Byrne, P.S. and Long, B.E.L. (1976) *Doctors Talking to Patients*. London: HMSO.

Cars, O., Mölstad, S. and Melander, A. (2001) Variation in antibiotic use in the European Union, *Lancet*, 357: 1851–3.

Christensen, D.B. (1978) Drug-taking compliance: a review and synthesis, *Health Services Research*, 6: 171–87.

Conrad, P. (1985) The meaning of medication: another look at compliance, *Social Science and Medicine*, 26: 29–37.

Consumers International (2002) *Credibility on the Web: An International Study of the Credibility of Consumer information on the Internet*. London: Office for Developed and Transition Economies (ODTE).

Denktas, S., Vogels, H.M.G., Niehof, T. *et al.* (1999) *Minderhedenmonitor*. Rotterdam: ISEO.

Deschepper, R., vander Stichele, R.H. and Haaijer-Ruskamp, F.M. (2002) Cross-cultural differences in lay attitudes and utilisation of antibiotics in a Belgian and a Dutch city, *Patient Education and Counselling*, 48: 161–9.

Edwards, A.M. and Elwyn, G. (2001) *Evidence-Based Patient Choice: Inevitable or Impossible?* Oxford: Oxford University Press.

European Commission (2001) Proposal for a Directive of the European Parliament and of the Council amending Directive 2001/83/EC on the Community code relating to medicinal products for human use (available from http://pharmacos.eudra.org/F2/review/doc/finaltext/011126-COM_2001_404-EN.pdf).

Fallsberg, M. and Hansen, E.H. (1995) *Håndkøbsmedicin – danske og europæiske perspektiver* [*Non-Prescription Medicines – Danish and European Perspectives*], Sundhedsstyrelsen (National Board of Health). Copenhagen: Schultz Information.

Gordis, L., Markowitz, M. and Lilienfeld, A.M. (1969) Studies in the epidemiology and preventability of rheumatic fever. V. A quantitative determination of compliance in children on oral penicillin prophylaxis, *Pediatrics*, 43: 173–82.

Hansen, E.H. and Launsø, L. (1988) Drugs and users – problems and new directions, *Health Promotion*, 3: 241–8.

Hansen, E.H., Holstein, B.E., Due, P. and Currie, C.E. (2003) International survey of self-reported medicine use among adolescents, *Annals of Pharmacotherapy*, 37: 361–6.

Harding, J.M. and Modell, M. (1985) How patients manage asthma, *Journal of the Royal College of General Practitioners*, 35: 226–8.

Haugen, Ø., Hjort, P.F. and Waaler, H.T. (1978) *Legemiddelforbruk i fylkene – store forskjeller, små forklaringer* [*Drug Utilization in the Counties – Wide Variations, Few Explanations*]. Oslo: NAVFs gruppe for helsetjenesteforskning.

Haynes, R.B., Taylor, D.W. and Sackett, D.L. (eds) (1979) *Compliance in Health Care*. Baltimore, MD: Johns Hopkins University Press.

Helman, C.G. (1990) *Culture, Health and Illness: An Introduction for Health Professionals*. London: Wright.

Hepler, C.D. and Strand, L.M. (1990) Opportunities and responsibilities in pharmaceutical care, *American Journal of Hospital Pharmacy*, 47: 533–43.

Hingson, R., Scotch, N.A., Sorenson, J. and Swazey, J.P. (1981) *In Sickness and in Health: Social Dimensions of Medical Care*. St Louis, MO: C.V. Mosby.

Hjelm, K., Bard, K., Nyberg, P. and Apelqvist, J. (2003) Religious and cultural distance in beliefs about health and illness in women with diabetes mellitus of different origin living in Sweden, *International Journal of Nursing Studies*, 40: 627–43.

Holme Hansen, E.H., Holstein, B.E. and Due, P. (2003) Time trends in medicine use among adolescents in ten industrialised countries, *European Journal of Public Health*, 13(suppl. 4): 43.

Jackevicius, C.A., Mamdani, M. and Tu, J.V. (2002) Adherence with statin therapy in elderly patients with and without acute coronary syndromes, *Journal of the American Medical Association*, 288: 462–7.

Larsen, B.O. and Hansen, E.H. (1985) The active medicine user, *Scandinavian Journal of Primary Health Care*, 3: 6–10.

Leeflang, R.L.I. (1994) *Zoeken naar gezondheid. Hulpzoekgedrag van personen van Nederlandse en Turkse herkomst [Looking for Health: Help Seeking Behaviour of Persons with Dutch and Turkish Background]*. Leiden: LIDESCO.

Ley, P. (1988) *Communicating with Patient: Improving Communication, Satisfaction and Compliance*. Cheltenham: Stanley Thornes.

Lüschen, G., Cockerham, W., van der Zee, J. *et al.* (1995) *Health Systems in the European Union*. München: R. Oldenbourg Verlag.

McGavock, H., Britten, N. and Weinman, J. (1998) *A Review of the Literature on Drug Adherence*. London: Royal Pharmaceutical Society of Great Britain.

Mischler, E.G. (1984) *The Discourse of Medicine: The Dialectics of Medical Interviews*. Norwood, NJ: Ablex.

Mölstad, S., Lundborg, C.S., Karlsson, A.-K. and Cars, O. (2002) Antibiotic prescription rates vary markedly between 13 European countries, *Scandinavian Journal of Infectious Diseases*, 34: 366–71.

Monane, M., Bohn, R.L., Gurwitz, J.H., Glynn, R.J. and Avorn, J. (1994) Non-compliance with congestive heart failure therapy in the elderly, *Archives of Internal Medicine*, 154: 433–7.

Payer, L. (1988) *Medicine and Culture: Varieties of Treatment in the United States, England, West Germany, and France*. New York: Henry Holt.

Procordia and Trygg Hansa SPP (1992) *Modern Families: A Comparative Study of Middle Class Families in Sweden, USA, Germany, and France*. Stockholm: Procordia & Trygg Hansa SPP (in Swedish).

Roth, H.P., Caron, H.S. and His, B.P. (1970) Measuring intake of a prescribed medication: a bottle count and a tracer technique compared, *Clinical Pharmacology*, 11: 228–37.

Royal Pharmaceutical Society of Great Britain (1997) *From Compliance to Concordance: Achieving Shared Goals in Medicine Taking*. London: Royal Pharmaceutical Society of Great Britain.

Schytte-Hansen, S. (2003) The Danes and over-the-counter drugs – opinions, behaviour and attitudes. Masters thesis, Danish University of Pharmaceutical Sciences.

Stevenson, F.A., Barry, C.A., Britten, N., Barber, N. and Bradley, C.P. (2000) Doctor–patient communication about drugs: the evidence for shared decision making, *Social Science and Medicine*, 50: 829–40.

Stewart, M. (1995) Studies of Health Outcome and Patient Centredness, in M. Stewart, J.B. Brown, W.W. Westen *et al.* (eds) *Patient Centred Medicine: Transforming the Clinical Method*. Thousand Oaks, CA: Sage.

Stewart, M., Brown, J.B., Weston, W.W. *et al.* (eds) (1995) *Patient Centred Medicine: Transforming the Clinical Method*. Thousand Oaks, CA: Sage.

Toop, L., Richards, D., Dowell, T. *et al.* (2003) *Direct to Consumer Advertising of Prescription Drugs in New Zealand: For Health or for Profit?* Otago, NZ: University of Otago.

van den Brink-Muinen, A., Verhaak, P.F.M., Bensing, J.M. *et al.* (1999) *The Eurocommunication Study: An International Comparative Study in Six European Countries on Doctor–Patient Communication in General Practice*. Utrecht: Nivel.

van den Brink-Muinen, A., van Dulmen, A.M., Bensing, J.M. *et al.* (2003) *Eurocommunication II: A Comparative Study Between Countries in Central and Western Europe on Doctor–Patient Communication in General Practice*. Utrecht: Nivel.

World Health Organization (1996) *Good Pharmacy Practice (GPP) in Community and Hospital Pharmacy Settings*, WHO/PHARM/DAP/96.1. Geneva: WHO.

ten

Financial incentives and prescribing

Tom Walley and Elias Mossialos

Introduction

Governments face many difficulties in containing prescribing costs – public health needs, demands by patients and doctors' desire to prescribe. Doctors are in a difficult position, acting both as agents for the patient in meeting the patient's health needs and sometimes demands, and also often as an agent of the third-party payer. Doctors themselves might have no direct interest in the cost of their prescribing, as they do not pay for the medicines themselves. While this allows them to advise their individual patients, it means that their advice might not accord with the policy of the third-party payer, or even with broader public health. Doctors are very susceptible to a range of influences, including sometimes inappropriate demand from patients: where patients can move easily between general practitioners, doctors may feel obliged to prescribe to meet any patient demand, real or perceived, lest they lose the patient from their panel, and ultimately lose income. Many countries have attempted to balance these influences with increased education, including academic outreach programmes. Some have gone further: where the third-party payer of medicines also pays for the doctor in some way, it may seek to use direct incentives to influence clinical behaviour and, in particular, prescribing. These incentives are the focus of this chapter (see Figure 10.1) and we need to consider whether this is an appropriate way to try to influence professional behaviour or whether it might result in more harm than good.

Incentives might be direct to the doctor, influencing his or her own income, or indirect, to provide a more collective benefit to a practice or the practice's patients (e.g. having a pharmacist funded to improve management of medicines generally). Incentives other than financial can be very broad, ranging from doctor empowerment to better care for patients. These might be considered as professional incentives. Incentives might be positive, rewarding behaviour in line

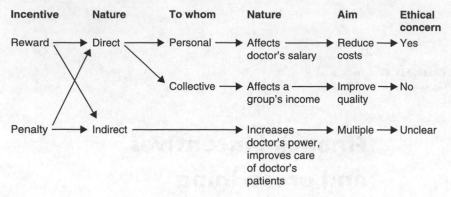

Figure 10.1 Taxonomy of incentives to influence clinical behaviour.

with the payer's policy, or negative, such as fines or loss of income or disempowerment. Incentives are inevitably a reflection of any health service, its structure and the prevailing professional and political ethic. It may be, therefore, that international experience in this area teaches us something general about doctors' behaviour, but does not provide any direct lessons for individual countries.

From the point of view of a third-party payer, containing costs by this method has some advantages: it moves the possibly unpopular cost-containment decision from the payer to the doctor, thus avoiding direct criticism from both doctor and patient; and it allows the doctor to be the judge of each clinical situation, thereby limiting the risk of harm to any one patient that a blanket sanction (e.g. withdrawal of reimbursement for a particular medicine) might cause. From the perspective of the patient or the doctor, there will be many misgivings about the motive behind such incentives.

The aims of incentives may be to reduce utilization of health care resources, transform clinical practice, improve quality of care or achieve a health target. Those that involve improving care might be seen as just rewards, and socially and professionally acceptable, while those that aim to cut costs at the expense of quality of care might be seen as corrupt. Perhaps as a result, the exact aim of an incentive is often not stated, or the overt statement is belied by the covert intention. Often, too, the objectives of incentives are all of these, and in assessing the outcome of an incentive it is unclear how to weight comparative success in different fields. For instance, a prescribing incentive might encourage identification of particular patients who need therapy (improving practice and hopefully clinical outcomes) while increasing overall costs due to increased drug use: this may undermine another endpoint, that of reducing the costs of prescribing. An example of this was the Indicative Prescribing Scheme (IPS) in England in 1990 (see below). Its objectives were described as 'placing [of] downward pressure on expenditure on drugs, particularly in those practices with the highest expenditure, but without in any way preventing people getting the medicines they need' (Department of Health 1990). The objectives, therefore, were both financial (easily measured) and improved quality (far more difficult to measure, and still difficult many years on).

It is often difficult to study such policy interventions in a European setting (though possibly easier in the more fragmented US systems, see Chapter 5), as they tend to develop quickly and are often all encompassing, leaving no time for adequate before and after data collection, nor any control group. Furthermore, such incentives are often introduced together with organizational changes, such as the introduction of the IPS alongside other interventions: the introduction of health authority medical advisers with an educational as well as a managerial agenda to improve prescribing, improved systems providing feedback on each doctor's prescribing, and other educational interventions. Therefore, it might be difficult to disentangle which element of these changes brought about a particular result.

Evidence from systematic reviews

A systematic review of the medical and economic literature of the effects of financial incentives (Chaix-Couturier *et al.* 2000) found that there were few randomized controlled trials, most studies being observational with a control group or before and after designs, or no control group at all. Most reported short-term rather than long-term results, and there was a wide range of methods used to assess the effects of the incentives, limiting the external validity of the conclusions. Some, mostly from the UK, examined prescribing and are considered further below.

The types of financial incentives were varied and ranged from those that were a part of the organized health service (fee per service, salary related to performance, fundholding, capitation funding, payments for targets achieved) to the morally dubious or even illegal (such as fee sharing, referral to services where the doctor had a financial share, etc.). Even with similar incentives, the results varied depending on a range of confounding factors, including the type and duration of disease treated, the diagnostic or therapeutic procedures involved, patient gender, or patient requirement or ability to pay. Other confounding factors were the nature of the doctors themselves: their age, education, experience, individual versus group practice, levels of competition and volume of activity. Finally, as mentioned above, many incentives were combined with a range of other non-financial incentives or measures, such as utilization review, peer pressure or educational activities (for instance, GP fundholding and incentive schemes in the UK and health maintenance organizations in the USA).

Chaix-Couturier *et al.* (2000) identified how such schemes of financial incentives can limit the quality or quantity of care:

- limited continuity of care, especially for patients with chronic illness;
- reduced ranges of services offered, especially preventive services;
- improper use of emergency services;
- reduced confidence on the part of patients;
- reduced time for teaching or research;
- multiplicity of guidelines or formularies recommending different courses of action for the same conditions;
- and, most importantly perhaps, a conflict of interest between the patient and

the physician, whereby the doctor ceases to act as the agent of the patient and acts more on their own account.

The authors' broad conclusions were that doctors did alter their clinical behaviour to obtain financial incentives but within limits: where there were fee per item payments, there was an increase in medical activity and doctors could influence patient demand, both in terms of quantity and in terms of the types of services demanded. On the other hand, switching from a fee per service to a salaried payment for doctors seemed to reduce provision of only the most elective of services, while the patterns of care for more severe conditions remained unchanged. The weakest element of these studies was their examination of the effects of these schemes on health outcomes: although results from individual studies are mixed, in general US studies show no consistent pattern of difference in overall health outcomes between patients in managed care and fee per service schemes.

This is generally reassuring for third-party payers – it seems that the doctor will continue to meet the more basic needs of the patient while cutting back on more discretionary and less necessary (or even unnecessary) care.

Several lessons can be drawn from this review:

1 Changes due to financial incentives do not result from the internal motivation of doctors to change practice and therefore are unlikely, on their own, to be an effective long-term tool for public health policies.
2 Incentives directed at physicians must not create a conflict of interest between their income and the quality of care provided. As such, the incentives themselves should not be limited to decreasing health service utilization, but must also be adjusted to encourage and reward quality and productivity. Furthermore, adjustment may be needed to avoid the dumping of high cost/more severely ill patients.
3 Disclosure of the incentives is necessary to maintain public trust in the doctors and in the payer, whether it be an insurance company or state.
4 Doctors need regular information on their use of resources and on what are the approved/cost-effective ways of managing particular conditions.
5 Incentives need to be simple, transparent and direct – a complex system is puzzling both for doctors and for payers and can create obscure perverse incentives.

Incentives ideally need to support the professional aspirations of doctors – improving health in the population and improving treatment for the individual patient, while maintaining their personal income. Incentives aimed at saving money are professionally acceptable if there is maintenance of quality and if it is explicit that savings go back into the health service, even where there is no direct gain to the doctor – that is, the gain is indirect, in helping to ensure health gain for patients. A variety of different types of incentives may be needed depending on circumstances and aims; for instance, a fee per item is highly likely to improve delivery in areas that are underserved, but would be inappropriate for areas already overserved.

Financial incentives and prescribing

Incentives related to prescribing might take many forms depending on the nature of the health service and of payments to doctors. One of the most studied is the use of prescribing budgets, either at the level of the individual doctor or practice [i.e. an indicative (rarely real) budget given to physicians to cover their prescribing over a given period], or a more collective real or indicative budget given to an organization or area.

In systems with a split between purchasers and providers, the purchasers can allocate budgets directly. Such budgets can take different forms. They can be 'hard' with penalties and rewards. The rewards can involve retention by the agent of some or all of any surplus made (UK fundholding). The penalties can take the form of requiring the agent concerned to repay any overspending out of subsequent years' allocation, or only partial reimbursement of overspending (Germany).

An alternative to hard budgets is target, indicative or 'shadow' budgets, where a record is kept of the costs of the transactions undertaken by the agent concerned, who is made aware of any overspending or underspending, but where no immediate penalties are applied and overspending is automatically met (e.g. current UK practice, see below). Such budgets are less likely to be effective instruments of cost control than hard budgets. 'Naming and shaming' practitioners who habitually overspend may affect behaviour, but the costs and benefits of such interventions in the medium term are not well researched (Mossialos and Le Grand 1999).

Some countries have introduced 'hard' or 'target' budgets for publicly funded pharmaceutical expenditure. If budgets are allocated to the relevant agents (doctors and/or pharmacists), and those agents have a strong incentive to spend within their budget (through penalties for overspending, through rewards for underspending, or both), then cost pressures may be contained. The budgets can be set at the level of the doctor, the practice or any higher level of health care organization. There could be an overall budget cap at government level, with the government committing itself to a fixed allocation for pharmaceutical spending. In this case, budgets are either agreed with the industry (Spain) or simply laid down by government (Greece, Italy, Portugal). The Dutch government is currently planning to introduce an overall pharmaceutical budget for health insurers by 2004. The expectation is that health insurers will become more active in purchasing pharmaceuticals and putting more pressure on doctors and pharmacists to increase cost-effective delivery of pharmaceutical care.

When governments self-impose budgetary restrictions, these have limited effect, since governments in general cannot (or will not) levy penalties on themselves. It is therefore not surprising that they have not been effective. In Spain, agreements between the government and the industry that limited the growth in social security expenditure on pharmaceuticals have not been respected, even though companies had to repay 56.7 per cent of the gross profit on any sales exceeding the fixed growth rate (Lopez-Bastida and Mossialos 2000). In 1994, the Italian government introduced a ceiling on public pharmaceutical expenditure. Nonetheless, budgets have regularly been exceeded (8.7 per cent in 1998,

11.6 per cent in 1999 and 16.5 per cent in 2000). Since 1998, the industry, wholesalers and pharmacists have been made responsible for paying to the government 60 per cent of the annual deficit. However, it is unclear whether this policy has been implemented (Donatini *et al.* 2001).

Other forms of incentive include payments or fines for adherence or non-adherence to treatment guidelines, best exemplified in France, or the achievement of targets that relate more to quality of prescribing rather than financial targets only, as also seen, but not well studied, in the UK. So far, most European countries have not pursued such approaches. In general, there are similar themes emerging from the use of such schemes across Europe: the need to examine costs in other areas than just prescribing, since an increase in prescribing costs may save money in other budgetary areas; reluctance on the part of doctors to participate in such schemes, often because they claim ethical concerns but sometimes, at least, because of issues around transfer of power to managers; and the need for good information systems.

United Kingdom

Prescribing budgets in the UK

In the UK, general practitioners (GPs) prescribe over 90 per cent of all medicines by volume and about 80 per cent by cost. Hospitals generally transfer most outpatient prescribing to the GP. All patients are registered with a named GP who are typically organized in practices of 1–10 GPs. General practitioners are paid largely on a fixed per capita basis with limited additional fee per item payments (e.g. for vaccinations). There is a fixed patient co-payment (£6.50 or approximately €10 from April 2003) for each item prescribed regardless of its cost, but there is an extensive range of exemptions to this charge affecting about half the population (based mainly on income and age). In practice, only about 15 per cent of prescriptions actually attract such a charge. There is a very accurate system of identifying prescribing spending by GPs, through the Prescribing Analysis and CosT (PACT) data (Majeed *et al.* 1997). This facilitates feedback to GPs on their spending and monitoring budgets.

In 1990, as part of widespread reforms to general practice, two schemes were set up involving prescribing budgets:

1 *GP fundholding.* Large well-organized practices could volunteer to receive a 'hard' or real budget to cover prescribing costs, elective surgery and non-medical practice staff. Any money saved in a part of the budget could be spent on other parts, or in other ways to benefit the patients of the practice. With each year, the regulations were relaxed so that more and more practices joined the scheme in annual 'waves'.
2 *The indicative prescribing scheme*, for all non-fundholding practices. Target or indicative budgets were set for the spending of a practice on drugs for a year. The GPs received regular feedback on their prescribing and their actual spending against their budget. There was a small incentive to keep within budget.

Prescribing budgets for both schemes were set in a similar manner, based on historical spending (i.e. the previous year's spending) plus an 'uplift' to allow for new drugs. This effectively rewarded the profligate and punished the more restrained prescribers. The non-prescribing parts of the fundholder budget had no such data and were often a 'best guess' and usually generous.

Other initiatives to improve prescribing while containing costs included better provision of independent therapeutic information to GPs, monthly feedback on their spending against their budget, and local prescribing advisers to monitor budgets and to deliver 'academic detailing' to help practices to manage their prescribing.

The two schemes fared very differently. The results were as follows:

Fundholding

For the first time, GP fundholders had the power to negotiate services with hospitals, a strong professional incentive that made the scheme very popular. The prescribing portion of the budget was by far the easiest in which money could be saved, often by a simple move to generic prescribing (i.e. prescribing by proper name so that the prescription could be dispensed using non-branded and less expensive preparations) or by simple therapeutic substitution (e.g. using the less expensive Nizatidine instead of the more expensive Ranitidine). Neither of these changes would be expected to impact on patient well-being.

These GPs had an almost personal incentive to contain their prescribing costs: although strictly the incentive was not directly financial to the GPs, in many early cases the savings were used to fund developments that would otherwise have had to come out of practice profits. However, the major incentives were professional, to improve the care of their patients, and personal, as GPs saw this as a means to take control of their own destinies and for primary care to direct the whole of the NHS. The GP fundholders, therefore, aggressively addressed their prescribing.

Harris and Scrivener (1996) found that the absolute cost of prescribing increased greatly in all practices between 1990 and 1996, though by 66 per cent for non-fundholders and by 56–59 per cent for fundholders (Figure 10.2). There was, therefore, a relative reduction in the costs of fundholders, compared with non-fundholders, reaching about 6 per cent over the first three years of fundholding. This was achieved by a reduction in the average cost per item prescribed (consistent with simple generic prescribing or therapeutic substitution) rather than by a decrease in the number of items dispensed which remained stable. The authors concluded that, in financial terms at least, fundholding had some success.

After the first three years of fundholding, however, the difference in the rate of increase in prescribing costs disappeared. This is explained by the fact that the reduction in the rate of increase in prescribing was due to a shift to generic prescribing or to simple therapeutic substitution. These changes could only happen once; thereafter, the rate of increase would be dictated in the fundholding, as in the non-fundholding practices, by new drugs coming onto the market or initiatives to truly improve treatment, which almost always involved more prescribing rather than less. The reductions in prescribing growth rate then seemed to cease, although the 'locked in' savings remained. There seemed to be

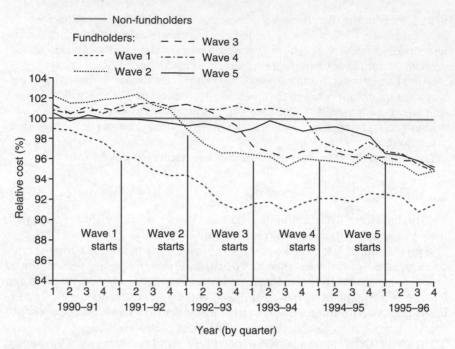

Figure 10.2 Cost per prescribing unit for each wave of fundholding general practices in England as a percentage of the cost for the continuing non-fundholders: before and after fundholding, 1990–91 to 1995–96, by quarter. Reproduced with permission from Harris and Scrivener (1996).

little or no strategic cost-reducing behaviour – that is, no fundamental change in prescribing behaviour, only in what was actually prescribed. Although no new areas for saving appeared, the existing savings were effectively locked into the system – that is, the savings made by a generic shift went on for as long as the generic was prescribed (Wilson *et al.* 1997).

Results were more mixed on whether fundholders restricted the use of new, more effective drugs; some suggested greater therapeutic conservatism (i.e. less inclination to prescribe new drugs) in fundholders than non-fundholders, but others showed no difference. Nor does there seem to have been any widespread cream skimming (i.e. selection of low-cost patients or adverse selection of high-cost patients so as to maximize the fundholding budget surplus) (Matsaganis and Glennerster 1994). Sometimes individual fundholders did behave in a bizarre way to optimize their own benefits; for example, making drastic over-night changes to prescribing when they became fundholders and so upsetting patients substantially. But most fundholders behaved in a more responsible way and introduced changes more gradually.

Overall, there was no evidence of poorer treatment by fundholders than non-fundholders; if anything, fundholders seemed to provide better care. However, this was due largely to the nature of the practices that became fundholders – these were well-organized practices, often working in more affluent areas.

Fundholding was driven by the market philosophy of the government of the day, and so was facilitated in every way (any budget overspends were usually quietly met by the health authority rather than coming out of the following year's budget as was intended, and budgets were often more generous to fund-holders than to non-fundholders). In the mid-1990s, there was a move away from historical funding to more equitable capitation based funding, although still not reflecting need (as late as 2003, long after the demise of fundholding, most primary care organizations were setting GP indicative prescribing budgets based up to 50 per cent on historic and 50 per cent on capitation or other need-oriented factors). This reduced the share of money for fundholders. Also, as the scheme extended to include 70 per cent of GPs, the advantages to the privileged few early fundholders were diluted. In 1997, the newly elected Labour government rejected the partial market approach created by the previous government, including GP fundholding. It slowly decreased incentives for fundholders until fundholding ceased completely in 1999, to be replaced by a range of new reforms that also carried some incentives for GP prescribing described below.

The major advantage of fundholding was its empowerment of GPs to direct the local health service, in what the government intended to become a primary care led NHS, rather than be the poor relative of hospital medicine. The major disadvantage was its fundamentally divisive effects, increasing differences in standards of care across the country and between rich and poor areas. In prescribing, fundholding contained the extent of the rise in the medicines bill. Another success was an increasing willingness by GPs to consider costs in their prescribing (Tobin and Packham 1999); this was a cultural change, markedly different from what was the case in 1990.

Gosden and Torgerson (1997) concluded that it was impossible to comment on the success or otherwise of GP fundholding. It had never been more than partial in its coverage of services. There were no data on patient outcomes, choice or equity, or on general efficiency, although these had been declared as aims of the scheme. The best studied aspect was prescribing, with the results reported above.

The Indicative Prescribing Scheme

This scheme faced many problems. There were few positive incentives for doctors to keep within their budget, and no real negative incentives, so most ignored doing so. The result was that in 1991–1992, 85 per cent of GP practices overspent their budget. By 1994, the Audit Commission concluded that the scheme 'has been somewhat discredited to date as a means of controlling expenditure'.

Part of the scheme had included the development of incentives for GP non-fundholders. These were collective – part of the money generated by any savings would be available for local projects. This element of the scheme was also largely ignored by GPs. In 1993, the government, impressed by the savings in prescribing costs by fundholding GPs, resurrected the scheme by allowing limited incentives to go directly to each practice. The targets for the incentive were not purely financial (an outturn 1–3 per cent below the practice target budget was usually expected), but often included a level of generic prescribing, use of a formulary or control of repeat prescribing. The details were determined locally. The payment was a maximum of £3000 per GP.

There has been no published report on the success or otherwise of these schemes nationally and their diversity would make such a study difficult. The only study to report the effects of one such local scheme (Bateman *et al.* 1996) concluded that 'The prescribing behaviour of non-fundholding general practitioners responded to financial incentives in a similar way to that of fundholding practitioners. The incentive scheme did not seem to reduce the quality of prescribing.' However, this study was flawed in many ways, unavoidably perhaps given the nature of the incentives the authors sought to assess. The 'savers' were defined after the event and there was no control group; the 'non-savers' were not an adequate control group, since it was not clear how many practices had tried to achieve savings but failed. The study is therefore, in part, tautological – 'savers' (i.e. those claiming the incentive reward) are defined *post hoc* as scheme participants – and hence the scheme was deemed successful. Anecdotally, these schemes were popular among GPs and were the basis of later schemes in primary care trusts.

UK developments 1999–2003

In 1999, GP fundholding was replaced by primary care trusts (PCTs), geographically determined groups of GP practices typically covering about 80,000–10,000 patients. These groups are composed of a wide variety of GPs, ranging from former enthusiastic first-wave fundholders to those philosophically opposed to all such market reforms. The PCT is responsible for purchasing a wide range of services (not just prescribing or primary care) from a single cash-limited budget held by the PCT, not by individual practices. Any benefits from prescribing savings are therefore largely collective and may benefit the gross overspender as well as the cautious prescriber. This reduces any incentive and undermines the support of the enthusiast for addressing prescribing. In addition, government-produced national service frameworks are driving prescribing in key areas (e.g. use of statins to prevent ischaemic heart disease), undermining any attempt to contain prescribing costs. As a result, almost every PCT is overspent on the prescribing element of the budget and has to take money from other services or offset it against future years to pay for prescribing.

Primary care trusts attempt to use peer pressure and to develop a sense of corporate affinity among GPs to control overall prescribing cost rises, while at the same time improving quality in particular areas of prescribing. Since all doctors in a PCT treat patients funded by the same budget, there is a corporate or professional incentive to constrain inappropriate cost rises in prescribing – wasteful prescribing will cut resources available for other patients. In contrast to the Indicative Prescribing Scheme, where a similar professional incentive was ineffective, peer pressure in a smaller group may reinforce this, and there is now a greater cultural acceptance among doctors of the need to consider the benefits of the wider population. In addition, PCTs are legally obliged to have a practice-level incentive scheme, similar to those used for non-fundholders in the past with practices' financial targets set against an indicative budget and usually a range of quality targets also (e.g. reduction in antibiotic or benzodiazepine use, or increase in numbers of patients appropriately treated with statins). Payments can be as high as £45,000 (approx €70,000) per practice. A recent review concluded that there is no clear pattern to these schemes and no evidence even of their financial effectiveness (Ashworth *et al.* 2002). Individual schemes are very diverse but key targets include keeping within budgets, adherence to targets for generic prescribing, review of repeat prescribing, and adherence to guidance for specific disease areas (Mason *et al.* 2003).

Ireland

In Ireland, approximately one-third of the population have 'medical cards' (largely based on income), which entitles them to all medical services and medicines free of charge. For other patients, medicines are often self-funded. For prescribing for the medical card patients, the government introduced a prescribing incentive scheme in 1993 whereby prescribers were set an indicative budget based on the national average spend per head of population and their number of patients; the GPs could receive half of all savings made against this budget for practice developments (Walley *et al.* 2000). This mechanism for setting budgets in effect rewarded low-cost prescribers without any need for them to change their practice. The results showed that 'savers' (and hence those who received the incentive payments) were always lower cost prescribers than non-savers. They contained their rate and costs of prescribing compared with the other groups; for example, the percentage rise in prescribing costs in the year after the introduction of the scheme was −7.9 per cent for savers and +7.3 per cent for large overspenders, respectively. This effect was short-lived, however, and was gone by the third year of the scheme (Figure 10.3).

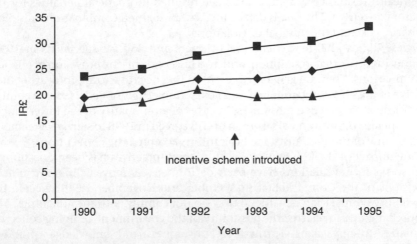

Figure 10.3 Effects of an incentive scheme on costs per patient in Ireland (groups subdivided retrospectively by performance against budget). ▲, savers; ◆, modest overspend; ■, large overspend. Reproduced with permission from Walley *et al.* (2000).

The national auditors estimated that IR£13.5 million was saved in the first year of the scheme and were broadly enthusiastic about it. The savings mechanism by which changes were made was therapeutic substitution or the use of alternative less expensive brands (generic prescribing in Ireland does not save money because of the lack of a national drug tariff). There was also a greater degree of therapeutic conservatism; that is, a reluctance among savers to use new drugs, which might be appropriate but may give some cause for concern. Again, this echoes some of the UK work. The use of the savings by GPs was not well supervised in the early years, allowing some to profiteer (payments of as much as IR£100,000 or €130,000 to one GP were alleged in the popular press). The scheme continues in a greatly modified form, with more quality assessment of prescribing and more supervision of the use of any savings.

In contrast with the UK, there is little emphasis on generic prescribing in Ireland, as there is no set price for generics and some branded preparations may actually be less expensive.

France

In France, most patients receive medicines funded by a health insurance fund. There are variable co-payments depending on the medicine, but many patients have top-up private health insurance to cover these. Regulatory practice guidelines (*références médicales opposables*, RMOs) were introduced by law in 1993. The National Agency for Accreditation and Health Care Evaluation (ANAES) produces practice guidelines (RMOs), which are recommendations on good practice that doctors are required to follow in accordance with agreements signed between their professional representatives and the health insurance funds in 1994, 1995 and 1997. Up until 1999, frequent or serious failure to comply with these recommendations, or non-compliance that was particularly expensive for the health insurance system, could have resulted in financial penalties for the doctor concerned. The fine is determined by a weighted combination of indices of harm, cost and the number of violations.

These RMOs (200 for general practitioners and 250 for specialists in 1998) mainly involve drug prescriptions and, to a lesser extent, the provision of medical examinations. They are generally presented in a negative form, indicating ineffective or possibly dangerous practice. For example: 'It is not advisable to employ two or more vaso-active substances, in cases of arteriopathy of the lower limbs'. Nonetheless, only one medical union of GPs agreed in 1998 to sign an agreement, while none of the specialists' medical unions accepted the convention.

The impact of the RMO policy on physicians' practices has been questioned, but so far few evaluations have been performed. Moreover, different judicial decisions of the Conseil d'Etat (in October and November 1999) rejected the possibility of physician penalties if they do not comply with the guidelines. The Conseil d'Etat also rejected the possibility of the government applying collective penalties to physicians. Furthermore, awareness and knowledge of RMOs among French family physicians seems to be weak. The difficulty of controlling physicians, the large number of RMOs and the lack of a relevant information system limit the credibility of this policy (Durieux *et al.* 2000a,b).

Since 1998, to promote gatekeeping, every general practitioner can become a 'referring doctor' for any patient willing to enter into the referral system. These GPs are paid a capitation fee (initially €23 and later €46 per patient) in addition to usual fees. In return, the GPs and their patients undertake: to keep to prices listed in the agreement; to use only the third-party payment system (to shelter patients from direct payments); to keep patients' medical records; to provide continuous service, ensuring continuity of care; to participate in public preventive programmes; to comply with practice guidelines; and to make efforts to contain drug costs, for instance by prescribing not less than 5 per cent generics (Sandier *et al.* 2003). To date, only about 10 per cent of GPs and 1 per cent of patients have accepted this system. The prescription of generics has increased, but only slightly. Generic sales due to 'gatekeeper' GP prescriptions were 3.32 per cent, compared with 2.4 per cent by other GPs (CNAMTS 2001). It seems unlikely that this scheme will either reduce overall health care costs or improve pubic health substantially.

Germany

Germany also operates a social security type system, with patients' medicines being paid by local sickness funds. Ten per cent of the population with the highest income are excluded from these schemes. Unlike the individual prescribing budgets in the UK, cash-limited prescribing budgets in Germany were set collectively, in 1993, for all GPs in a district. A collective penalty was applied for any overspend of the budgets. In the first year following the implementation of drug budgets, there was a 11.2 per cent decrease in the number of prescriptions and an 18.8 per cent reduction in sickness funds' expenditure for medicines (Busse and Howerth 1999) (Figure 10.4). Only about 60 per cent of the total reduction was due to changes in doctors' prescribing behaviour; the other 40 per cent was due to price cuts, increases in user charges and the reference price system. No sanctions were imposed in 1994 or 1995, but in 1996 sickness funds claimed back money from nine regions that had overshot their budget by up to 11.3 per cent.

The effects of this on quality of care are hotly debated. Busse (2000) claims that the initial reduction in drug expenditure was mainly attributable to a change in practice by doctors who had previously prescribed drugs of higher quality and greater cost simply to prescribing cheaper drugs. Junger *et al.* (2000) showed that the drug budget had no relevant long-term impact on drug prescribing for diabetic patients, and others did not document any consistent pattern between medication changes and cost-effective prescribing practices attributable to medication budgeting in Germany (Weltermann *et al.* 1997). Some doctors, pharmacists and the pharmaceutical industry representatives claimed that silent rationing, in terms of infrequent prescription of drugs for certain conditions (i.e. for Alzheimer's disease), took place (MMW 2001). Some (Schoffski and Graf von der Schulenburg 1997) also argue that the number of referrals and hospital admissions increased significantly after the introduction of a drug budget in Germany, but others argue that the evidence for this is uncertain (Delnoij and Brenner 2000).

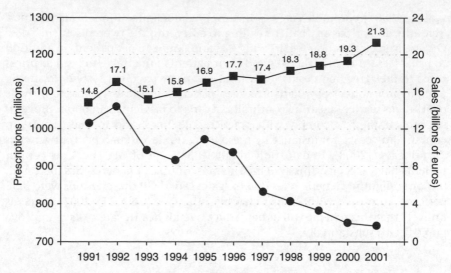

Figure 10.4   Prescribing costs (■, in billions of euros) and number of prescriptions (●, millions) funded by sickness funds in Germany, 1991–2001.
Source: Busse and Howarth (1999).

In 1998 soft budgets replaced hard budgets, but in 1999 the coalition government reintroduced hard budgets, only to abolish them again in 2001. In this year, drug expenditure grew by 11.2 per cent (Presse- und Informationsamt der Bundersregierung 2002). The reason for the 1998 and 2001 abolition of the hard budgets was that the schemes proved difficult to operate (Delnoij and Brenner 2000). Data for overspending were delivered too late to allow doctors to change their prescribing (Dietrich 2000); moreover, many questioned how fines could be allocated to each doctor, since no individual budgets existed. Several lawyers argued that collective fines and claw backs from doctors who have been rational prescribers but who happened to work in an overspending region, were a breach of Article 3(1) of the German Basic Law addressing equality and equal treatment (Jacker 2000).

Since 2001, target budgets have been set for individual doctors, taking into account the regional budget, the doctor's specialization, and age and case-mix structure of treated patients. If a doctor is thought to overprescribe, the regional associations of doctors must review whether this is justified by specific circumstances or whether the doctor has been inefficient. In the latter case, the doctor will be warned on his or her prescribing and stricter controls will apply in the following two years. If the overprescribing is considerable, a pay back will be imposed. However, doctors can object to the committee's decisions and it is difficult to agree on criteria when overspending shall be deemed justified and when not (Korzilius 2001). Recent studies suggest that there is still wasteful prescribing in Germany (Sperschneider and Kleinert 2002).

Spain

In Spain, INSALUD (the National Health Insurance Institute), which covers 38 per cent of the population, now offers financial incentives to health centres whose spending is below a target budget and whose doctors meet guidelines of good clinical practice. Part of the savings are passed on to those individual GPs (up to €1540 per year) who prescribe at least 6 per cent generics. Some regional health authorities apply similar schemes, while others reported making direct offers to GPs to cut costs. However, most doctors did not adhere to their targets, claiming to be more concerned about providing high-quality pharmaceutical care to their patients than keeping within their budgets. In Catalonia, primary care doctors receive €3000 per year if they keep within their budgets and increase the volume of generics but without reducing the number of their prescriptions. In Navarra, primary care doctors receive €2400 a year if they meet their budget targets. In addition, 50 per cent of the savings revert to the primary care health centres where the doctors work. None of the schemes operating in Spain has been properly evaluated yet.

Italy

The 1992 NHS reforms introduced expenditure targets per GP and incentives for GPs to achieve their targets. The prevailing approach, a gain-sharing scheme whereby GPs keep a percentage of the savings as an income supplement, has been heavily criticized. Critics emphasize that the scheme applies only to drug expenditure as opposed to overall expenditure (including referrals and diagnostic services) and may distort appropriate prescribing because of the conflict of interest of GPs to increase their income (Fattore and Jommi 1998); these arguments are similar to those in the UK. Implementation was left to the regional administrations and local health units but only a few regions and local health units have implemented these policies. Furthermore, the impact of this scheme, where it has been implemented, has yet to be evaluated.

Other European countries

Pilot schemes are underway looking at financial incentives in Sweden and the Netherlands. In Sweden, these are operated by the local county councils, which, for instance, have offered small bonuses targeting the use of proton pump inhibitors. In the Netherlands, some health insurers offer small bonuses to doctors, for instance for prescribing all oral contraceptives in accordance with an approved protocol. There is also an experimental scheme in Limburg where GPs are receiving an extra payment of up to €6018 in return for savings achieved by increased generic and decreased benzodiazepine prescribing. This scheme seems successful so far, based on very early results.

The ethics of incentives

Financial incentives that seem to reward the limiting of care may pose ethical problems for the doctor. This has been best considered in the American literature. The USA has a diversity of health care systems, ranging from entirely fees for services charged to patients, third-party payer systems where insurance companies, health maintenance organizations (HMO) or the government are the payer, to totally salaried schemes. As such, there is a wide diversity of systems for paying doctors and many schemes involve some degree of incentives related to prescribing, or following guidelines. This has led to study and debate on the ethics of these incentives.

Research in the USA also illustrates the effectiveness of incentives, particularly when they are personal to the doctor and affect his or her income (Hillman 1990). The question of whether doctors would allow such incentives to harm patients is less clear. Many find themselves in a system where they are paid bonuses for reduced clinical spending and cost-conscious gatekeeping, and are discouraged from telling patients about expensive treatment options. All of these are justified by the payers as an affirmation of the physician's moral responsibility and role in stewardship and, therefore, ethical practice. However, a clash of ethics persists between Hippocratic (do the best for each individual patient) and societal or utilitarian (do the best for the whole patient population) principles.

Most HMOs use positive and negative incentives to ensure compliance with treatment or investigation guidelines; in one survey, 17 per cent of doctors thought these were so restrictive that they were harmful to patient care (Grumbach *et al.* 1998). In another survey (Sulmasy *et al.* 2000), only 17 per cent thought that incentives to doctors to limit patient access were ethically acceptable and only 6 per cent that it was acceptable to hide such incentives from patients.

There has been only limited similar work in European countries where the nature of the health services and views on the balance between individual and collective welfare may differ. It may be, for instance, that in a cash-limited public service, patients are more accepting of implicit rationing. Bateman *et al.* (1996), in their study of incentive schemes in the UK, noted that a number of GPs thought the schemes were unethical. Similar responses were common in the early days of GP fundholding, and in both cases represent a limited view of the aims of the schemes as being to limit health care utilization rather than to make more efficient use of resources. The GPs who expressed such views cannot be blamed for this – the aims of the schemes were often not clearly stated and in practice, both at health authority level and in practices, the emphasis was often on cash saving rather than on using the savings to enhance other services. This was, in turn, the result of the tight budgets and regular overspends where instead of expanding services, savings disappeared just to keep the *status quo*. An Irish study suggested that patients were far more interested to know about the incentive scheme than doctors were to tell them (Walley *et al.* 2001).

The issues here are important. Clearly the US doctors were disturbed in part by the ethical implications but perhaps also by loss of personal and professional autonomy. In the UK, the dilemma is not dissimilar to that experienced by doctors within a primary care trust, where expensive treatment for one patient may limit treatments for others. The degree of loss of autonomy is less severe than that experienced by some of the US doctors, and the societal ethic is perhaps better established in the UK NHS than in the fragmented US system. There are, of course, also social, cultural and legal differences between the systems. This area has not been well explored in Europe and warrants further work. In the meantime, it is important to make any incentives transparent to all stakeholders (as required in some US states by law), and possibly to limit the risk of individual patient harm and excessive enthusiasm by an individual doctor by using collective rather than individual incentives, even though these may be less effective.

Conclusions

Incentives have considerable power to change prescribing practice. Incentives that are personal and individual are more effective but probably less acceptable professionally or ethically than group incentives. Incentives could be rewards or penalties. In practice, the penalties have been more difficult to enforce. Incentives could be used to contain cost alone, but never by inhibiting clinically acceptable behaviour. Incentives can be better used to reward or encourage good performance. The most effective incentives are simple to understand and achievable. Incentives are most effective at changing the detail rather than the broad thrust of clinical practice – that is, what a doctor prescribes rather than whether a doctor prescribes.

The nature of incentives range from the UK approach – almost all incentive and almost no disincentive – to the punitive approach taken by the Germans and increasingly by the French. Cynically, it might be argued that any interference with doctors' salaries is very influential, but the British experience argues that GPs are interested in the power to use resources innovatively for the benefit of their patients, and that reducing prescribing is seen professionally as an acceptable way to free up the necessary resources. However, there are dangers in such incentives, which must be transparent and carefully monitored lest they promote perverse results, such as increased referral of patients to hospitals, thus shifting costs away from the physician's budget but increasing overall health care costs. The cheaper therapies may not necessarily be more cost-effective in the long term. Further study of the clinical outcomes of patients in such schemes is needed.

References

Ashworth, M., Golding, S., Shepherd, L., Majeed, A. and Sullivan, F. (2002) Prescribing incentive schemes in two NHS regions: cross sectional survey. Commentary: Prescribing incentive schemes – more evidence is needed of how they work, *British Medical Journal*, 324: 1187–8.
Audit Commission (1994) *A Prescription for Improvement: Towards More Rational Prescribing in General Practice*. London: HMSO.

Bateman, D.N., Campbell, M., Donaldson, L.J., Roberts, S.J. and Smith, J.M. (1996) A prescribing incentive scheme for non-fundholding general practices: an observational study, *British Medical Journal*, 313: 535–8.

Busse, R. (2000) *Health Care Systems in Transition: Germany*. Copenhagen: European Observatory on Health Care Systems.

Busse, R. and Howerth, C. (1999) Cost containment in Germany: twenty years experience, in E. Mossialos and J. Le Grand (eds) *Health Care and Cost Containment in the European Union*. Aldershot: Ashgate.

Chaix-Couturier, C., Durand-Zaleski, I., Jolly, D. and Durieux, P. (2000) Effects of financial incentives on medical practice: results from a systematic review of the literature and methodological issues, *International Journal for Quality in Health Care*, 12: 133–42.

CNAMTS (2001) *Les médicaments remboursés par le régime d'Assurance maladie au cours du premier semestre 1999 et du premier semestre 2000 (MEDICAM)*. Paris: CNAMTS.

Delnoij, D. and Brenner, G. (2000) Importing budget systems from other countries: what can we learn from the German drug budget and the British GP fundholding?, *Health Policy*, 52: 157–69.

Department of Health (1990) *Improving Prescribing*. London: HMSO.

Dietrich, E.S. (2000) Arzneimitteldaten: das Drama der späten Lieferung. *Deutsches Ärzteblatt*, 97: A3321.

Donatini, A., Rico, A., D'Ambrosio, M.G. *et al.* (2001) *Health Care Systems in Transition: Italy*. Copenhagen: European Observatory on Health Care Systems.

Durieux, P., Chaix-Couturier, C., Durand-Zaleski, I. and Ravaud, P. (2000a) From clinical recommendations to mandatory practice: the introduction of regulatory practice guidelines in the French healthcare system, *International Journal of Technology Assessment in Health Care*, 16: 969–75.

Durieux, P., Gaillac, B., Giraudeau, B., Doumenc, M. and Ravaud, P. (2000b) Despite financial penalties, French physicians' knowledge of regulatory practice guidelines is poor, *Archives of Family Medicine*, 9: 414–18.

Fattore, G. and Jommi, C. (1998) The new pharmaceutical policy in Italy. *Health Policy*, 46(1): 21–41.

Gosden, T. and Torgerson, D.J. (1997) The effect of fundholding on prescribing and referral costs: a review of the evidence, *Health Policy*, 40: 103–14.

Grumbach, K., Osmond, D., Vranizan, K., Jaffe, D. and Bindman, A.B. (1998) Primary care physicians' experience of financial incentives in managed-care systems, *New England Journal of Medicine*, 339: 1516–21.

Harris, C.M. and Scrivener, G. (1996) Fundholders' prescribing costs: the first five years, *British Medical Journal*, 313: 1531–4.

Hillman, A.L. (1990) Health maintenance organizations, financial incentives, and physicians' judgments, *Annals of Internal Medicine*, 112: 891–3.

Jacker, A. (2000) Alternativen zu Arzneimittelbudgets, *Pharmazeutische Industrie*, 62(10): 740–43.

Junger, C., Rathmann, W. and Gianni, C. (2000) Prescribing behavior of primary care physicians in diabetes therapy: effect of drug budgeting, *Deutsche Medizinische Wochenschrift*, 125: 103–9.

Korzilius, H. (2001) Arzneimittelbudget: die Zeit danach, *Deutsches Ärzteblatt*, 98: A2844.

Lopez-Bastida, J. and Mossialos, E. (2000) Pharmaceutical expenditure in Spain: cost and control, *International Journal of Health Services Research*, 30: 597–616.

Majeed, A., Evans, N. and Head, P. (1997) What can PACT tell us about prescribing in general practice, *British Medical Journal*, 315: 1515–19.

Mason, A., Towse, A., Drummond, M. and Cooke, J. (2003) *Influencing Prescribing in Primary Care Led NHS*. London: Office of Health Economics.

Matsaganis, M. and Glennerster, H. (1994) The threat of 'cream skimming' in the post-reform NHS, *Journal of Health Economics*, 13: 31–60.

MMW (2001) Erhebliche Defizite bei der Arzneimittelversorgung. *MMW-Fortschritte der Medizin*, 143: 43.

Mossialos, E. and Le Grand, J. (eds) (1999) *Health Care and Cost Containment in the European Union*. Aldershot: Ashgate.

Presse- und Informationsamt der Bundersregierung (2002) *Sozialpolitische Umschau*. Berlin: Presse- und Informationsamt der Bundersregierung.

Sandier, S., Polton, D. and Paris, V. (2003) *Health Care Systems in Transition: France*. Copenhagen: European Observatory on Health Care Systems.

Schoffski, O. and Graf von der Schulenburg, J.M. (1997) Unintended effects of a cost-containment policy: results of a natural experiment in Germany, *Social Science and Medicine*, 45: 1537–9.

Sperschneider, T. and Kleinert, S. (2002) Germany's sick health-care system, *Lancet*, 360: 1758.

Sulmasy, D.P., Bloche, M.G., Mitchell, J.M. and Hadley, J. (2000) Physicians' ethical beliefs about cost-control arrangements, *Archives of Internal Medicine*, 160: 649–57.

Tobin, M.D. and Packham, C.J. (1999) Can primary care groups learn how to manage demand from fundholders? A study of fundholders in Nottingham, *British Journal of General Practice*, 49: 291–4.

Walley, T., Murphy, M., Codd, M., Johnston, Z. and Quirke, T. (2000) Effects of a monetary incentive on primary care prescribing in Ireland: changes in prescribing patterns in one health board 1990–1995, *Pharmacoepidemiology and Drug Safety*, 9: 591–8.

Walley, T., Murphy, M., Codd, M., Johnston, Z. and Quirke, T. (2001) Effects of a monetary incentive on primary care prescribing in Ireland: attitudes and perceptions of health care professionals and patients, *European Journal of General Practice*, 7: 92–8.

Weltermann, B., Martin, C., Adl, S. *et al.* (1997) Prescribing practice for beta blockers at patient discharge to ambulatory care: a health care economic evaluation in a cardiology patient sample with special reference to drug budgeting, *Gesundheitswesen*, 59: 258–61.

Wilson, R.P., Hatcher, J., Barton, S. and Walley, T. (1997) General practice fundholders' prescribing savings in one region of the United Kingdom, 1991–1994, *Health Policy*, 42: 29–37.

chapter eleven

Regulating pharmaceutical distribution and retail pharmacy in Europe

David Taylor, Monique Mrazek and Elias Mossialos

Introduction

Medicines distribution spans the links in the pharmaceutical 'value chain' between manufacturers and patients (Figure 11.1). The primary actors in this process are wholesalers, as well as pharmacists working in community and hospital settings. This chapter focuses on wholesaling and community pharmacy, and the multifaceted sets of regulation that govern what those employed in these areas do, how and where they do it, and how they are remunerated.

The present pharmaceutical distribution system allows almost everyone in Western Europe (the focus of this chapter) reasonable access to modern medicines, and advice about their safe use. Yet from an analytical perspective, key questions to be addressed relate to the extent to which current regulations serve to inhibit or promote competition in this sector, and whether or not this benefits or imposes needless costs on consumers. Developing understanding of this requires comparative data on the costs and quality of both medicines distribution and pharmaceutical care (Hepler and Strand 1990) in different countries, and insight into the tensions inherent in the role of community pharmacists as both private retailers and health professionals expected to work increasingly closely with other clinicians in the delivery of well-integrated health care in European Union (EU) countries. Other core questions relate to:

- the continuing evolution of pharmaceutical and other relevant technologies such as information and communications technology (ICT) based therapeutic decision support, prescription/dispensing monitoring and patient record systems, and the ways in which individuals, health care systems and

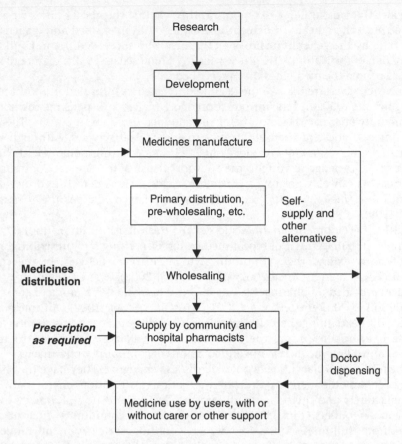

Figure 11.1   The pharmaceutical value chain.

communities learn to use established and innovative treatments to best effect;

● the nature of the economic incentives created for actors in the medicines supply chain by regulatory provisions affecting factors such as pharmacy ownership, medicine prices and dispensing fees;

● the abilities required by patients and other pharmaceutical distribution chain customers to make informed choices, and so drive service improvement through competition as opposed to regulation; and

● the political, social and financial forces that contribute to regulatory innovation or stasis.

There are about 120,000 community pharmacies across the EU (Paterson *et al.* 2003b), which supply in the order of 80 per cent by volume and value of all pharmaceuticals used in member states. Throughout most of mainland Europe, the historic role of pharmacists in ensuring the safe manufacture and supply of medicines has traditionally been separate from the part played by the medical profession in diagnosing illness and determining treatment. English experience provides the most notable exception to this, via first the apothecaries who, in the eighteenth and early nineteenth centuries, both prescribed and dispensed, and then by the general medical practitioners who succeeded them. Until the formation of the National Health Service (NHS) in the late 1940s, many English GPs dispensed the medicines they prescribed.

However, given trends like the decline of medicines formulation in pharmacies since the 1950s and the introduction of original pack dispensing, the role of community pharmacists is now being re-examined throughout Europe. There is growing awareness of their ability to provide clinical services. Although still sometimes seen as 'merely retailers' outside hospital settings, pharmacists have extensive knowledge relating to the appropriate use of medicines. Community pharmacists can play an important role in fields such as detecting drug interactions and side-effects and facilitating appropriate medicines use (Chamba *et al.* 1999).

Further developments in areas such as the treatment of minor illnesses and pharmacist management of repeat medication dispensing and prescribing may significantly extend their contribution to health care delivery in the coming decade (Cabinet Office 2002; Watson *et al.* 2002). There is evidence that services provided by pharmacists can improve outcomes in a range of contexts (Anderson 2000, Bernsten *et al.* 2001; Kansanaho *et al.* 2002). Although the debate over extending their clinical role is beyond the scope of this chapter, it is relevant to understanding the significance of regulatory provisions such as those controlling the ownership and locations of community pharmacies.

The role of pharmaceutical wholesalers is also changing. They have traditionally been 'middle-men' in the pharmaceutical distribution chain, between manufacturers and pharmacists, dispensing doctors and non-pharmacy over-the-counter outlets. Most medicines dispensed by community pharmacists come from 'full-line' wholesalers, which continuously carry a full range of products. But other types of wholesaler include 'pre-wholesalers' (agencies acting for pharmaceutical producers who need support in supplying bulk orders to wholesalers), short-line wholesalers carrying just a selected product range, and parallel importers operating within the EU's borders.

The lines between manufacturers, wholesalers and community pharmacies become blurred in cases where there is vertical integration between them. With increasing consolidation and competition, questions like those relating to the size of wholesalers' margins become progressively more complex. As in other areas of the pharmaceutical market, the distribution of medicines in the EU is controlled by an intricate web of supranational and national regulations, together with requirements of local professional bodies and health service payers and providers. The specifics of legislation differ between the member states. But the activities covered include trading in medicines, their labelling and the maintenance of records, which, in part, serve to facilitate product recalls when necessary. There are also regulations on whether a medicine should be supplied with or without a prescription, by whom and to whom.

The primary objective of regulating pharmaceutical distribution is conventionally taken to be to protect the public's interests in safety and access to medicines. The secondary, sometimes conflicting, aims of regulation include: protecting private interests (and the financial viability or operational integrity of pharmacies and wholesalers); promoting service/care quality; limiting distribution and overall pharmaceutical costs; and promoting increased consumer choice.

As a professional group, community pharmacy has long sought to maintain a strong monopoly over the supply of both prescribed and over-the-counter medicines, to control the number and location of pharmacies, and to confine pharmacy ownership to its members. In much of Europe, only pharmacists can purchase or establish pharmacies, and in many instances a pharmacist cannot own or be responsible for more than one pharmacy. Such regulations inhibit the formation of large managed pharmacy chains such as those most typically found in the UK and North America. This may to an extent protect the public's interests in professional care standards. However, it might also serve to protect 'rent-seeking' by wholesalers and pharmacy owners through inhibiting competition, and so increase prices and restrict consumer choice (Philipsen and Faure 2002).

The wholesaling sector

There has been significant consolidation of pharmaceutical wholesalers in Europe in the last decade, affecting not only the distribution of market share but also the strategic orientation of the surviving firms. In 2001, there were 346 wholesalers providing a full-line service in the EU (GIRP 2002; Harris 2002; Long 2002) compared with approximately 600 in the early 1990s (Macarthur 1996a); of the latter, 70 per cent were based in Italy and Spain. In France, for instance, there were over 150 wholesalers at the start of the 1960s, compared with 13 regional and national full-line suppliers in 2002.

The impact of this process has been such that in many EU member states two-thirds or more of the market is now supplied by the three largest wholesalers operating in the locality concerned. In 2003, the actual percentages varied from about 40 per cent in Spain and Italy, a little over 60 per cent in Germany, 75 per cent in France and 85 per cent in the UK (Long 2002). The German company Gehe (now Celesio AG) alone in 2002 distributed over 20 per cent of the €80 billion worth of pharmaceuticals consumed in the EU. Such concentration suggests that further consolidation could, in an increasing number of instances, be limited by competition policy.

Three other major wholesalers also operate at a pan-European level: Pheonix, Tamro and Alliance Unichem. National level examples of important wholesalers include Alliance Santé in France, OPG and Brocacef in the Netherlands, Kronans Droghandel in Sweden, and Alleanza Salute Italia and Adivar in Italy. The latter has been unusual in being directly owned by a pharmaceutical manufacturer, Angelini. Recently, the European Court of Justice has become involved in instances where individual drug companies have sought to establish exclusive supply arrangements with individual wholesalers.

Although major wholesalers purchase both generic and branded (including patented) pharmaceuticals throughout the EU and as legally permitted from other sources, relationships between pharmacists and wholesalers are normally conducted within national boundaries. That is, even in the case of transnational pharmaceutical wholesalers, pharmacy customers in any one state are normally supplied via the locally based subsidiary. This is not least because of differing controls on product price mark-ups. With the exception of the Netherlands and Denmark (in Denmark it is illegal for wholesalers to offer discounts to pharmacies, while in the former wholesalers' margins are determined by market forces), all European countries impose limits on drug wholesalers' margins, either via statutorily defined mechanisms or through established practice with the public health care sector. Permitted wholesaler margins vary significantly between EU states (LIF 2002), although differences in discounting to pharmacies (plus local VAT policies) to a degree reduce the apparent disparities. Table 11.1 provides an overview of EU medicine pricing and spending levels.

As described in Chapter 6, there has been an increase in parallel importing across the EU. Initially, wholesalers in countries such as Germany were reluctant to take part in this trade, for fear of both driving down overall earnings and harming relationships with pharmaceutical companies. Parallel importing remains opposed by pharmaceutical industry-related interests, and recent action in the European Court of Justice has challenged the ability of the European Commission to force pharmaceutical manufacturers in Europe to supply unlimited volumes of medicines to companies known to be involved in parallel exportation (Olswang 2001). But parallel trading in medicine is now well established and involves many, if not all, the main European wholesalers.

Providing a full-line pharmaceutical wholesaling service entails overcoming major logistical challenges, because of the volume of product presentations and active substances available. For example, in Norway (which has traditionally had the most restricted range of medicines available in Western Europe) the

Table 11.1 Medicine retail price structures and overall costs in EU member states

Country	VAT (% price)	Pharmacy (% price)	Wholesaler (% price)	Manufacturer (% price)	Pharmaceutical expenditure, % GDP (year)
Austria	16.7	24.1	7.5	51.8	1.3 (1999)
Belgium	5.7	29.2	8.5	56.6	1.4 (1997)
Denmark	20	23.4	4.1	52.5	0.8 (2000)
Finland	7.4	26.6	2.6	63.3	1.0 (2000)
France	5.2	26.2	3.8	64.8	1.9 (2000)
Germany	13.8	27.3	7.7	51.2	1.3 (1998)
Greece	7.4	24	5.5	63.1	1.5 (2000)
Ireland	0.0	33	10.1	57	0.6 (2000)
Italy	9.1	20.4	6.7	63.8	1.9 (2001)
Luxembourg	2.9	30.9	8.7	57.5	0.7 (1999)
Netherlands	5.7	20.2	10.8	63.4	1.0 (2000)
Portugal	4.8	19	8.4	67.8	2.0 (1998)
Spain	3.8	26.8	6.7	62.7	1.4 (1997)
Sweden	0.0	20	2.4	77.6	1.0 (1997)
UK	0.0	17.3	10.3	72.4	1.1 (1997)

Source: Paterson *et al.* (2003b).

number of drug presentations (prescription and over-the-counter) supplied was about 4000 in the mid-1990s. They contained around 800 active substances. The equivalent figures for Germany were 70,000 and more than 3000, respectively. At the same time, there are in any one region or country hundreds if not thousands of pharmacy outlets to be served, each of which will normally expect to order and receive medicines at least twice a day.

In some EU countries, short-line wholesalers offer pharmacists a limited range of products at competitive prices. One effect of this is likely to have been to accelerate consolidation in the full-line sector. However, where there is a perceived public interest in obliging all wholesalers to offer a full-line service, as in France and Italy, short-line wholesalers are prohibited. A system of primary pharmaceutical stockholders (depositaries) supplying secondary national and regional wholesalers has evolved in France and Italy to allow the latter to meet full-line service obligations.

Wholesaling developments in Europe have in the last few decades been driven by the pursuit of economies of scale associated with the rationalization of warehousing facilities, computerization and the use of electronic record-keeping and data interchange systems for ordering medicines and optimizing stocks. This is relevant from a regulatory policy viewpoint because the market power and competencies of the surviving wholesalers have been strengthened, and they are now in a position to take a stronger leadership role in the overall pharmaceutical distribution chain.

Vertical integration between wholesalers and established pharmaceutical companies in Europe has often been prohibited under national regulation because of the perceived need for objectivity in the drug purchasing–pharmacy supply relationship. However, where regulations permit integration between wholesalers and pharmacies, it has become a common strategic response by the former to consolide and decrease margins in their sector. It can allow advantages such as opportunities to develop self-produced or especially contracted 'own brand' lines in relatively protected settings, and to balance earnings at each point along the pharmaceutical product distribution chain from manufacture to endpoint sale.

One example of a long-standing vertically integrated company is Boots The Chemist, which combines capabilities in manufacturing, medicines purchasing, distribution and retailing within a single organization. In the UK, Boots owns over 1100 pharmacy outlets. It has a gross annual turnover of €7.5 billion. Another key example is that of the wholesaler Gehe/Celesio. It owns 1750 pharmacies across Europe, in large part as a result of its acquisition of the Lloyds group in the UK in the 1990s.

Recent legal changes in Norway (and Iceland) have permitted the vertical integration of pharmacy chains owned by wholesaling companies there (Anell and Hjelmgren 2002), although the Norwegian legislation sets a limit on the percentage of the pharmacy market that can be controlled by any one company. Elsewhere in Europe, pharmacists combine together in various voluntary ways to gain some of the advantages of 'chaining' without sacrificing the principle of individual pharmacy ownership. For example, Plus Pharmacie (which was originally organized by a major wholesaler) acts as a purchasing group in France, while in Belgium there is a relatively strong tradition of social/cooperative ownership of both pharmacies and wholesalers by Mutuelles. Against this, the Netherlands has tried to weaken the previously close relationship (the so-called 'golden chain') between manufacturers, wholesalers and pharmacists by decreasing the maximum reimbursement price through a reference price scheme, and consequently reducing the size of the discounts along the distribution chain (de Vos 1996).

Community pharmacy

The average populations served by community pharmacies in Western European states in 2001 are shown in Figure 11.2. In most European countries, community pharmacists outnumber their hospital colleagues by between 12 : 1 (Belgium, Denmark) and 25 : 1 (Spain, Germany). In the Netherlands and the UK, this ratio is about 6 : 1. In population per pharmacy terms, Southern European nations have more pharmacies than those of the north, although in countries like Denmark, Sweden and Norway the figures normally quoted do not include branch pharmacies and other prescription distribution points.

In the Scandinavian countries and the Netherlands, qualified pharmacy staff other than pharmacists play a more important role in dispensing over-the-counter and prescription medicines than that currently permitted elsewhere in

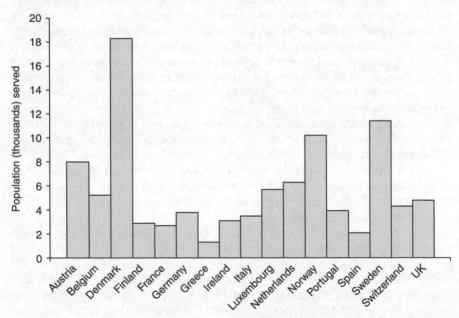

Figure 11.2   Population served by an average community pharmacy in Western European countries, 2001 (from Macarthur and Grubert, 2002; based on GIRP and OECD data).

the EU. They work with greater autonomy, which permits pharmacists to delegate more work and may, for example, allow them to leave their premises to undertake other tasks while medicines are being dispensed.

There are direct regulations on pharmacists to population ratios in many European nations. Restrictions on GP/doctor dispensing, which is more prevalent in Switzerland, the Netherlands and the UK than other parts of Europe, represent another key form of intervention. Box 11.1 provides further information on the diverse patterns of EU member state controls on pharmaceutical distribution.[1] Additional relevant regulatory measures relate to the management of pharmacies and their branches, the extent of the immediate pharmacist involvement required in dispensing prescription medicines and selling over-the-counter products, and the ability of pharmacists to practise in member states other than those where they obtained their qualification.

The comparison of pharmacy service provision in France and the UK offered in Box 11.2 highlights differences that reflect not only high rates of medicines consumption in France, but also the impact of national regulations on pharmacy ownership. Similar controls on pharmacy ownership are in place in Germany. Some 40 per cent of all pharmacies in the EU in 2001 were located in France and Germany.

Elsewhere in Europe, the chaining of pharmacies is tending to become more prevalent. Norway has already been referred to, and chaining is also permitted in varying forms and to varying degrees in Belgium, Ireland, Italy, the Netherlands and the UK. Since deregulation, the population to pharmacy ratio in Norway has decreased. The only remaining restriction on pharmacy locations is that they must be physically separated from the prescribing practice (Mossialos and Mrazek 2003).

In the Netherlands, strong relationships exist between pharmacies and dominant local insurers. These may help to ensure continuity of patient care, but also act as a barrier to market entry for new pharmacies. There are also differences across the EU in terms of where and how medicines can be sold. In Denmark, Germany, the Netherlands, Norway and the UK, some non-prescription medicines are available outside licensed pharmacies in locations such as drug stores, ordinary retail shops and supermarkets. The development of mail order and online pharmacies is another factor that has a significant potential to impact on pharmacy service structures and medicine costs.

The most significant developments in this last context have taken place in Switzerland (with the formation of companies such as Apotheke zur Rose, www.aporose.ch, and Apotheke Schweiz, www.apotheke-schweiz.ch), the UK (www.pharmacy2u.co.uk) and the Netherlands (www.0800docmorris.com). DocMorris has sought to supply not only the Dutch market, but also (controversially) the larger German market. Most German health insurance funds favour mail order and online pharmacy as a way of lowering prescription expenditures.

But it is opposed by many pharmacists, whose representative bodies have sought to enforce legislation which demands that most medicines must be dispensed in a conventional pharmacy. A recent preliminary ruling by the European Court of Justice in the case of the Deutscher Apothekerverband versus DocMorris (by the Advocate General) suggested that banning the latter's mail

Box 11.1 The regulation of community pharmacy in EU member states

Field	*Regulatory approaches*
Pharmacy licensing, and contracting to provide reimbursable medicines	Pharmacies must be licensed in all EU and EFTA states. The agencies responsible for this range from the French Départements and German Länder through to the Inspectorate for Public Health in the Netherlands, the National Medicines Agency in Finland (and recently Norway), the national health departments of countries such as Belgium, Denmark and Portugal, and the Royal Pharmaceutical Society in Britain and the College of Pharmacists in Spain. In Sweden, the Apoteksbolaget (owned by the state and the Swedish Pharmaceutical Association) has since 1970 had total control of pharmaceutical supply. However, having a licence does not universally entitle a pharmacy to dispense medicines reimbursed by local or national health care providers. In the Netherlands, for instance, contracts have to be negotiated with health care insurers, whose attitudes may be influenced by pharmacists already providing services within the locality. In the UK, NHS authorities have since the late 1980s decided if it is in the public's interest that a new NHS dispensing contract should be granted.
Pharmacy numbers, and the location of new pharmacies	Germany is the largest European nation where pharmacists are free – subject to possible pressures from their professional peers – to open a new pharmacy in any locality where there is sufficient trade to support it. Elsewhere, there are national or (in the case of Sweden, the UK and Ireland) service criteria for regulating the number of pharmacies relative to population numbers and locality type. For instance, in Italy, towns with a population of less than 12,500 have one pharmacy for every 5000 people; larger towns are permitted one pharmacy per 4000 inhabitants.
Pharmacy ownership	Except in Belgium, Ireland, the Netherlands, Sweden (where all pharmacists are Apoteksbolaget employees) and the UK, only pharmacists or partnerships of pharmacists can own pharmacies. Similarly, in most of the EU, a pharmacist cannot own or be responsible for the operation of more than one pharmacy.
Selling pharmacies	In most EU states the sale of pharmacies is subject to restrictions, the most frequently occurring forms of which relate to the period for which they have been

open. For example, in France, Belgium and Austria, there normally has to be a 5-year period before sale is possible. In Italy, the equivalent period is 3 years and in Portugal it is 2 years. Luxembourg grants two types of pharmacy concession, transferable or non-transferable, while in Denmark pharmacies cannot be sold; when their owners reach 70, their licences expire and are reallocated by the Ministry of Health. When pharmacy owners die, the sale of pharmacies may, even where permissible, be subject to further regulation. For example, in Germany, a surviving spouse may retain the pharmacy until she [*sic*] remarries; the children may do so until their 23rd birthday. If the youngest child studies pharmacy, the transfer period may be extended until he [*sic*] completes his studies. In Greece, widows can retain a pharmacy for a period of up to 5 years; children may do so until they are aged 18.

Monopoly over the sale of pharmaceuticals and para-pharmaceutical products	In most EU member states, pharmacists retain a strong monopoly over the supply of not only prescribed but also veterinary and over-the-counter medicines and, in some cases, other para-pharmaceutical goods. France provides an example of a nation where this is particularly evident. At the other end of the spectrum, countries such as the Netherlands (which requires patients to register with individual pharmacies) allow less qualified druggists to supply a full range of over-the-counter medicines. There are more *drogisterij* (drug stores) in the Netherlands than pharmacies. In the UK, general sales list (GSL) over-the-counter medicines can be supplied by any retailer; only pharmacy (P) over-the-counter medicines have to be supplied under the supervision of a pharmacist. (In the USA, all over-the-counter medicines have the same status as UK GSL pharmaceuticals).
Advertising	Across Europe, the public advertising of prescription, as opposed to over-the-counter pharmaceuticals, is prohibited. But there are inconsistencies between which medicines are so classified between member states. There are in addition further controls on advertising of services and over-the-counter medicines by pharmacists in and outside their pharmacies in most member states, imposed by a range of statutory and professionally mediated mechanisms. The objectives of such interventions ostensibly relate to promoting public safety, but they may also serve to inhibit competition and curb demands for better treatment.

Box 11.2 Community pharmacy in France and the UK

In France, there are over 2500 people per community pharmacy. There are almost twice that number in the UK. Similarly, there are over 50,000 community pharmacists in France, compared with 30,000 (including significant numbers of part-time employees) in England. Because legislation prohibits multiple ownership of pharmacies in France while allowing it in the UK, there are some 27,000 pharmacist owners and co-owners of pharmacies in the former, compared with around 4000 individual and corporate owners in the UK. Other differences relate to the criteria that define whether a new pharmacy is permitted; the strength of the pharmacy monopoly over the sale of medicines and allied goods; the range of other non-pharmaceutical goods available in pharmacies; the system for reimbursing dispensed medicines; and the extent of community pharmacy competition.

The French market is characterized by one of the strongest monopolies over medicinal and para-pharmaceutical product supply in the world. There are statutory provisions dating back to the 1940s on when new pharmacy licences are allowed, and relatively high overall pharmacy earnings.

In the UK, NHS authorities have discretionary powers to decide on new pharmacy contracts permitting public reimbursement of dispensed prescriptions. However, UK competition authorities favour the removal of all such restrictions (Office of Fair Trading 2003). The NHS payment system penalizes pharmacists who do not purchase medicines as cheaply as possible (see main text). Other actors in the medicines supply chain are subject to similar pressures, and approaching 80 per cent of all NHS prescriptions are now written generically.

Independent pharmacy numbers are decreasing in the UK, which has the advantage of a low-cost system increasingly dominated by supermarkets and large chains with superior purchasing power. In France, where independent professional pharmacy service providers have been protected from both market competition and a monopsonist health care payer, there is a more costly but in some ways more respected and valued pharmacy service.

One possible interpretation of these observations is that the British regulatory system has defended public interests against those of pharmacy owners. It might alternatively be argued that the UK approach has served 'big pharmacy business' interests to a questionable degree, albeit that current NHS developments aimed at promoting integrated 'one-stop' centres, which combine medical, nursing and pharmaceutical services and free pharmacists to spend more time on clinical care rather than dispensing, appear set to change radically the community pharmacy business model.

order service outright will not be judged in the European public interest, provided that regulations on medicines advertising to the public have not been broken and the company is providing appropriately authorized treatments (European Commission 2003).

The payment of pharmacists, generic substitution and cost control

Community pharmacists have a potentially important role to play in controlling pharmaceutical expenditures through dispensing (or persuading prescribers to select) the cheapest multi-sourced (generic) medicine available (see Chapter 14). In many EU countries, generic medicine dispensing is allowed only if the prescription is written using the generic name of the product. Use of lower-cost generic products is a direct requirement in some states, but is more typically promoted through financial incentives. In Denmark, for example, pharmacists are required to substitute the least expensive reference priced product to stay within their permitted dispensing budgets. In Germany, pharmacists are in appropriate circumstances required to dispense from the lowest-cost one-third of available generic versions.

In the Netherlands and the UK, as in Ireland and Sweden, pharmacists are paid a fixed fee per item dispensed. In the case of the British NHS, pharmacists are additionally reimbursed a fixed amount to meet the ingredient cost of each type of medicine dispensed. This offers them an incentive to demand discounts from wholesalers. A simultaneous scheme operates to 'claw back' (on an averaged basis) some of the profits that the pharmacists accrue from this. Those with high medicine purchasing costs relative to other pharmacies with a similar dispensing volume are penalized.

The Netherlands also operates a form of profit claw-back on pharmacists' earnings from drug price discounts. But if a cheaper product from a reference price cluster is dispensed, the pharmacist can charge the insurance fund one-third of the difference between the reference price and the retail price of the dispensed product, on top of the fixed dispensing fee. Since 1990, France has had a 'smooth declining margin'. The permitted pharmacy mark-up declines for each successive increase in the price of each medicine provided. This partly de-links the level of the pharmacy mark-up from the price of the prescribed drug. French pharmacists have also, from 1998, been entitled to a beneficial margin for dispensing from an official list of substitutable generics.

In other EU countries (Austria, Germany, Belgium, Finland, Greece, Italy, Portugal and Spain), pharmacists' profits are normally directly linked to the price of the product dispensed. This makes it attractive to supply more expensive medicines. To the extent that regulatory and linked remuneration schemes give pharmacists and/or other professionals a perverse incentive to use higher cost medicines (or, alternatively, as with some reference price schemes, effectively impose 'price floors'; Puig-Junoy 2003), questions exist as to why such arrangements continue to exist in many parts of the EU.

Analysis: the future of pharmaceutical supply and its regulation in the EU

A recent analysis of the economics of four liberal professions, one of which was community pharmacy, in the EU member states concluded that economic benefits tend to be gained by highly regulated professions at the expense of consumer welfare (Paterson *et al.* 2003a). The findings of this major study were in respect of pharmacy less clear-cut than those drawn in some other contexts – complicating factors range from the extent to which other controls limit pharmaceutical costs to a lack of meaningful data on pharmaceutical care quality. However, it highlighted concerns that high levels of regulation inhibit competition between pharmacies and restrict opportunities for mergers or new forms of service provision (such as supermarket-based pharmacies), which might benefit some sections of the public.

Despite the fact that increased pharmacy sector competition might also reduce service levels to other, perhaps more vulnerable, members of the community, policy makers across Europe appear to be becoming increasingly convinced of its potential advantages. Perhaps in part because of the dramatically expanded range of medicines that has become available to treat illnesses in the past 50 years, community pharmacy has remained relatively unchanged in recent decades. By contrast, since the 1960s pharmaceutical wholesaling has emerged as an increasingly dynamic force in the pharmaceutical supply chain. Mergers in this sector appear likely to continue, nationally and trans-nationally. Notwithstanding current and possible future regulatory changes applying to pharmaceutical pricing and the ownership and operation of hospital and community pharmacies, such a trend may well have a major impact on other parts of the medicines supply and value-adding chain.

Assuming controls permit it, integrated wholesaler and community pharmacy service companies are likely to grow further. New or enlarged mail order 'clicks and mortar' cross-border pharmacy operations will also emerge. Combined with other developments in the health sector, this may eventually cause the established business model underpinning community pharmacy to cease to be viable.

In some EU contexts, a combination of new government policies, changing professional aspirations and rising public expectations (regarding not only health care, but also the maintenance of good health) could be sufficient to drive a major transition in the role of community pharmacy towards a more clinical orientation in the next five to ten years (Taylor and Carter 2002). In the case of the UK, restrictions on medical manpower availability, coupled with both a political desire to improve NHS service delivery and increased public funding for health care, could help facilitate such a change.

However, across Europe as a whole there are many factors inhibiting progress in such directions. In addition to high levels of surplus medical manpower in some countries, they include:

1 The nature of the logistical and economic challenges involved in safely supplying 5 billion plus individual prescription items a year (calculation based on Office of Health Economics 2003) to the European population, and

facilitating appropriate self-medication. Although the use of robotic dispensing machines and home delivery services may reduce costs at the margin, there will still be considerable demand for face-to-face pharmaceutical advice and care. In the foreseeable future, the fixed costs of the latter will remain significant, regardless of any apparent savings made in the distribution of selected types of medicine to selected groups of patients. Similarly, the costs of training and deploying new types of dispensing labour and extending pharmacists' education and training will also be considerable.

2 The fact that the current forms of pharmacy service found across the EU (for example, the Scandinavian approach, the Dutch and British models, southern European pharmacy) are deeply embedded in local cultural structures, and broader health care provisions. This in itself generates resistance to change, and can conceal differences in approaches to service provision that are greater than is commonly understood. For example, regulations relating to the supply of prescription-only medicines by pharmacists appear to have been more strictly enforced in northern Europe than in parts of Southern Europe. Pharmacists there have *de facto* been able to provide a wider health care service than strictly imposed regulatory controls would have permitted.

3 The strength of the professional and allied bodies that protect existing pharmacy interests. Pharmacy worldwide has a long history as a self-regulating profession, and well-developed capabilities in fields such as lobbying in Brussels and the individual member states. In practice, this means that pharmacy owners and other established groups are better represented than young and/or employee pharmacists. This by itself represents a significant barrier to 'transformational' changes in regulation and service delivery. In instances where the interests of community pharmacy establishments coincide with those of other groups, such as national or international pharmaceutical manufacturers, the resultant synergies may have particular political potency and could partly explain apparent regulatory perversities.

4 Lack of consistent public pressure for better pharmacy services, and of a coherent political vision of how pharmaceutical and other forms of health care should in the future be improved. There appears to be a growing consensus that all forms of medicine use and healthy living demand significant self-care skills, and that pharmacists are well placed to move on from traditional models of professional care towards establishing equal, supportive rather than infantilizing relationships with service users. In countries like Canada, where there are established examples of innovations such as community pharmacy access to service user health/medication records and on-line remuneration systems, pharmacy service providers have arguably already moved some way towards this end. Nevertheless, paternalistic attitudes still dominate many Europeean decision-making bodies. An apparent concern for public safety and protection could on occasions conceal a desire to preserve the *status quo*, and to inhibit developments that might in fact benefit community pharmacy service users.

Given such realities, together with variables such as the desire of member states to retain individual competencies in the area of health care, the most probable prospect for the future of pharmacy service regulation is one of piecemeal evolution rather than dramatic revolution. This prospect is also made likely by the fact that even if relatively rapid reform were to prove practically possible in the near future, the level of evidence available makes it difficult to calculate which types of change would ultimately prove to be in the European public's best interests.

Simplistic assumptions about the extent to which less regulated competition would or would not be desirable should be avoided. Bias in either direction is undesirable. For example, analyses linking the levels of competition and market concentration in wholesaling and/or community pharmacy and the prices paid by consumers or communities for over-the-counter or prescription medicines should not be accepted uncritically. This is not least because the relationships between such factors and others like public health improvement rates are in many parts of Europe mediated by a complex set of social and political variables associated with the expression of social solidarity. Increased competition might serve to undermine the latter, so that the unintended consequences of policy changes designed to improve access to affordable medicines might ultimately outweigh their benefits to poorer service users.

Additional concerns range from the extent to which 'pharmaceutical literacy' can be achieved in the general population to anticipated trends towards more individually tailored preventive as well as curative therapeutic approaches. It also remains to be demonstrated that were, for example, profit-driven, vertically integrated wholesaler/pharmacy chains and other large retail organizations to gain control of most of the pharmaceutical distribution chain, how far they would in practice strive to minimize costs to consumers, and be motivated to provide better pharmaceutical care for groups like older, less affluent health service users who now represent the main users of modern medicines.

Nevertheless, in the final analysis a regulatory strategy for pharmaceutical supply that aims to combine the advantages of scale in pharmaceutical wholesaling and competitive consumer retailing with the benefits of professionally delivered personal care may be able to offer medicine (and health service) users further value. Seen from this perspective, an ideal European pharmaceutical supply future might pragmatically conflate the expertise found in companies such as Celesio, Boots and other successful health care and consumer goods and services providers with some of the safeguards for independent professional excellence embedded in current community pharmacy regulations in countries such as France and the Netherlands. Achieving this is in time likely to involve reductions rather than increases in the volume and extent of regulatory controls imposed on the ownership and operation of community pharmacies.

Note

1   Information on pharmacy regulation across Europe is available from the European Commission and organizations such as the Groupement Pharmaceutique de l'Union Europeenne (www.pgeu.org; European Commission 2002).

References

Anderson, C. (2000) Health promotion in community pharmacy: the UK situation, *Patient Education and Counselling*, 39: 285–91.

Anell, A. and Hjelmgren, J. (2002) Implementing competition in the pharmacy sector: lessons from Iceland and Norway, *Applied Health Economics and Health Policy*, 1(3): 149–56.

Bernsten, C., Bjorkman, I., Caramona, M. *et al.* (2001) Improving the well-being of elderly patients via community pharmacy-based provision of pharmaceutical care: a multi-centre study in seven European countries, *Drugs and Aging*, 18(1): 63–77.

Cabinet Office UK (2002) *Making a Difference: General Practitioners Report*, June. Regulatory Impact Unit, Public Sector Team (available from http://www.cabinet-office.gov.uk/regulation/PublicSector/ReducingGPPaperwork2.pdf).

Chamba, G., Bauguil, G. and Gallezot, J. (1999) The role of the French community pharmacist in drug dispensing, *Pharmacy World and Service*, 21(3): 142–3.

de Vos, C.M. (1996) The 1996 pricing and reimbursement policy in the Netherlands, *Pharmacoeconomics*, 10(suppl.): 75–80.

European Commission (2002) *Conditions for the Operation of a Community Pharmacy in the Member States*. European Commission DG Internal Market Working Document XV/E/8115/4/97-EN.

European Commission (2003) Press Release No. 16/03: Opinion of Advocate General Stix-Hackl in Case C-322/01. Reference for a preliminary ruling in the case of *DeutscherApothekerverband e.V.* v. *0800 DocMorris NV and Jacques Waterval* (available from www.pict-pcti.org/news_archive/03/03Mar/ECJ_031103.htm) (accessed June 2003).

GIRP (2002) Available from www.girp.org (Accessed January 2003).

Harris, J. (2002) Presentation to the British Association of Pharmaceutical Wholesalers Conference, June 2002, Belfast. *Scrip Daily News Alert*, item 35309.

Hepler, C.D. and Strand, L.M. (1990) Opportunities and responsibilities in pharmaceutical care, *American Journal of Hospital Pharmacy*, 47: 533–43.

Kansanaho, H., Isonen-Sjolund, N., Pietila, K., Airaksinen, M. and Isonen, T. (2002) Patient counselling profile in a Finnish pharmacy, *Patient Education and Counselling*, 47: 77–82.

Lægemiddelindustriforeningen (LIF) (2002) *Tal and Data* (available from http://lif.albatros.dk/) (accessed 30 January 2003).

Long, D.M. (2002) Presentation to the International Federation of Pharmaceutical Wholesalers Conference, September 2002, Monaco (available from www.ifpw.com/2002GMM/presentations/).

Macarthur, D. (1996a) *Drug Distribution in Europe: Trends and Driving Forces*. Waltham, MA: Decision Resources Inc.

Macarthur, D. (1996b) Parallel trading of medicines: the case for a fair deal, *Consumer Policy Review*, 11(1): 6–10.

Macarthur, D. and Grubert, N. (2002) *Online Pharmacies in Europe: Current Situation, Future Prospects, and Possible Impact*. Spectrum Life Sciences Series. Waltham, MA: Decision Resources Inc.

Mossialos, E. and Mrazek, M. (2003) *The Regulation of Pharmacies in Six Countries*. London: Office of Fair Trading.

Office of Fair Trading UK (2003) *The Control of Entry Regulations and Retail Pharmacy Services to the UK: A Report of an OFT Market Investigation*, January. London: OFT (available from www.oft.gov.uk).

Office of Health Economics (2003) *Compendium of Health Statistics, 2002*. London: OHE.

Olswang (2001) Available from www.olswang.com/eu/legal_news/20010314_bayer.html (accessed June 2003).

Paterson, I., Fink, M., Ogus, A. *et al.* (2003a) *Economic Impact of Regulation in the Field of Liberal Professions in Different Member States. Final Report – Part 1*. Study for the European Commission. Vienna: Institute for Advanced Studies (HIS).

Paterson, I., Fink, M., Ogus, A. *et al.* (2003b) *Economic Impact of Regulation in the Field of Liberal Professions in Different Member States. Final Report – Part 2*. Study for the European Commission. Vienna: Institute for Advanced Studies (HIS).

Philipsen, N.J. and Faure, M.G. (2002) The regulation of pharmacists in Belgium and the Netherlands: in the public or private interest?, *Journal of Consumer Policy*, 25: 155–201.

Puig-Junoy, J. (2003) *Incentives for Pharmaceutical Reimbursement Reforms in Spain*. Barcelona: Research Centre for Health and Economics, Pompeu Fabra University.

Taylor, D.G. and Carter, S.L. (2002) *Realising the Promise: Community Pharmacy in the New NHS*. London: The School of Pharmacy, University of London, with the Social Market Foundation and the College of Health.

Watson, M.C., Bond, C.M., Grimshaw, J.M. *et al.* (2002) Educational strategies to promote evidence-based community pharmacy practice: a cluster randomised control trial, *Family Practice*, 19(5): 529–36.

twelve

Hospital pharmacies

Steve Hudson

The role of pharmacists and the function of hospital pharmacies

The developments in the field of hospital pharmacy internationally share common trends in the direction of services. These can be summarized as: initiatives in provision of medicines information as drug treatments have become more complex; participation in quality and cost control measures as treatment decisions have become grounded in the evidence base; and more patient-centred services as pharmacists seek to develop their role in individual patient care. These changes have occurred in various ways in different countries. There is a lack of specific information on particular initiatives in individual European countries, because many developments remain unpublished. Nevertheless, certain national trends affecting developments, such as structural changes in education and government endorsement of new roles of pharmacists, can be identified to highlight differences between countries.

Many of the services to support the better use of medicines offered by hospital pharmacies are common to most European countries. However, the extent of inclusion of the hospital pharmacist's role in individual patient care is most evident in the UK where the hospital pharmacist population is the largest in the European Union (EU) – some 20 per cent of the total pharmacist population compared with 4–7 per cent in most other EU countries (EAHP 2002). This demographic fact has the effect of providing the UK with a much wider range of models of clinical pharmacy services than other countries and the opportunity to start to research those models as developed services. Equally, in terms of the identification of best practice, it is likely that countries with smaller numbers of hospital pharmacists will have developed compensating alternative mechanisms for influencing the ways medicines are used in clinical areas. This chapter includes evidence from different EU countries, although detailed comparisons are outside the scope of the review. Since there is limited retrievable published data on services provided in different EU countries, the description of the role and function of the hospital pharmacy service draws from experience in the UK setting together with the author's recognition of some of the key distinctions in clinical service developments in the member countries of the EU. The foregoing description is intended to represent the common direction of hospital pharmacy services in the EU. Within this common direction, wherever pertinent, particular differences of approach among the EU countries will be identified.

Historical perspective

Up until perhaps two decades ago, there had been an expectation that hospital pharmacies should retain a large capability to manufacture medicines in bulk to meet specialized local requirements. The necessary manufacturing facilities have also traditionally been used for economic purposes to offer an alternative in-house source of bulk products such as disinfectants, topical medicines and infusions. This emphasis on preparation and quality assurance of product lines, which has traditionally also included certain dressings and other surgical items, has rooted the skill mix of the hospital pharmacy team in quality system procedures such as documentation and environmental control.

The past 30 years has seen a number of factors changing the role and function of hospital pharmacies. The increase in the sophistication and extent of use of the intravenous route has been mirrored by the shift of the bulk preparation of infusion fluids to the pharmaceutical industry. At the same time, the need for specialized products has emerged. That has created a very large demand for individually dispensed, aseptically prepared medicines – typically exemplified by intravenous nutrition cocktails of nutrients, electrolytes and vitamins. The use of such products, being prepared for individual patients, has led to the need for the pharmacist to build effective working relations with the end-users – in the case of intravenous nutrition products, that has included prescribers, nurses, dietitians and biochemists. Similar changes have occurred in the use of other medicines prepared aseptically, such as intravenous antimicrobial agents, anaesthetic and pressor agents in intensive care, analgesics and cytotoxic drugs. Each group of drugs that has placed special requirements on the traditional preparatory role of the hospital pharmacist has also created a need for closer working relations at ward level. The consequence has also been multidisciplinary collaboration with other clinical support services such as microbiology and biochemical laboratory scientists. These changes arising from an increased emphasis on providing products to suit individual patients' needs have occurred internationally, at the same time as the drug industry has adapted to meet the provision of most of the bulk supplies of medicinal products. Technical advances in pharmacotherapy have therefore shifted the application of pharmacy facilities and skills in the direction of identifying and responding to specific drug use problems and to contributions to individual patient care.

The shift to safe, effective and economic use of medicines

Hospital pharmacy services in many European countries have developed a range of initiatives at institutional level to support the safe, effective and economic use of medicines in hospitals. This function has developed as multidisciplinary committees have emerged as the means of formulating drug use policies to help control budgetary spend and to address the need to ensure safe and effective ways of using drugs. Such committees have brought pharmacists into closer formal working relationships with medically trained clinical pharmacologists and hospital medical specialists to devise hospital policies. Such committees have typically been referred to as Drugs and Therapeutics Committees and the development of hospital formularies has been an important way of implementing institution-wide influence over drug use (Cotter and McKee 1997; Thurmann *et al.* 1997; Fijn *et al.* 1999b, 2000). The earliest motive for that influence has been to help control costs. The size of expenditure on antimicrobials, which has grown from 10 per cent to over 15 per cent of hospital drug budgets, has made antimicrobial prescribing guidelines the forerunners of the comprehensive hospital formularies (Gould and Jappy 2000). In Scotland, the national cooperation of Drugs and Therapeutics Committees is illustrated by the development of the Scottish Medicines Consortium, in which clinical pharmacists contribute to national drug evaluations and drug use policy. The consortium of Drugs and Therapeutics Committees seeks to reduce duplication of effort in interpretation of the evidence base in medicines evaluation and to provide national equity of access to new medicines.

In all EU countries, the hospital pharmacy service has needed to respond to shorter hospital stays of patients, greater mobility of patients being transferred from one clinical setting to another and an increase in day-case procedures. These changes in delivery of health care have placed an increased emphasis on discharge arrangements and emphasized the need to bridge hospital and primary care services (Himmel *et al.* 1996). Links with primary care in the UK have been led by government policy requiring attention to continuity of care to improve the experience of the patient on their journey through the health care system (Scottish Executive 2002). In the UK, initiatives to improve the logistics and quality of the supply and use of medicines, 'medicines management', have been adopted widely. These initiatives in turn are affecting the delivery of professional supervision and advice through clinical pharmacy services. The function of the hospital pharmacy service as it responds to changes in society, changes in the health care professions and changes in patterns of delivery of health services will be examined.

Medicines information services

The advances in pharmacotherapy have created a demand for medicines information services within hospitals. Those services in many hospital pharmacies, which now form an internationally recognized sub-specialty in hospital pharmacy, have developed out of paper-based systems of cataloguing manufacturers' information on drug products (Follath *et al.* 1990). Specialized national and international databases have been developed to focus on the need to support drug treatment decisions within the hospital, both at individual patient care and institutional levels. In Europe, the medicines information support role has mirrored that in the USA, as it has developed from a personal, telephone-based enquiry system into a wider supporting system for formulary development and implementation (Mullerova and Vlcek 1998). Medicines information services based in hospitals have built on local networks to form national cooperative groups sharing enquiry response capacity, building specialized databases and collaborating with government and industry agencies (Taggiasco *et al.* 1992; Scala *et al.* 2001).

The developments in medicines information provision have occurred internationally, driven by the same expansion in the volume and complexity of drug use. The developments have been particularly marked in economies where the pressures on drug expenditure have required the pharmaceutical industry's sources of information to be balanced by an independent health care sector of medicines information provision. Medicines information services have grown to have a variable impact on local formulary developments. In a number of countries, the function has developed to provide nationally published drug evaluations and to participate in the managed entry of new drugs at hospital, regional and national levels (Taggiasco *et al.* 1992).

Clinical pharmacy services

The increased demand for information and advice on medicines has been met by an extension of the pharmacy service onto the hospital wards. This extension has been led, since the 1960s, by changes in the role of the hospital pharmacist in the USA. In the USA, the development of clinical pharmacy services has emerged from the application of individual pharmacists' skills in patient care settings (Bond *et al.* 2002). Technical developments such as the use of plasma concentration measurements to assist dosing adjustment – therapeutic drug monitoring – have drawn individual pharmacists closer to support bedside decision making. Recognition of the potential impact on patient care of complications to drug therapy, such as drug interactions, drug administration problems, patient compliance, patient educational needs and adverse drug effects masquerading as clinical symptoms associated with natural disease, has expanded the demand for pharmacists to function within patient care settings. At the same time, in the US model, there has been a focus on the pharmacy providing medicines in ready-to-use forms and an expansion of pharmacy personnel by the assumption of greater responsibility for administration of drugs to individual patients at ward level. This has led in the USA to many models where a large pharmacy staff presence in patient care areas provides a round-the-clock service (Bond *et al.* 2002). An additional driver has been the greater use of unit dose packaging and distribution systems in the USA, which have facilitated not only patient safety but also the individualized billing of patients' consumption of medicines.

Clinical pharmacy services over the past 30 years have emerged as a significant element of hospital pharmacy activity in the UK (Cotter *et al.* 1994), reflecting similar changes worldwide, especially in North America, Australia and New Zealand. In Europe, because of the differences in the numbers of hospital pharmacists, the balance of ward-based or clinical-based services to centralized pharmacy clinical support services varies and is rapidly changing as the educational formation of the pharmacist as a clinical practitioner develops through changes in university curricula. For example, in the Netherlands, Germany, the UK, Ireland and Norway, new curricula in new schools of pharmacy or major curriculum revisions in existing schools are underpinning the trend to recognize clinical pharmacy as a discipline.

The range of international service models has extended to the inclusion of pharmacists within multidisciplinary ward and ambulatory care teams. In advanced clinical pharmacy service models, pharmacists have relocated – to be based for the majority of their time in the clinical setting. Those service models have allowed the development of specialist clinical roles that integrate the pharmacist's contributions to individual patient care with the institution-wide contributions to the evidence-based use of medicines and to risk management.

Clinical pharmacy has developed in EU countries in many different ways, often arising out of localized developments. In certain countries (Denmark, Ireland, Greece and the UK), it has been underpinned by postgraduate courses at university master's level. In Germany and the UK, the educational underpinning is reflected in nationally agreed changes in the basic university curriculum. In some countries, a postgraduate hospital pharmacy specialization programme (such as in Belgium, France, Italy, the Netherlands, Portugal and Spain) has provided a means of expanding clinical pharmacy training, although the content of such programmes in this respect is varied.

Medicines use in hospitals: quality and budgetary control

In those countries where clinical pharmacy services have become established, the institution-wide development of drug policies has been informed by clinical pharmacists working in medical specialties. Pharmacists' experience in the patient care setting is able to both inform the hospital policy and help to implement it. In the UK, over 80 per cent of hospital pharmacists practise in patient care areas and half of them spend more than 50 per cent of their time on clinical activities (UK Audit Commission 2001). The population of hospital pharmacists is at least twice that in most other European countries. The number of clinical pharmacists has expanded sufficiently in many major UK hospital centres to provide wide coverage of hospital specialties. This resource of expertise has allowed Drugs and Therapeutics Committees to function through the input of individual clinical pharmacists contributing to the work of the medicines information centres. As clinical guidelines are gaining prominence as clinical tools, the emphasis on cost-effective use of medicines is being balanced by the need to address quality of disease management.

The conduct of clinical audit systems by individual professions has helped the clinical audit concept develop into a multidisciplinary effort, coordinated by hospital-wide committees in which hospital pharmacists play a role (Cotter *et al.* 1993; Panton and Fitzpatrick 1996; Cunney *et al.* 2003). The management of medicines use in hospitals can be informed by pharmacy-based review of the use of particular drugs by means of a drug-focused audit of use compared against specific drug recommendations in the formulary. Clinical audit is a more integrated approach in which quality of care is evaluated by multidisciplinary audit of the management of specific procedures or conditions against quality standards expressed in clinical guidelines. Hospitals find a place for both types of approach to the examination of quality of medicines use. Audit methodology is being developed as part of a developing research culture in health service delivery, which is reflected in the expansion of health services research within each of the health care professions.

Managing risk

The function of the clinical pharmacist in the patient care setting has become recognized within hospital risk management strategies (Bond *et al.* 2002). Pharmacists' close familiarity with medicines use in discrete clinical environments in which they work allows them to focus on the types of medicines use known to carry particular risks. The assignment of a clinical pharmacist, with a clear focus on medicines use, to a clinical area allows work practices involving those medicines to be scrutinized. The model of routine prescription monitoring on daily ward visits has been shown to identify prescribing errors in 1.5 per cent of prescriptions written (Dean *et al.* 2002) in the UK. However, it is not possible to generalize from individual studies, since variations in the operational definitions of services means a lack of standardization of the prescribing problem-solving role. The pharmacist working in a clinical area can help work practices to be adapted to safeguard both patients and staff, since handling medicines has health and safety implications.

In some hospital pharmacy models in Europe and North America, the 'satellite pharmacy' concept has been part of the risk management strategy. Small pharmacy units on hospital floors allow preparations for individual patients, including parenteral products, to be made close to the point of end-use. These models have been developed in the Netherlands, Germany, the UK and in some Nordic countries – in particular hospitals, rather than generally. Such models bring a closer clinical liaison role to pharmacy technicians and pharmacists with 'prescriptionist' training; the latter make up the majority of the pharmacist population in some Nordic countries. In those countries where the hospital pharmacy staff mix contains a relatively small proportion of pharmacists with the 'independent professional' level of education (such as Finland, Norway and Sweden), the provision of patient-centred services relies on models in which the clinical pharmacist acts partly through a team of support staff. The 'satellite pharmacy' model provides a means of delivering clinical pharmacy problem identification and problem solution through that team effort.

In countries such as the UK, where clinical pharmacy services have developed through individual pharmacists becoming part of ward-based teams, the continued expansion of services is already limited by manpower problems. Those problems require greater use of pharmacy technicians and other pharmacy support staff. It is clear that the common problem in most European countries is a shortage of pharmacists to develop new models of individual patient care across all specialties. There is an opportunity for different countries to share experiences in developing new teamwork approaches to drug use controls at ward level, as electronic systems in health care emerge. The prospect of widespread adoption of electronic prescribing offers to improve efficiency of quality assurance in medicines use and the capacity for teamwork within the pharmacy as well as within the hospital.

Pharmacovigilance

The voluntary reporting of unwanted drug effects provides the basis for pharmacovigilance of adverse effects to newer agents and serious reactions to established drugs. Hospital pharmacists in clinical settings and in medicines information centres in a number of European countries have evolved local connections into regional and national pharmacovigilance systems, often working closely with clinical pharmacologists. Examples of highly developed pharmacovigilance systems can be found in the Netherlands, France, the UK and Norway (van Boxtel and Wang 1997). The provision of feedback to clinicians is aimed at improving the quality and quantity of adverse drug reaction reports. The reporting of adverse effects by hospital pharmacists directly into such systems is evident in a number of countries, and in the UK this remains an area of continuing professional development as pharmacists become more closely involved with individual patient care (Green *et al.* 1999).

Medication errors

Medication errors are estimated to affect approximately 5 per cent of oral doses administered in hospitals, based on European evidence, and they affect a higher percentage of intravenous doses. Cultural and operational differences between different European countries are likely to reveal quite different findings that may require different responses from hospital pharmacists (Taxis *et al.* 1999; Taxis and Barber 2003). Voluntary reporting in a 'no-blame' culture provides a means of monitoring patient misadventures and medication errors. Hospital pharmacists have cooperated in the development of methods for surveillance by which clinical staff are encouraged to self-report incidents of wrong drug, dose errors or errors from the route of administration (Department of Health 2001a). 'Near misses' reported in this way allow local risk management teams to address patient safety issues by identifying the need to introduce better safeguards in the handling of particular drugs in certain clinical areas. Similar near miss reports of dispensing errors offer a means for identifying areas of activity of particular clinical risk in the dispensing operations of the hospital pharmacy service.

In the UK, local initiatives in medication error risk management are benefiting from a nationally coordinated strategy that has derived from the wider recognition of the concept of 'clinical governance' in health care. Clinical governance is a term that places responsibility for effective clinical outcomes at a corporate level and so demands organizational structures within hospitals to formalize methods for continuous improvement in delivery of services. The risk of medication errors is likely to be amenable to reduction by a range of automation initiatives in hospital prescribing, administration and dispensing of medicines (Bates 2000).

Procurement and financial planning

Medicines procurement involves direct supply from manufacturers and contractual arrangements with wholesalers. Procurement by hospital pharmacies in many EU countries takes place through regional purchasing groups (EAHP 2002) and national tendering of contracts to suppliers. In some countries, this is coupled with negotiated arrangements with local wholesalers. Hospitals wherever possible often seek to arrange contacts through cooperative purchasing with other hospitals in order to secure the best purchasing power through consortium arrangements.

Hospital pharmacies operate within an economic environment in which governments play a major role directly or indirectly in the strategic management of health care delivery. The hospital pharmacy service has constantly to play a role in providing information and advice to finance directors, because of the relative size of drug budgets and their importance within non-staff hospital expenditures. Drug budget overspending is a common problem due to higher inflationary pressure within health care in general and the costs attached to constant innovation in the drugs sector in particular.

Hospital pharmacy developments have been funded from cases made by pharmacy managers that expansion in a clinical pharmacy service to a particular specialty may justify itself in terms of control of medicines costs, while delivering improvements in safety and effectiveness. Increasingly in established clinical pharmacy services in the UK, the pharmacist's role at specialty level is required to provide information in the forecasting of drug budgetary spend and to help to develop strategies to control annual expenditure.

Pharmaceutical care as a unifying concept in medicines use

While hospital pharmacists have been responding to the opportunities to provide clinical pharmacy services through centralized (pharmacy-based) and decentralized (patient-centred) initiatives, the concept of 'pharmaceutical care' has emerged to describe the goals of both types of service developments. Pharmaceutical care has been variously defined both as a system and as a form of pharmacy practice focused on achieving better patient outcomes by attention to the quality of the processes in drug therapy provision (Hepler and Strand 1990; American Society of Health System Pharmacists 1996; UK Clinical Pharmacy Association 1996; Cipolle *et al.* 1998). Regardless of differences in particular literature definitions, pharmaceutical care serves to describe the application of mechanisms that constitute a quality system of safe and effective drug therapy.

Pharmaceutical care has become adopted internationally by pharmacists as a concept that is relevant to both the hospital setting and the community setting. It therefore allows hospital pharmacists to review their role and function not only in terms of inpatient services, which is where their traditional focus in Europe has always been, but also to ambulatory care settings within hospitals, where US pharmacists have been most innovative. Pharmaceutical care is becoming accepted at policy-making levels among politicians in some EU countries (see, for example, Scottish Executive 2002). As a concept, pharmaceutical care has been particularly useful in guiding the development of improved use of medicines in chronic disease management and therefore in primary care. When the goals of improved medicines use are described in terms of the achievement of pharmaceutical care, hospital pharmacists are obliged to take a wider view. That view includes addressing medication-related issues in the transfer of care before and after the patient's hospital stay and the continuity of care in the use of medicines as patients are referred around the whole health care system. Attention to pharmaceutical care means, to pharmacists, closer working in treatment delivery and an inclusion in treatment modification and adjustment. The future direction for patient-centred hospital pharmacy services may vary considerably in different European countries as new services demand pharmacy staff focusing on handling clinical information as much as medicinal products. Individual countries will respond to demands for new patient services by different staff mixes. Nordic countries, with the availability of 'prescriptionists', are able to respond to opportunities to develop pharmaceutical care by developing the 'prescriptionist' role within the clinical pharmacy team role. The response in the UK is reflected in the movement of the UK 'pharmacy technician' into patient care areas within the emerging medicines management programmes.

Medicines management programmes

The medicines management programmes that are now being implemented in UK hospitals are resulting in the restructuring of ward-based services (Department of Health 2001b; UK Audit Commission 2001). The restructuring initially centres on a redefinition of the pharmacy assistant role (pharmacy technician in the UK) at ward level with greater individual patient contact and supervision of medicines-handling on wards. The programmes are designed to allow greater use of patients' own medicines when they come into hospital and greater use of commercial original packs to retain the manufacturer's product information within the EU requirements (European Community Directive 92/27). A further advance in medicines management among hospital inpatients is the establishment of systems to allow patient self-administration of their own medication while in hospital. Such systems address present risks, while potentially exposing patients to new ones. The introduction of medicines management systems therefore requires cautious implementation, with appropriate safeguards and under pharmacy staff supervision. The use of patient self-administration offers the prospect of better introduction of new medication while the patient is in hospital. The new systems of medicines management will therefore help to address the need for better patient education, while the patient is self-administering a new drug in hospital, to ensure continuity of treatment after discharge (Lowe *et al.* 1995).

Effective relationships with primary care

The transfer of patient care between hospital specialist and community physician is acknowledged as a major weakness in health care systems generally and in pharmaceutical care in particular. Drug histories conveyed between community physicians and hospital specialists show a high incidence of inaccuracies (Mageean 1986; Holmes *et al*. 1994). Information sent to the community physician after hospital discharge is also frequently incomplete in respect of details of treatment changes, diagnoses and patient follow-up requirements (Mottram *et al*. 1994; Soloman *et al*. 1995; Brackenborough 1997). The communication failures risk poor patient compliance, errors in dosage adjustment and inadequate monitoring of unwanted effects. The frequent delay in transfer of information from hospital to community threatens the continuity of medication changes initiated by hospital specialists during inpatient stays and after outpatient consultations (Sandler *et al*. 1989).

Improving secondary–primary care communications

Attempts to remedy the general problem of post-discharge communication of medication information via the hospital pharmacy have been demonstrated using specialized pharmacy documentation (Burns *et al*. 1992; Cromarty *et al*. 1998). The recognition of the importance of multidisciplinary coordination in chronic disease management (Wagner 2000) has led to a focus on the need to improve shared care arrangements. The aim is to improve the patient's self-management role in diseases such as diabetes, chronic respiratory disease, heart failure, coronary heart disease and rheumatoid arthritis. The reduction in hospital re-admission rates is one objective that has been achieved through improved chronic disease management.

Arrangements to facilitate secondary to primary care transfer have been developed by hospital pharmacists working with nurse specialists in certain 'transmural' programmes, which are well developed in the Netherlands and in Finland for instance. These programmes involve interventions to improve patient education, to provide a hospital contact point for transfer of information and in certain cases follow-up by home visits from a specialist team member (usually a nurse or a pharmacist). When the effects of improved secondary–primary care communication on pharmaceutical care issues have been formally evaluated, a reduction in prescribing discrepancies has been associated with the introduction of a transfer letter between hospitals and community pharmacists (Duggan *et al*. 1998; Kelly *et al*. 2001).

Improving primary–secondary care pharmacist cooperation

With increasing emphasis on day care, the role of the pharmacy services in supporting the sharing of care by the hospital specialist and community physician is becoming more important and is reflected in new local models in various European countries. The rate of progress in the widespread adoption of new models is dependent on the development of mechanisms for professional reimbursement of pharmacists. An important driver is the potential for such services to reduce hospital re-admission rates and therefore help to lower overall costs to third-party payers in chronic disease management.

The need to implement clinical guidelines in chronic disease management is stimulating the linkage of hospital and primary care systems for addressing quality of medicines use. Drugs and Therapeutics Committees are needing to operate across the primary–secondary care interface (Himmel *et al.* 1996). The local use of new medicines by community physicians, in cardiovascular disease and gastroenterology for example, is known to be greatly influenced by local hospital specialist prescribing. The development of formularies that are agreed across primary and secondary care has been driven by the need to control costs in primary care prescribing, especially costs associated with the promotion of new medicines by the pharmaceutical industry. The primary–secondary care joint formulary approach is leading to increased emphasis on quality of prescribing and the promotion of adherence of prescribing decisions to national and local guidelines.

In the UK, a new form of clinical pharmacy practice is emerging in primary care, where primary care pharmacy specialists are employed to play a liaison role in implementing improved medicines management by working with community physicians, community pharmacists, hospital pharmacists and medical specialists. Pharmacists in the UK are developing roles working directly with community physicians in health centres in ways that make those roles analogous to the hospital clinical pharmacist roles working within clinical specialties (Scottish Executive 2002).

Conclusions

In countries where clinical pharmacy was established before the 1990s, the educational infrastructure has since become more responsive to preparing pharmacists for the role as clinical pharmacists. This educational support is reflected in undergraduate and/or postgraduate courses and in continuing professional development programmes. In Europe, although many clinical pharmacy models have generally been constrained by much smaller hospital pharmacist populations than in the USA, countries such as France, Spain, Ireland and the UK have been prominent in developing educational structures in support of clinical pharmacy services. The UK has a hospital pharmacy workforce some two to four times larger than most other European countries and has been in a better position to provide patient care services across a range of clinical specialties. The international evidence base, relating to clinical pharmacy services provided at the individual patient care level, shows that local clinical pharmacy models have emerged in most European countries. However, there are still only a few countries in which hospital clinical pharmacy models are widespread or their future suitably underpinned by clinical pharmacy education and training programmes at undergraduate or postgraduate levels.

Pharmaceutical care as a term referring to quality of medicines use has become relevant to health care professionals other than pharmacists, as quality of medicines use has become increasingly widened into a team responsibility. In the UK in 2003, there has been legal expansion of pharmacists' and nurses' roles to include prescribing. This is allowing multidisciplinary systems for drug treatment individualization within formal agreements with physicians. This widening of prescribing rights is likely to have a major impact on the range of models of pharmacy practice in Europe, in both hospital and community settings. The extension of prescribing responsibilities to other professions will lead to new models of delivering medicines to patients that are intended to improve treatment optimization, efficiency of delivery and convenience. The pharmaceutical care concept, therefore, means to prescribers potentially better success in drug therapy management by a wider team effort in the continuous processes of monitoring for unwanted effects, assessment of drug effectiveness and patient education (Wagner 2000).

Pharmacists in hospitals and in the community are recognizing the goals of pharmaceutical care as mandates to develop their own clinical practice in support of overall patient care. Pharmacists' control over treatment provision places them in a position to oversee the use of medicines by patients in both hospital and community settings. The prospect of the continuity in medicines provision and quality assurance becoming a reality is likely to be dependent upon health care systems implementing computer tools to achieve effective communication between health care professionals. Such tools are slowly emerging in the form of electronic prescribing in both hospital and community settings.

Medicines usage continues to offer challenges to hospitals and to society as a whole. The future of hospital pharmacy services has been demonstrated to be in developing the clinical pharmacy role as a means of delivering quality assured use of medicines. The advancement of the function of the hospital pharmacy in the quality and efficiency of medicines use will require schools of pharmacy to respond by appropriate shifts in the education of the pharmacist as a clinical practitioner.

In this chapter, the directions of change in hospital pharmacy in Europe have been described. Individual countries present different health care environments, barriers and opportunities. The desire for harmonization within the EU will be reflected in hospital pharmacies pursuing similar roles and functions, but through different models to suit the clinical settings and manpower differences in the various countries of Europe. The mobility of pharmacists and students within the EU is likely to continue to increase and that will influence the process of harmonization through a sharing of educational opportunities and a sharing of best practice.

References

American Society of Health System Pharmacists (1996) *Guidelines on Standardized Method for Pharmaceutical Care*, 53: 1713–16.

Bates, D.W. (2000) Using information technology to reduce rates of medication errors in hospitals, *British Medical Journal*, 320: 788–91.

Bond, C.A., Raehl, C.L. and Franke, T. (2002) Clinical pharmacy services, hospital pharmacy staffing, and medication errors in United States hospitals, *Pharmacotherapy*, 22: 134–47.

Brackenborough, S. (1997) Views of patients, general practitioners and community pharmacists on medicines-related discharge information, *The Pharmaceutical Journal*, 259: 1020–3.

Burns, J.M.A., Sneddon, I., Lovell, M., MacLean, A. and Martin, B.J. (1992) Elderly patients and their medication: a post-discharge follow-up study, *Age and Ageing*, 21: 178–81.

Cipolle, R.J., Strand, L.M. and Morley, P.C. (1998) *Pharmaceutical Care Practice*. New York: McGraw-Hill.

Cotter, S.M. and McKee, M. (1997) Models of hospital drug policy in the UK, *Journal of Health Services Research and Policy*, 2: 144–53.

Cotter, S., McKee, M. and Barber, N. (1993) Hospital pharmacists' participation in audit in the United Kingdom, *Quality in Health Care*, 2: 228–31.

Cotter, S.M., Barber, N.D. and McKee, M. (1994) Survey of clinical pharmacy services in United Kingdom National Health Service hospitals, *American Journal of Health Systems Pharmacy*, 51: 2676–84.

Cromarty, E., Downie, G., Wilkinson, S. and Cromarty, J.A. (1998) Communication regarding discharge medicines of elderly patients: a controlled trial, *The Pharmaceutical Journal*, 260: 62–4.

Cunney, A., Williams, D. and Feely, J. (2003) Prescription monitoring in an Irish hospital, *Irish Medical Journal*, 96: 20–3.

Dean, B., Schachter, M., Vincent, C. and Barber, N. (2002) Prescribing errors in hospital inpatients: their incidence and clinical significance, *Quality and Safety in Health Care*, 11: 340–4.

Department of Health (2001a) *Building a Safer NHS for Patients: Implementing 'An Organisation with a Memory'*. London: Department of Health.

Department of Health (2001b) *Medicines Management Framework*. London: Department of Health.

Duggan, C., Feldman, R., Hough, J. and Bates, I. (1998) Reducing adverse prescribing discrepancies following hospital discharge, *International Journal of Pharmacy Practice*, 6: 77–82.

EAHP (European Association of Hospital Pharmacists), Standing Committee of the Hospitals of the European Union (2002) *Survey Report: Hospital Pharmacies in the European Union*, Leuven, May (available from www. hope.be).

Fijn, R., Brouwers, J.R., Knaap, R.J. and De Jong-Van Den Berg, L.T. (1999a) Drug and Therapeutics (D&T) Committees in Dutch hospitals: a nation-wide survey of structure, activities, and drug selection procedures, *British Journal of Clinical Pharmacology*, 48: 239–46.

Fijn, R., De Jong-Van Den Berg, L.T. and Brouwers, J.R. (1999b) Rational pharmacotherapy in the Netherlands: formulary management in Dutch hospitals, *Pharmacy World and Science*, 21: 74–9.

Fijn, R., Engels, S.A., Brouwers, J.R., Knaap, R.J. and De Jong-Van den Berg, L.T. (2000) Dutch hospital drug formularies: pharmacotherapeutic variation and conservatism, but concurrence with national pharmacotherapeutic guidelines, *British Journal of Clinical Pharmacology*, 49: 254–63.

Follath, F., Meier, C. and Grimm, E. (1990) Computer assisted drug information, *Schweizerische Medizinische Wochenschrift*, 120: 1845–8.

Gould, I. and Jappy, B. (2000) Trends in hospital antimicrobial prescribing after 9 years of stewardship, *Journal of Antimicrobial Chemotherapy*, 45: 913–17.

Green, C.F., Mottram, D.R., Rowe, H. and Brown, A. (1999) Adverse drug reaction monitoring by United Kingdom hospital pharmacy departments: impact of the introduction of 'yellow card' reporting for pharmacists, *International Journal of Pharmacy Practice*, 7: 238–46.

Hepler, C.D. and Strand, L.M. (1990) Opportunities and responsibilities in pharmaceutical care, *American Journal of Health Systems Pharmacy*, 47: 533–43.

Himmel, W., Kron, M., Hepe, S. and Kochen, M.M. (1996) Drug prescribing in hospital as experienced by general practitioners: East versus West Germany, *Family Practice*, 13: 247–53.

Holmes, G.K.T., Crisp, P. and Upton, D.R. (1994) Letter, *British Medical Journal*, 289: 497.

Kelly, J., Forrest, F. and Hudson, S. (2001) A patient-held medication record and a patient medication profile to support the continuity of acute cancer care, *International Journal of Pharmacy Practice*, 9(suppl.): R40.

Lowe, C.J., Raynor, D.K., Courtney, E.A., Purvis, J. and Teale, C. (1995) Effects of self-medication programme on knowledge of drugs and compliance with treatment in elderly patients, *British Medical Journal*, 310: 1229–31.

Mageean, R.J. (1986) Study of discharge communications from hospital, *British Medical Journal*, 293: 1283–4.

Mottram, D.R., Slater, S. and West, P. (1994) Hospital discharge correspondence – how effective is it?, *International Journal of Pharmacy Practice*, 3: 24–6.

Mullerova, H. and Vlcek, J. (1998) European drug information centres – survey of activities, *Pharmacy World and Science*, 20: 131–5.

Panton, R. and Fitzpatrick, R.J. (1996) The involvement of pharmacists in professional and clinical audit in the UK: a review and assessment of their potential role, *Journal of Evaluation of Clinical Practice*, 3: 193–8.

Sandler, D.A., Heaton, C., Garner, S.T. and Mitchell, J.R. (1989) Patients' and general practitioners' satisfaction with information given on discharge from hospital: audit of a new information card, *British Medical Journal*, 299: 1511–13.

Scala, D., Bracco, A., Cozzolino, S. *et al.* (2001) Italian drug information centres: benchmark report, *Pharmacy World and Science*, 23: 217–23.

Scottish Executive (2002) *Strategy for Pharmaceutical Care in Scotland*. Edinburgh: Scottish Executive.

Solomon, J.K., Maxwell, R.B. and Hopkins, A.P. (1995) Content of a discharge summary from a medical ward: views of general practitioners and hospital doctors, *Journal of the Royal College Physicians*, London, 29: 307–10.

Taggiasco, N., Sarrut, B. and Doreau, C.G. (1992) European survey of independent drug information centers. *Annals of Pharmacotherapy*, 26: 422–8.

Taxis, K. and Barber, N. (2003) Ethnographic study of incidence and severity of intravenous drug errors, *British Medical Journal*, 326: 684–7.

Taxis, K., Dean, B. and Barber, N. (1999) Hospital drug distribution systems in the UK and Germany – a study of medication errors, *Pharmacy World and Science*, 21: 25–31.

Thurmann, P.A., Harder, S. and Steioff, A. (1997) Structure and activities of hospital drug committees in Germany, *European Journal of Clinical Pharmacology*, 52: 429–35.

UK Audit Commission (2001) *Spoonful of Sugar: Medicines Management in NHS Hospitals*. London: Audit Commision.

UK Clinical Pharmacy Association (1996) Statement on pharmaceutical care, *The Pharmaceutical Journal*, 256: 345–6.

van Boxtel, C.J. and Wang, G. (1997) Some observations on pharmacoepidemiology in Europe, *Netherlands Journal of Medicine*, 51: 205–12.

Wagner, E. (2000) The role of patient care teams in chronic disease management, *British Medical Journal*, 320: 569–72.

thirteen

Influencing demand for drugs through cost sharing

Sarah Thomson and Elias Mossialos

Introduction

The use of cost sharing in health care is often controversial, generating academic debate about its effectiveness as a policy tool and political debate about its feasibility. Economic theory underlies arguments put forward on both sides of the debate.

Neo-classical economists claim that the use of health services exceeds socially beneficial levels when health care costs are fully covered by insurance. Insurance reduces the marginal cost – to individuals – of using health services because it effectively lowers the price of these services to zero. Consequently, insured individuals will make use of as much health care as they would if the health care were free; that is, more than if they had to pay for it at the point of use (Arrow 1963; Pauly 1968). This 'extra' utilization is considered to be excessive if the marginal cost – to society – of providing additional health services outweighs the marginal benefit accruing to society from the use of these services, resulting in a loss of social welfare.[1] Cost sharing combats social welfare loss by restoring the price signal negated by insurance, thereby reducing 'excess' utilization.

In economic terms, excess utilization does not refer exclusively to the use of services that are either unnecessary or potentially harmful (Kutzin 1998). Nevertheless, it is often argued that the existence of a price signal will selectively discourage the use of health services that provide little value to the individual and prevent the negative effects of consuming too much health care. The case for cost sharing therefore rests on the assumption that it will enhance micro-efficiency (i.e. health care will be more effective) and macro-efficiency (i.e. health care costs will be contained) if it does not lower health status or lead to increased consumption of other health care resources.

Cost sharing can also be used to encourage more cost-effective patterns of utilization. This is achieved by conveying price signals to individuals to opt for certain types of health care or follow a particular system of referral or, via individuals, to providers responsible for prescribing treatment (Brandt *et al.* 1980). The implication is that providers will be more cost-conscious if they know that patients are subject to cost sharing.

Other arguments in support of cost sharing focus on its potential to mobilize resources and raise revenue to sustain and expand the provision of health care, particularly in countries where public budgets are under pressure or funding health care through other means is politically sensitive (Brandt *et al.* 1980; Kutzin 1998). While this may lower equity in funding health care, equity in the receipt of benefits would be preserved if the revenue raised were to be targeted at poor people or spent on tackling inequality in the health care system.

However, the diverse nature of health care 'goods' and the existence of information asymmetries in the health care market have led some economists to question both the appropriateness of using the neo-classical economic model to measure welfare loss and the ability of cost sharing to achieve efficiency gains (Evans 1984; Kutzin 1998; Rice 1998). Arguments about inefficiency arising from excess utilization are based on the assumption that individuals are well-informed about their own need for health care and are able to distinguish between effective and ineffective or harmful treatment. Moreover, the neo-classical economic model assumes that supply and demand are independently determined, but because health care providers are usually better informed than patients, often acting as patients' agents, they have considerable potential to influence both the type and quantity of health services used (Evans 1984). In practice, most decisions about the use of health services are made by providers and are not based on patients' individual assessment of potential benefits. For example, a US study found that higher co-payments for prescription drugs were associated with lower expenditure on drugs when doctors did not have any financial incentive to control drug spending, but had little impact when doctors had financial incentives to control drug spending (Hillman *et al.* 1999).[2] In both cases, lower expenditure ultimately resulted from reductions in utilization. However, due to information asymmetries, it would appear preferable for the prescribing doctor to make decisions about which types of drugs patients can do without. The neo-classical economic model also fails to take into account the travel, time and psychological costs that individuals may incur when using health services (Brandt *et al.* 1980).

Overall, the theoretical case for using cost sharing as a means of reducing excess utilization is weak, particularly when cost sharing is applied to health services that are used as a result of a provider's recommendation, referral or prescription (Chalkley and Robinson 1997). Furthermore, cost sharing is unlikely to contain health care costs in the long term, as spending on health care is primarily driven by supply-side factors (Evans and Barer 1995). Additionally, the revenue-raising potential of cost sharing may be limited by the existence of protection mechanisms, high transaction costs, fraud or providers' reluctance to enforce user charges (Brandt *et al.* 1980; Evans and Barer 1995).

Finally, the welfare gain arising from insurance – that is, protection from the risk of financial loss due to ill health – may outweigh the welfare loss arising from excess utilization. By shifting the financial burden away from population-based risk-sharing arrangements towards out-of-pocket payments by individuals, cost sharing erodes the third-party payer principle and reduces equity in funding health care (Chalkley and Robinson 1997; Creese 1997). Cost sharing also reduces equity in access to health care, as those with low incomes are most likely to be discouraged from using health services, while those in poor health will suffer most from lower levels of use. Attempts to exempt these groups of people from cost sharing are not always successful (Brandt *et al.* 1980) and the claim that any extra revenue raised can be directed towards people with low incomes or in poor health may be difficult to substantiate in practice.

As a consequence of persisting debate about the theoretical and practical advantages and disadvantages of cost sharing, the introduction of user charges for health services in Western Europe has often been accompanied by opposition from different groups.[3] In spite of political opposition, however, governments across Western Europe have increasingly applied cost-sharing policies in the health sector, particularly to pharmaceuticals, reflecting a wider attempt to contain public expenditure on health care that began in the late 1980s and continued throughout the 1990s (Mossialos and Le Grand 1999). Some form of cost sharing for prescription drugs can now be found in all Western European countries, resulting in rising levels of private expenditure on drugs, as a proportion of gross domestic product (GDP), relative to public expenditure.[4] Prescription charges have not been subject to as much political opposition as charges for other types of health care, perhaps due to the fact that users of more expensive drugs – for example, drugs for chronic illnesses – are often exempt from charges, so the financial cost to the individual is usually small. For similar reasons, the market for over-the-counter drugs has not stimulated significant political debate.[5]

In this chapter, we review the possibility of influencing demand for prescription drugs in Western European health care systems – thereby increasing micro- and macro-efficiency – through the use of cost sharing. We also consider the potential impact of prescription charges on access to health care and health status. Much of the evidence drawn on originates from North America, which is indicative of a bias in the literature, but evidence from Western Europe is reviewed where it is available.

Prescription charges in Western Europe

Direct forms of cost sharing include:

- flat-rate payments, which are fixed fees per item prescribed or per prescription;
- co-insurance based on a fixed percentage of the total cost of a good or service;
- deductibles, which require the user to bear a fixed quantity of the cost, with any excess borne by the statutory health care system; deductibles can apply to specific cases or to a period of time (usually a year).

Co-insurance is the most common form of cost sharing for prescription drugs in Western Europe.[6] Flat-rate co-payments are applied per prescription in Austria (€4.07) and the UK (£6.30 or €8.80) and in combination with other forms of cost sharing in Finland, Germany and some regions in Italy. In Germany, flat-rate co-payments vary according to pack size. Deductibles are used in Denmark, Ireland and Sweden and combined with co-insurance in Finland and

Switzerland. In the Netherlands, deductibles apply to people who are excluded from statutory health insurance and purchase substitutive private health insurance (Kasje *et al.* 2002).[7]

Reference pricing is an indirect form of cost sharing that has been applied in several Western European countries, notably Germany and the Netherlands (Kanavos and Reinhardt 2003). The reference price refers to the maximum price for a group of equal or similar drugs that the insurer will reimburse the user. If the actual price exceeds the reference price, the user must pay the difference. In practice, the European experience of reference pricing suggests that it rarely acts as a cost-sharing mechanism because drug manufacturers adapt their prices to coincide with the reference price.[8]

In many countries, cost sharing is accompanied by mechanisms to protect the finances of vulnerable groups of people. Protection mechanisms can take the form of reduced rates, exemptions, discounts for pre-paid charges, annual caps on expenditure, tax relief, the substitution of private for public prescriptions by doctors, and the substitution of cheaper or generic drugs by doctors and/or pharmacists. Protection mechanisms may apply to particular groups of people or to particular types of product – for example, essential drugs or drugs for chronic or life-threatening illnesses.

Significant population groups are exempt from cost sharing in several Western European countries. Reduced rates or exemptions commonly relate to one or more of the following:

- *Clinical condition*: diabetics in Sweden, pregnant women in the UK and people with specified chronic illnesses in Ireland, Finland, Spain and the UK.
- *Level of income*: all those with low incomes in Austria, Belgium, Germany, Ireland and the UK and older people with low incomes in Greece.
- *Age*: older people in Belgium, Ireland, Spain and the UK and children in Germany and the UK.
- *Type of drug*: drugs for chronic illnesses in Portugal, drugs for life-threatening illnesses in Belgium, both types of drug in Greece and effective drugs in France.

Some governments employ caps on the amount individuals pay out-of-pocket as a result of cost sharing for prescription drugs, either caps per prescription or annual caps (sometimes referred to as out-of-pocket maximums). Annual caps apply to families with higher incomes in Ireland, to the whole of the population in Sweden and Norway, and to chronically ill people in Denmark, Finland and Germany. Caps per prescription are applied to people with chronic illnesses in Spain (Mossialos and Le Grand 1999; Noyce *et al.* 2000). The Austrian government applies an annual cap on all health care-related spending for families with low incomes.

Out-of-pocket expenditure on health care can be deducted from taxable income in Portugal, which tends to benefit families with higher incomes (Pereira 1995). Individuals who are not exempt from cost sharing in Ireland can claim tax relief at the marginal rate on drug spending up to €780 a year. Again, the value of this relief will be higher for those with higher incomes.

The availability of complementary private health insurance covering the cost of prescription charges is another form of protection mechanism. This type of private health insurance is widespread in France and can also be found in Belgium, Denmark, Ireland, Italy and Sweden (Mossialos and Thomson 2002). More recently, it has also been introduced in Central and Eastern European countries such as Croatia and Slovenia. However, its availability may have distributional implications: it only removes price signals and alleviates the financial burden of cost sharing for those who can afford to purchase it. Complementary private health insurance raised equity concerns in France during the 1990s because the 15 per cent of the population without this type of coverage largely consisted of unemployed people, younger and older people and people with low incomes. In 2000, the French government addressed these concerns by making complementary private health insurance available free of charge to individuals with low incomes (Mossialos and Thomson 2003).

The impact of prescription charges on efficiency and equity in health care systems

This section reviews North American and Western European evidence of the impact of cost sharing for prescription drugs. Evidence from North America is based on a recent systematic review of the literature on the impact of prescription charges and related outcomes in OECD countries (Lexchin and Grootendorst 2002). Due to its unique experimental status, the findings of the RAND study, a randomized controlled trial undertaken in the USA during the 1970s, are sometimes discussed separately (Newhouse and The Insurance Experiment Group 1993).[9] The European studies reviewed in this section were identified using databases (PubMed, EconLit and IBSS) and through hand and internet searches. Published studies focusing on Western Europe are easily outnumbered by those focusing on North America. They also tend to be observational in design and do not generally employ sufficient controls, which reduces the strength of their evidence.[10] Taken together, however, the findings of the studies under review do provide tentative answers to a range of policy questions concerning:

- the size of reductions in demand in response to prescription charges;
- the effect of these reductions on expenditure and health status;
- the extent of substitution by over-the-counter products or generic drugs; and
- the distributional impact of prescription charges, both in terms of income and the provision of health services.

Does cost sharing reduce utilization?

Evidence from North America suggests that prescription charges can lead to significant reductions in the use of prescription drugs. Lexchin and Grootendorst (2002) found that prescription charges led to a decrease in the use of prescription drugs in all population groups studied, although studies that looked at elderly people in general found that prescription charges had a moderate effect on demand in this group. The RAND study found that expenditure on prescription drugs was 60 per cent higher for individuals with access to free care than for those subject to a 95 per cent co-insurance rate (Leibowitz *et al.* 1985). However, the observed decrease in expenditure was a consequence of higher user charges for all types of health care, not just for prescription drugs (Leibowitz *et al.* 1985). If user charges for prescription drugs alone had varied, price elasticities[11] may have been lower – a hypothesis that is supported by the finding that the use of drugs by participants diagnosed with hypertension was almost insensitive to the level of co-insurance (Keeler *et al.* 1985).

Western European studies also suggest that cost sharing reduces the utilization of prescription drugs, although there is some variation in estimates of own-price elasticity. For example, the own-price elasticity of drug consumption in Spain between 1978 and 1985 was found to be –0.13 (Puig Junoy 1988). However, other studies have found that, during the same period, about 30–40 per cent of prescriptions for retired individuals, who were exempt from prescription charges, were in fact purchased on behalf of non-exempt family members (Lopez Bastida and Mossialos 2000). The relatively low sensitivity to price estimated by Puig Junoy (1988) may therefore be partly explained by the effect of substitution between different population groups. Analyses of UK data from 1969 to 1985 reveal own-price elasticities between –0.15 and –0.64 (Lavers 1989; O'Brien 1989; Smith and Watson 1990; Ryan and Birch 1991; Hughes and McGuire 1995). A Belgian study found that prescription drug consumption was sensitive to price in most cases, with own-price elasticities ranging from 0.0 to –0.6 depending on user characteristics and drug categories (van Doorslaer 1984).

An Italian study found that cost sharing did not have any effect on total utilization of prescription drugs, although it found that cost sharing led to a shift in utilization from partially to fully reimbursed products (Brenna *et al.* 1984). A more methodologically rigorous study of one region in Italy found that the introduction of cost sharing was associated with a reduction in pharmaceutical spending, but the impact declined over time (Hanau and Rizzi 1986). More recently, estimates of the own-price elasticity of cardiovascular drugs in 11 districts in Italy were in the range –0.26 to –0.36 (Anessi 1997).

Between 1988 and 1990, a deductible was applied to prescription drugs in Denmark, so that consumption below an annual maximum amount of DKK800 was no longer reimbursed by the statutory health care system. A national survey conducted in January 1990, combined with interviews at pharmacies in December 1989 and April 1990, found that 14 per cent of the population had exceeded the limit (Hansen *et al.* 1991). By the end of December 1989, 53 per cent of patients at pharmacies had exceeded the limit. More than 90 per cent of patients bought the prescribed drug, while fewer than 10 per cent asked their doctor to prescribe a cheaper drug. Overall, the introduction of the deductible reduced pharmaceutical consumption by only 2–3 per cent, but it was abolished at the beginning of 1991, in response to widespread public resistance, and replaced by a system of co-insurance (Christiansen *et al.* 1999).

In Sweden, significant increases in prescription charges were introduced in 1997. Various survey-based studies found that the increases did reduce utilization and that low-income groups were most sensitive to price (see below) (National Board of Health and Welfare 1997; Elofsson *et al.* 1998; Lundberg *et al.* 1998; Burström 2002). A study of the impact of an increase in prescription charges on public expenditure on pharmaceuticals in Iceland in 1997 found that the increase did not lead to a significant reduction (Almarsdottir *et al.* 2000). However, this was partly due to the fact that community pharmacies absorbed most of the increase in cost sharing, so the effect of the reform on users was not substantial.

Dutch researchers examining the impact of prescription charges and changes in regulation on the use of anti-hypertension drugs in the Netherlands found that at the end of the period under investigation (i.e. 1986), the number of prescriptions per 1000 people was about 9 per cent lower than could have been expected during a period without changes in charges or regulation (Starmans *et al.* 1994). However, the decrease caused by the prescription charge was accompanied by a 14 per cent increase in the number of units per prescription, leading the authors to conclude that the use of antihypertensives was not sensitive to a charge per prescription (as opposed to a charge depending on pack size). Cost sharing for all health services used by people insured by the statutory health insurance scheme was introduced in 1997 in the form of co-insurance combined with an annual cap on out-of-pocket expenditure, but the policy was abandoned in 1999 because it was deemed to be ineffective – that is, it did not have much impact on drug utilization – and the costs associated with administering the policy were considered to be too high (Kasje *et al.* 2002).

Does cost sharing increase micro-efficiency?

It is argued that prescription charges can be used to increase micro-efficiency both by reducing 'excess' or 'unnecessary' utilization and by encouraging the consumption of cheaper or more cost-effective drugs. However, the RAND study found that increased cost sharing had the same impact on the utilization of effective and ineffective or medically inappropriate treatment, including the consumption of prescription drugs (Lohr *et al.* 1986; Foxman *et al.* 1987). The study also found that over-the-counter drugs complement prescription drugs, rather than substituting for them (Leibowitz 1989). These results are supported by Lexchin and Grootendorst's review, which found that prescription charges reduced the use of both essential and 'discretionary' drugs (Lexchin and Grootendorst 2002).

Western European evidence concerning the ability of prescription charges exclusively to reduce unnecessary utilization is inconclusive, perhaps because studies are unable to distinguish between user and provider responses to cost sharing (see below for further discussion of provider responses).

Lundberg examined the hypothetical rather than observed effect of prescription charges on the use of drugs among different socio-economic groups in Sweden, finding that increased charges would result in a greater relative reduction in the consumption of discretionary drugs, such as antitussives, than essential drugs, such as those used for menopause (Lundberg *et al.* 1998). If prescription charges were to be doubled, 40 per cent of antitussive users would reduce their consumption, compared with only 11 per cent of menopause drug users.

A Danish study found that the increase in co-payments for antibiotics as a result of the deductible introduced in 1988 (see above) had a significant impact on the prescribing patterns of general practitioners (GPs), resulting in a decrease of 13 per cent in the consumption of antibiotics (measured in defined daily doses) in North Jutland county between 1995 and 1996 (Steffensen *et al.* 1997). The impact was high for broad-spectrum antibiotics – for example, the consumption of tetracyclines fell by 42 per cent – while the consumption of narrow-spectrum penicillins remained stable.

Dutch researchers used focus groups to explore Dutch GPs' perceptions of the impact of different types of out-of-pocket payment for drugs on their prescribing behaviour in relation to the following conditions: mild hypertension, hormone replacement therapy, the prevention of osteoporosis, dyspepsia and hayfever (Kasje *et al.* 2002). They found that cost sharing did not normally influence GPs' prescribing, partly because GPs did not consider any type of out-of-pocket payment to be problematic for patients or to influence demand,[12] partly because they felt that reference pricing was more of an issue for pharmacists, who were more likely to encounter complaints from patients, and partly because the selection of drugs at their disposal for the conditions under study were all fully reimbursed by the statutory health insurance scheme. However, the existence of out-of-pocket payments did influence their behaviour when prescribing to patients whom they knew to have low incomes. Other Dutch researchers (see above) found that the use of antihypertensive drugs was not sensitive to a charge per prescription and had no effect on prescribing, concluding that this type of prescription charge was ineffective in reducing the use of inappropriate drugs (Starmans *et al.* 1994).

Belgian researchers were not able to find evidence to suggest that prescription charges acted as an incentive for doctors to substitute cheaper for more expensive peripheral vasodilators or for pharmaceutical firms to use price as a means of competition (van Doorslaer 1984).

Differential charges – sometimes referred to as tiered charges – can be used to encourage a more 'rational' use of prescription drugs. In Western Europe, they tend to be applied on the basis of a drug's therapeutic importance and/or severity of disease rather than on the basis of estimates of cost-effectiveness. For example, co-insurance rates for prescription drugs in France vary depending on whether drugs are classified as 'effective' or not, while reduced co-insurance rates apply to drugs for chronic and/or life-threatening diseases in Belgium, Greece and Portugal. Although there is no evidence of the impact of this type of differential charge on micro-efficiency, it is likely to be low.

Another type of differential charge aims to encourage users and providers to substitute generic for branded drugs. It is widely applied in North America, but does not feature in Western Europe (Mrazek and Mossialos 2000). However, evidence from North America suggests that the introduction of this type of differential charge might increase micro-efficiency. US studies that assessed the impact of charges applied exclusively to branded prescription drugs found that they led to a decrease in the use of branded drugs and an increase in the use of generic drugs (Weiner *et al.* 1991; Hong and Shepherd 1996; Motheral and Henderson 1999). A recent US study found that differential charges were also associated with a significant shift from non-preferred to preferred branded drugs (Rector *et al.* 2003).

Does cost sharing increase macro-efficiency?

As noted in the Introduction, cost sharing is unlikely to contain health care costs in the long term because spending on health care is primarily driven by supply-side factors. Several factors limit the potential for prescription charges to reduce expenditure or at least contain expenditure growth, so that the overall effect of increased prescription charges on expenditure is difficult to estimate. However, it may well be negative. US studies reviewed by Rice and Morrison (1994) were not able to show that cost sharing for health services in general reduced health care costs in the long term, particularly where insurers and providers already had strong incentives to contain costs and prevent the provision of unnecessary health services. In their review, Lexchin and Grootendorst (2002) found that while prescription charges reduced the use of drugs, savings in drug costs were heavily outweighed by additional expenditure in other parts of the health care system, such as doctor visits, inpatient care, emergency departments, nursing homes and mental health services – that is, not only was there no net gain in savings due to cost sharing, cost sharing may actually have increased spending on health care overall.

European studies also show that prescription charges are unlikely to reduce expenditure on drugs in the long term. In Sweden, for example, a significant increase in prescription charges in 1997 lowered expenditure in 1998, but since then expenditure has continued to grow at the same pace as before the increase (Persson and Guzelgun 1998). Another study found that the Icelandic statutory health insurance scheme did not experience a substantial decrease in reimbursement costs after increases in prescription charges came into effect (see above) (Almarsdottir *et al.* 2000). Research carried out in Italy reveals that regions with cost sharing for drugs have achieved low levels of growth in pharmaceutical spending, accompanied by a shift from public to private spending, but that regions with supply-side policies – particularly efforts to control prescribing behaviour and outpatient dispensing in hospitals – have achieved equally low levels of growth without any shift from public to private spending (Fattore and Jommi 2003).

The limited effect of cost sharing for prescription drugs on expenditure in the medium to long term may be linked to providers' sensitivity to the financial incentives facing their patients. Providers may respond to rises in charges per prescription by increasing the size of prescriptions, as has been the case in the UK (Hinchliffe 1959). A similar phenomenon has been observed in Germany, resulting in the current link between prescription charge and pack size, and in the Netherlands (see above) (Starmans *et al.* 1994). Evidence from the USA suggests that overall expenditure does not decrease following the introduction of cost sharing for some but not all of a provider's patients because the provider is able to increase the treatment he or she prescribes to other patients (Fahs 1992). This type of response to cost sharing may occur in Western Europe if providers are responsible for treating patients with different types of insurance entailing different levels of cost sharing.

Cost sharing may fail to curb expenditure if increased prescription charges lead to higher prices for over-the-counter substitutes – although this is unlikely in competitive over-the-counter markets – or result in the development of more expensive conditions by those who forego prescription drugs. The imposition of prescription charges could encourage inappropriate patterns of utilization, as Lexchin and Grootendorst (2002) demonstrate in their review of the literature. Evidence from France suggests that those without adequate health insurance coverage are more likely to make regular use of hospital emergency departments for routine care (Lang *et al.* 1997). In addition, prescription charges will not have much impact on levels of expenditure where it is possible to purchase complementary private health insurance to cover their cost (see above). Finally, implementing prescription charges may generate extra costs (Brandt *et al.* 1980). In the Netherlands, the costs associated with implementing a new cost-sharing policy in 1997 were considered to be too high and the policy was subsequently abandoned in 1999 (Kasje *et al.* 2002).

Does cost sharing have any impact on health status?

Lexchin and Grootendorst's (2002) review found that the impact of prescription charges on utilization of essential and discretionary drugs and other health services varied. While several studies of older people did not find that prescription charges had any effect on the use of other health services, a Canadian study found that increases in prescription charges resulted in a 9 per cent and 15 per cent fall in the use of discretionary and essential drugs, respectively, and that the fall in the use of essential drugs led to a 117 per cent increase in hospitalizations and doctor visits and a 77 per cent increase in emergency department visits (Tamblyn *et al.* 2001). The study also found that relatively modest increases in prescription charges targeted at welfare recipients resulted in larger reductions in the use of drugs than observed for older people, and similar increases in the rate of adverse events.

The RAND study found that there were only small differences in health status between those receiving 'free' care and those subject to cost sharing, but it did not estimate the long-term health effects of reductions in utilization as a result of increased cost sharing (Brook *et al.* 1983). It also found that people with specific conditions amenable to diagnosis and treatment benefited from free care. With regard to prescription drugs, the RAND study found that people with higher levels of education used more over-the-counter drugs and spent a larger proportion of their drug budget on such products, which suggests that poorer people have less access to self-care with over-the-counter drugs and that prescription charges may therefore lead to a greater overall negative effect on their health status (Leibowitz 1989).

Western European studies have not assessed the impact of prescription charges on health status.

Does cost sharing have any distributional impact?

The distributional impact of prescription charges appears to have important implications for equity. Lexchin and Grootendorst (2002) found that reductions in the consumption of prescription drugs were linked to income for elderly people and non-elderly people with low incomes. Own-price elasticities were higher for elderly people with low incomes. In all the studies reviewed, prescription charges for non-elderly people with low incomes resulted in considerable decreases in utilization. Non-poor and non-elderly people were least sensitive to price.

Although the RAND study only found small differences in health status between those receiving 'free' care and those subject to cost sharing, cost sharing appeared to affect people in low-income groups and those in poor health disproportionately (Brook *et al.* 1983; Lurie *et al.* 1984, 1986). The study also found that cost sharing led to a substantial reduction in the percentage of non-elderly adults with low incomes and children in low-income families who sought highly effective care for acute conditions (Lohr *et al.* 1986). Furthermore, the improvements in health status associated with free care were greater for people with low incomes. However, people in the lowest third of the income distribution used the fewest antibiotics, regardless of whether they were subject to cost sharing or not, which suggests that access to prescription drugs may be restricted by further barriers, both financial and non-financial in nature (Foxman *et al.* 1987).

After prescription charges were increased in Sweden in 1997, a survey carried out by the National Board of Health found that about 8 per cent of all households who had a prescription in 1997 refrained from collecting drugs from the pharmacy at least once for financial reasons (National Board of Health and Welfare 1997). Following on from this, a further study surveyed 8200 people living in the Stockholm area to assess the extent to which they refrained from seeking primary care due to its cost (Elofsson *et al.* 1998). Between 1970 and 1995, charges for GP visits in this area increased three times faster than the consumer price index. The study found that not seeking care was strongly correlated with self-assessed financial status. More than 50 per cent of those who described their financial status as poor reported that they had foregone seeking care on at least one occasion, compared with about 22 per cent overall. Unemployed people, students, foreign nationals and single mothers were over-represented in the 'poor' group. Those who claimed to have foregone seeking primary care had a lower perception of their health status and a higher degree of general pain, chronic illness and disability than those who did not forego care. A study of the hypothetical effect of prescription charges on the use of drugs among different socio-economic groups in Sweden found that price sensitivity was greatest for people in poor health – 33 per cent of whom would reduce their consumption, compared with only 20 per cent of those who rated their health as excellent – and decreased as educational level, age and income increased (Lundberg *et al.* 1998). Those most likely to reduce their consumption of prescription drugs were young people, unemployed people and those with low health status, educational level and income. These results are supported by Burström's (2002) study of inequalities in health care utilization in Sweden during the 1990s. Burström found that, in 1996–1997, people in the lowest income quintiles reported to a greater extent than in 1988–1989 that they had needed but not sought medical care in the three months prior to the interview.

A Belgian study of the effect of prescription charges (see above) found that, in general, employed people and their dependants were more responsive to price than non-active people such as pensioners, widows, invalids and orphans (van Doorslaer 1984). However, while non-active insured people with higher incomes did not respond to the increase in prescription charges, non-active people with a household income below a certain level were very sensitive to price.

French research shows greater variation by socio-economic status in the use of doctor visits and drugs than in the use of hospital care, which may be explained by the fact that hospital care is fully reimbursed by the statutory health insurance scheme, whereas other types of care are not (Jourdain 2000).

Does cost sharing raise revenue?

Evidence from the UK suggests that the revenue-raising potential of prescription charges is negligible, at least where extensive protection mechanisms are in place. It has been estimated that a 10 per cent increase in the UK prescription charge would raise the revenue generated from 4.8 per cent of NHS total expenditure on drugs in 1997 to 5.1 per cent (Hitiris 2000). However, prescription charges only account for a small proportion of total expenditure on health care in the UK, which may not be the case in other countries. The NHS also exempts a large proportion of the population from prescription charges. Nevertheless, the additional transaction costs associated with the collection of prescription charges and the implementation of protection mechanisms are likely to reduce the net amount of revenue raised. Fraud may also limit the extent to which cost-sharing policies contain costs or raise revenue (see the Spanish example above).

Discussion and conclusions

The more reliable evidence presented in this chapter originates from studies carried out in a North American context, which gives rise to questions about its generalizability to a Western European context. To date, research focusing on Western Europe has been hindered by a paucity of relevant data. In future, governments should consider investing in the collection of appropriate information so that studies can make use of individual rather than aggregate data (Gerdtham and Johannesson 1996). Researchers should design studies that are sufficiently controlled and are better able to distinguish between provider and user responses, between the responses of different population groups and between responses to different types of prescription drugs.

In spite of the lack of rigorous local research into the efficiency and equity implications of prescription charges, some form of cost sharing for prescription drugs can be found in all Western European countries. However, there is considerable variation in the type and level of prescription charges applied and in the nature and extent of protection mechanisms in place. Prescription charges are much higher in some countries than in others and the financial burden they place on different population groups may therefore be substantial.

While cost-sharing policies do have some impact on the utilization of prescription drugs, evidence shows that the demand for prescription drugs is relatively insensitive to price, at least for non-vulnerable groups of people. Price sensitivity is higher for heavy users of prescription drugs and people with low incomes, which suggests that income protection mechanisms should focus on these population groups. Exemption systems should be based on a clearly defined notion of 'need' and consistently applied. The Swedish practice of imposing a prescription drug deductible on all except those with diabetes provides an example of a poorly designed policy that exacerbates rather than allays concerns about equity (Hjortsberg and Ghatnekar 2001). At the same time, however, the presence of an annual cap on out-of-pocket spending on prescription drugs provides the Swedish population with protection against catastrophic risk. Means-tested exemptions may reduce the regressivity of prescription charges, but if exemptions essentially protect non-employed people, the burden of paying for prescription charges will be borne by the working population, which probably already contributes significantly to funding health care.

The type of prescription charge imposed may also affect the equity and efficiency implications of cost sharing. Marginal cost pricing in the form of co-insurance provides users with greater incentives to curb utilization. With respect to equity, any form of cost sharing that requires the user to pay first and be reimbursed at a later date may disadvantage people with low incomes. This effect is compounded when people are unable to afford complementary private health insurance. Deductibles may be more detrimental to equity than flat-rate fees or co-insurance because poorer people may not be able to afford the initial financial outlay required. At the same time, co-insurance involves a greater degree of financial risk, as the cost of the treatment, and therefore the amount the user is required to pay, may not be known in advance. However, the monetary amounts involved may be relatively small for prescription drugs, at least for non-heavy users. In some cases, flat-rate fees per prescription actually exceed the cost of the drugs prescribed. Where this is the case, providers may already resort to alternative means of protecting users, such as substituting private for NHS prescriptions, as in the UK.

Evidence from North America suggests that Western European governments could consider greater use of differential charges, both to encourage the substitution of cheaper or generic for more expensive or branded drugs and to stimulate the use of drugs with proven cost-effectiveness. In the USA, the use of differential charges to direct both users and providers towards more cost-effective pharmaceutical products may be important as an antidote to direct-to-consumer advertising. In Western Europe, differential charges are more likely to be used to encourage generic substitution, in which case they need to be accompanied by incentives targeted at pharmacists.

It is difficult to estimate the full economic impact of cost sharing. Even though prescription charges appear to reduce the utilization of prescription drugs, they do not appear to stabilize pharmaceutical expenditure in the long term or result in sustained reductions in the rate of expenditure growth. This is partly due to the existence of explicit protection mechanisms – including the availability of complementary private health insurance in some Western European countries – and implicit protection mechanisms employed by doctors and pharmacists. But it may also be due to changes in patterns of utilization in response to cost sharing – for example, the substitution of other health care goods and services for prescription drugs – and changes in health status arising from inadequate access to prescription drugs.

The political (in)feasibility of imposing supply-side controls and influencing doctors' prescribing behaviour may explain why so many Western European governments continue to apply cost sharing to a form of health care in which utilization is predominantly dependent on prescription by licensed providers. Nevertheless, because supply-side factors are primarily responsible for driving health care costs and the health care market is subject to asymmetrical information, policy tools applied to providers and other actors in the pharmaceutical sector might be more effective in enhancing micro- and macro-efficiency without reducing equity.

Notes

1 However, the social benefits conferred by the use of some health services – for example, the prevention and treatment of a communicable disease – exceed private benefits. The introduction of cost sharing for these services would therefore result in a socially sub-optimal level of utilization.

2 See Chapter 10 for a discussion of the impact of financial incentives targeted at providers on prescribing patterns.

3 For a discussion of opposition to the introduction of cost sharing for health services in France, Germany, Sweden and the UK, see Robinson (2002) and Ullrich (2002).

4 During this period, however, some countries experienced an increase in levels of public expenditure on drugs – for example, Ireland, Italy and Spain. Overall, there is little research into the impact of shifts in sources of pharmaceutical funding on health outcomes. See the Introduction for a further discussion of expenditure trends.

5 See Chapter 15 on over-the-counter drugs.

6 For up-to-date information on specific cost-sharing arrangements in different countries, see the European Union's MISSOC website (MISSOC 2003).

7 In Western Europe, private health insurance can be classified as substitutive (providing cover that would otherwise be available from the state), complementary (providing cover for services excluded or not fully covered by the state, including cover for statutory user charges) or supplementary (providing cover for faster access and increased consumer choice).

8 See also Chapter 6 for a discussion of the impact of fixed reimbursement levels on the price of drugs.

9 The RAND study has been criticized for its lack of generalizability, its sample inclusion criteria, its length, the range of health outcome measures it used and the income-related ceiling it imposed on its subjects' out-of-pocket expenditure. The study sample excluded large and vulnerable sections of the population: those over 62 years of age and those too disabled to work, but it has been noted that relatively healthy adults under the age of 62 are less likely to require or benefit from medical care than the very young, the elderly or the disabled (Brook *et al.* 1983). The extent of cost sharing was limited by an income-related ceiling on out-of-pocket expenditure defined as a percentage of family income, which would have afforded poorer households greater protection than rich households. Cost sharing not related to income would have caused disproportionate reductions in use by poor people. While the RAND study suggests that cost sharing is associated with a decrease in total health

expenditure, it was not actually designed to show whether cost sharing would lead to an overall system-wide reduction in utilization and costs (Evans and Barer 1995).

10 See Chapter 5 for a full discussion of methodological issues.

11 Elasticity of demand is a measurement of the change in demand for a good or service caused by (a) a change in the price of that good or service (own-price elasticity), (b) a change in the price of another good or service (cross-price elasticity) or (c) a change in the income of the person demanding the good or service (income elasticity).

12 Particularly where co-insurance with an annual cap was concerned, as patients were not always aware of individual drug costs because charges were paid cumulatively at the end of the year.

References

Almarsdottir, A.B., Morgall, J.M. and Grimsson, A. (2000) Cost containment of pharmaceutical use in Iceland: the impact of liberalization and user charges, *Journal of Health Services Research and Policy*, 5(2): 109–13.

Anessi, E. (1997) *The Effect of User Charges on the Utilisation of Prescription Medicines in the Italian Health Service*. Philadelphia, PA: University of Pennsylvania.

Arrow, K.J. (1963) Uncertainty and the welfare economics of medical care, *American Economic Review*, 53(5): 941–73.

Brandt, A., Horisberger, B., von Wartburg, W.P. and Abel-Smith, B. (eds) (1980) *Cost-Sharing in Health Care*. Berlin: Springer-Verlag.

Brenna, A., Grossi, M. and Lucioni, C. (1984) *L'effetto del ticket moderateur sui farmaci: presupposti economici ed analisi statistica*. Pavia: La Goliardica.

Brook, R.H., Ware, J.E., Jr., Rogers, W.H. *et al.* (1983) Does free care improve adults' health? Results from a randomized controlled trial, *New England Journal of Medicine*, 309(23): 1426–34.

Burström, B. (2002) Increasing inequalities in health care utilisation across income groups in Sweden during the 1990s?, *Health Policy*, 62(2): 117–29.

Chalkley, M. and Robinson, R. (1997) *Theory and Evidence on Cost Sharing in Health Care: An Economic Perspective*. London: Office of Health Economics.

Christiansen, T., Enemark, U., Clausen, J. and Poulsen, P. (1999) Health care and cost containment in Denmark, in E. Mossialos and J. Le Grand (eds) *Health Care and Cost Containment in the European Union*. Aldershot: Ashgate.

Creese, A. (1997) User fees: they don't reduce costs and they increase inequity, *British Medical Journal*, 315: 202–3.

Elofsson, S., Unden, A.L. and Krakau, I. (1998) Patient charges – a hindrance to financially and psychosocially disadvantaged groups seeking care, *Social Science and Medicine*, 46(10): 1375–80.

Evans, R.G. (1984) *Strained Mercy: The Economics of Canadian Health Care*. Toronto: Butterworths.

Evans, R.G. and Barer, M.L. (1995) User fees for health care: why a bad idea keeps coming back (or, what's health got to do with it?), *Canadian Journal on Aging*, 14(2): 360–90.

Fahs, M.C. (1992) Physician response to the United Mine Workers' cost-sharing program: the other side of the coin, *Health Services Research*, 27(1): 25–45.

Fattore, G. and Jommi, C. (2003) The regulation of the pharmaceutical market in Italy. Paper presented at the *Institute of Social Security (IKA) Seminar on Pharmaceuticals Policies in Europe*, 28–29 May, Athens.

Foxman, B., Valdez, R.B., Lohr, K.N. *et al.* (1987) The effect of cost sharing on the use of antibiotics in ambulatory care: results from a population-based randomized controlled trial, *Journal of Chronic Disease*, 40(5): 429–37.

Gerdtham, U.G. and Johannesson, M. (1996) The impact of user charges on the consumption of drugs: empirical evidence and economic implications, *Pharmacoeconomics*, 9(6): 478–83.

Hanau, C. and Rizzi, D. (1986) Econometria dei provvedimenti pubblici sull'assistenza farmaceutica: il caso dell'Emilia Romagna, *Economia Pubblica*, 3: 177–83.

Hansen, H., Jensen, C.H. and Rasmussen, N.K. (1991) The distribution effects of the Danish 800 crown rule: preliminary results of the DIKE study, *Ugeskr Laeger*, 153(20): 1436–7 (in Danish).

Hillman, A.L., Pauly, M.V., Escarce, J.J. *et al.* (1999) Financial incentives and drug spending in managed care, *Health Affairs (Millwood)*, 18(2): 189–200.

Hinchliffe, H. (1959) *Final Report of the Committee on the Cost of Prescribing*. London: HMSO.

Hitiris, T. (2000) *Prescription Charges in the United Kingdom: A Critical Review*. Discussion Papers in Economics No. 2000/04. York: University of York.

Hjortsberg, C. and Ghatnekar, O. (2001) *Health Care Systems in Transition: Sweden*. Copenhagen: European Observatory on Health Care Systems.

Hong, S.H. and Shepherd, M.D. (1996) Outpatient prescription drug use by children enrolled in five drug benefit plans, *Clinical Therapy*, 18(3): 528–45.

Hughes, D. and McGuire, A. (1995) Patient charges and the utilisation of NHS prescription medicines: some estimates using a cointegration procedure, *Health Economics*, 4(3): 213–20.

Jourdain, A. (2000) Equity of a health system, *European Journal of Public Health*, 10(2): 138–42.

Kanavos, P. and Reinhardt, U. (2003) Reference pricing for drugs: is it compatible with US health care?, *Health Affairs*, 22(3): 16–30.

Kasje, W.N., Timmer, J.W., Boendermaker, P.M. and Haaijer-Ruskamp, F.M. (2002) Dutch GPs' perceptions: the influence of out-of-pocket costs on prescribing, *Social Science and Medicine*, 55(9): 1571–8.

Keeler, E.B., Brook, R.H., Goldberg, G.A., Kamberg, C.J. and Newhouse, J.P. (1985) How free care reduced hypertension in the health insurance experiment, *Journal of the American Medical Association*, 254(14): 1926–31.

Kutzin, J. (1998) The appropriate role for patient cost sharing, in R.B. Saltman, J. Figueras and C. Sakellarides (eds) *Critical Challenges for Health Care Reform in Europe*. Buckingham: Open University Press.

Lang, T., Davido, A., Agay, D.B.E., Viel, J.F. and Flicoteaux, B. (1997) Using the hospital emergency department as a regular source of care, *European Journal of Epidemiology*, 13: 223–8.

Lavers, R.J. (1989) Prescription charges, the demand for prescriptions and morbidity, *Applied Economics*, 21(8): 1043–52.

Leibowitz, A. (1989) Substitution between prescribed and over-the-counter medications, *Medical Care*, 27(1): 85–94.

Leibowitz, A., Manning, W.G. and Newhouse, J.P. (1985) The demand for prescription drugs as a function of cost-sharing, *Social Science and Medicine*, 21(10): 1063–9.

Lexchin, J. and Grootendorst, P. (2002) *The Effects of Prescription Drug User Fees on Health Services Use and Health Status: A Review of the Evidence*. Toronto: University of Toronto.

Lohr, K.N., Brook, R.H., Kamberg, C.J. *et al.* (1986) Effect of cost sharing on use of medically effective and less effective care, *Medical Care*, 24(9 suppl.): S31–S38.

Lopez Bastida, J. and Mossialos, E. (2000) Pharmaceutical expenditure in Spain: cost and control, *International Journal of Health Services*, 30(3): 597–616.

Lundberg, L., Johannesson, M., Isacson, D.G.L. and Borgquist, L. (1998) Effects of user charges on the use of prescription medicines in different socio-economic groups, *Health Policy*, 44(2): 123–34.

Lurie, N., Ward, N.B., Shapiro, M.F. and Brook, R.H. (1984) Termination from Medi-Cal – does it affect health? *New England Journal of Medicine*, 311(7): 480–4.

Lurie, N., Ward, N.B., Shapiro, M.F. *et al.* (1986) Termination of Medi-Cal benefits: a follow-up study one year later, *New England Journal of Medicine*, 314(19): 1266–8.

MISSOC (2003) *Social Protection in the EU Member States and the European Economic Area: Situation on January 1st 2002 and Evolution*, Brussels, European Commission (available from http://europa.eu.int/comm/employment_social/missoc/index_en.html).

Mossialos, E. and Le Grand, J. (1999) Cost containment in the EU: an overview, in E. Mossialos and J. Le Grand (eds) *Health Care and Cost Containment in the European Union*. Aldershot: Ashgate.

Mossialos, E. and Thomson, S. (2002) Voluntary health insurance in the European Union: a critical assessment, *International Journal of Health Services*, 32(1): 19–88.

Mossialos, E. and Thomson, S. (2003) Access to health care in the European Union: the impact of user charges and voluntary health insurance, in M. Morgan (ed.) *Access to Health Care*. London: Routledge.

Motheral, B.R. and Henderson, R. (1999) The effect of a copay increase on pharmaceutical utilization, expenditures, and treatment continuation, *American Journal of Managed Care*, 5(11): 1383–94.

Mrazek, M.F. and Mossialos, E. (2000) Increasing demand while decreasing costs of generic medicines, *Lancet*, 356: 1784–5.

National Board of Health and Welfare (1997) *Can Households Afford Medicine? Results from a Survey Conducted in October 1997*. Stockholm: National Board of Health and Welfare.

Newhouse, J.P. and The Insurance Experiment Group (1993) *Free For All? Lessons from the RAND Health Insurance Experiment*. Cambridge, MA: Harvard University Press.

Noyce, P.R., Huttin, C., Atella, V. *et al.* (2000) The cost of prescription medicines to patients, *Health Policy*, 52(2): 129–45.

O'Brien, B. (1989) The effect of patient charges on the utilisation of prescription medicines, *Journal of Health Economics*, 8(1): 109–32.

Pauly, M.V. (1968) The economics of moral hazard: comment, *American Economic Review*, 58(3): 531–7.

Pereira, J.A. (1995) *Equity, Health and Health Care: An Economic Study with Reference to Portugal*. York: University of York, Department of Economics and Related Studies.

Persson, A. and Guzelgun, Z. (1998) Taxes, premiums, user charges: financing from the point of view of consumers, *Developments in Health Economics and Public Policy*, 7: 255–72.

Puig Junoy, J. (1988) Gasto farmaceutico en Espana: effectos de la participacion del usuario en el coste, *Investigaciones Economicas*, 12(1): 45–68 (in Spanish).

Rector, T.S., Finch, M.D., Danzon, P.M., Pauly, M.V. and Manda, B.S. (2003) Effect of tiered prescription copayments on the use of preferred brand medications, *Medical Care*, 41(3): 398–406.

Rice, T. (1998) *The Economics of Health Reconsidered*. Chicago, IL: Health Administration Press.

Rice, T. and Morrison, K.R. (1994) Patient cost sharing for medical services: a review of the literature and implications for health care reform, *Medical Care Review*, 51(3): 235–87.

Robinson, R. (2002) User charges for health care, in E. Mossialos, A. Dixon, J. Figueras and J. Kutzin (eds) *Funding Health Care: Options for Europe*. Buckingham: Open University Press.

Ryan, M. and Birch, S. (1991) Charging for health care: evidence on the utilisation of NHS prescribed drugs, *Social Science and Medicine*, 33(6): 681–7.

Smith, S. and Watson, S. (1990) Modelling the effect of prescription charge rises, *Fiscal Studies*, 11: 75–91.

Starmans, B., Janssen, R., Schepers, M. and Verkooijen, M. (1994) The effect of a patient charge and a prescription regulation on the use of antihypertension drugs in Limburg, the Netherlands, *Health Policy*, 26(3): 191–206.

Steffensen, F.H., Schonheyder, H.C., Tolboll Mortensen, J., Nielsen, K. and Toft Sorensen, H. (1997) Changes in reimbursement policy for antibiotics and prescribing patterns in general practice, *Clinical Microbiology and Infection*, 3(6): 653–7.

Tamblyn, R., Laprise, R., Hanley, J.A. *et al.* (2001) Adverse effects associated with prescription drug cost-sharing among poor and elderly persons, *Journal of the American Medical Association*, 285(4): 421–9.

Ullrich, C.G. (2002) Managing the behavior of the medically insured in Germany: the acceptance of cost-sharing and risk premiums by members of the statutory health insurance, *Journal of Health and Social Policy*, 15(1): 31–43.

van Doorslaer, E. (1984) The effects of cost sharing on the demand for prescription drugs in Belgium, *Acta Hospitalia*, 24(3): 69–81.

Weiner, J.P., Lyles, A., Steinwachs, D.M. and Hall, K.C. (1991) Impact of managed care on prescription drug use, *Health Affairs (Millwood)*, 10(1): 140–54.

fourteen

The off-patent pharmaceutical market

Monique Mrazek and Richard Frank

Introduction

The standard assumption is that price competition in pharmaceutical markets is weak. In general, pharmaceutical markets do suffer from some peculiarities in supply and demand that lead to market failure, and market regulations then aim at securing more efficient resource allocation. The generalizations about on-patent pharmaceutical markets do not necessarily hold in the off-patent pharmaceutical market. After patent expiration, a significant barrier to entry is removed and multiple generic equivalents of the original brand can enter and compete for market share. In theory, generic equivalents are close to perfect substitutes for the original brand, and can be expected to compete on price. Although there may be some residual loyalty for the original brand after patent expiration, there is evidence from the USA that this does not limit off-patent competition. The off-patent pharmaceutical market often differs on the demand side as well, because the financial incentives for physicians, pharmacists and patients to use generics increase product selection based on cost awareness. The characteristics of the off-patent pharmaceutical market create a potential for price competition, and this can be encouraged or stifled by regulations or other market interventions.

The size of the generics market has grown in a number of European Union (EU) countries over the past few years and is expected to continue to grow in the near future. This is due to support for the development of a competitive generics market at the supranational level, as well as member states' own initiatives to contain drug costs. The report by the High Level Group on Innovation and Provision of Medicines (2002) recommended that the EU institutions and member states should work towards ways of improving the penetration of generic medicines. As Figure 14.1 shows, in relation to total prescriptions, the generics markets in Germany, Denmark, the Netherlands and the UK are quite

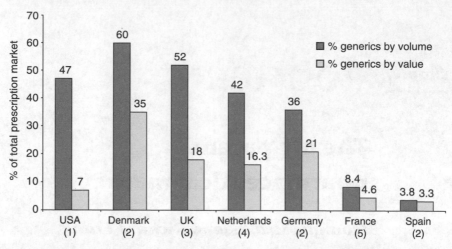

Figure 14.1 Sales of generics in selected EU countries and the USA by value and volume, 2001. Volume to value ratios: USA, 6.7; Denmark, 1.7; UK, 2.9; Netherlands, 2.6; Germany, 1.7; France, 1.8; Spain, 1.2. *Sources and notes*: (1) Pharmaceutical Research and Manufacturers of America (2002) (note: US data are for 2000); (2) European Generic Medicines Association (2003); (3) Department of Health (2002a); (4) Foundation for Pharmaceutical Statistics (2002); (5) CNAMTS (2003a) (note: French data are for 2002 and include reimbursed medicines only).

well developed in terms of volume; these countries have had policies of promoting the use of off-patent drugs for a number of years. The generics markets in other EU countries, like France and Spain, are in comparatively early stages of development.[1] The world's largest generics drug market is that of the USA, which has evolved through a series of legislative and health system developments since the 1970s. Interestingly, the ratio of volume to value in generic medicines is highest in the USA (with a ratio of 6.7), followed by the UK (2.9) and the Netherlands (2.6). Denmark, Germany, France and Spain have volume to value ratios lower than 2 (see Figure 14.1). The difference between the volume and value of generics reflects a number of factors, including the extent of generic entry and the penetration of branded generics, price differences between original brands and generics, price regulation of on-patent and off-patent drugs, as well as the extent of product selection based on price. This chapter examines the comparative development and regulatory approaches to promoting generic drug use across the EU and in the USA.

The European off-patent pharmaceutical market

As with the on-patent market, the regulation and structure of the EU off-patent pharmaceutical markets are influenced by both national and supranational policy developments and legislation. At the supranational level, legislation is in place giving market authorization to generic medicines through a mutual recognition procedure since 1998. One problem with this procedure has to do with differences in the summary of product characteristics for the originator product among EU countries (see Chapter 4). While most regulators have now accepted that originator products are similar across the EU despite not being identical to the originator in the country where the registration is sought, France nevertheless requires that the generic product be the bioequivalent of the local original brand, thus slowing the generic's entry (Atkinson 2002).

The EU pharmaceutical legislation, amended in 2004, includes provisions affecting generic products. One amendment concerns the harmonization of the period of data exclusivity across the EU – which was previously six or ten years depending on the country – and now is eight years data exclusivity plus two years of market exclusivity, adding another year for new indications authorized during the first eight years of data exclusivity. The implication of lengthening the exclusivity period will be to delay market entry of a generic to ten years. However, as the last two years are market exclusivity only, this introduces a 'Bolar-type' provision reducing the time to generic entry after the end of the patent and/or exclusivity period. The name originates from the 1984 US case of *Roche Products Inc.* (originator firm) v. *Bolar Pharmaceutical Co.* (generic firm), and refers to permitting applicants for authorization of a generic product to carry out the necessary tests prior to the end of the patent or data exclusivity period on the reference originator product, which was not previously permitted under EU legislation.

Policies that have influenced the penetration of generic medicines in national pharmaceutical markets have evolved within the context of national health care systems. One argument for the slow development of competitive generic markets in a number of EU countries is the presence of well-developed branded generic markets. In part, this is due to the absence of policies to promote the use of unbranded generics, but it is also due to several EU countries (Greece, Italy, Portugal, Spain) not having had product patent protection until the early 1990s, enabling low-priced branded generic versions to flourish.

Countries that have experienced greater penetration of generics into their markets generally have implemented policies favouring their use (generic substitution, financial incentives targeting physicians, pharmacists or patients, etc.). Depending on the policies in place, EU generics markets can be differentiated as either branded (Germany) or commodity (Netherlands, UK) generics markets. It is important to mention that concerns about the safety and quality of generics have often influenced their use in the EU (Peterson 2000; Delporte 2002; Hellstrom and Rudholm 2003). There is also a concern about the extent to which approaches promoting generic medicines infringe on prescribing freedom. The remainder of this section examines the approaches used to promote generic medicines within the EU, as well as factors affecting their cost.

Physician incentives

Table 14.1 shows some of the common approaches used across the EU to target physicians' prescribing behaviour and promote generic medicines. Countries often use multiple policies to encourage the prescription of generic medicine. In the UK, for example, the prescription of medicines using the generic name,

Table 14.1 Physician incentives used to promote generics in the EU

Method	Country
Generic name prescribing encouraged or required	Finland, France, Germany, Ireland, Italy, Luxembourg, Netherlands, Portugal, Spain (some regions), UK
Prescribing budgets	Germany, Italy, Ireland, UK
Pay agreement linked to prescribing	Spain (local schemes), Netherlands (local scheme in Limburg)
Dissemination of information to promote generics	Belgium, Italy, Ireland, Portugal, UK
Prescribing guidelines	France, Netherlands, Portugal, UK
Monitoring prescribing	Austria, Belgium, Denmark, Luxembourg, Netherlands, UK

accounting for more than 74 per cent of all prescriptions (Department of Health 2002a), is encouraged through formularies that list products by their generic name at the practice level, and through PRODIGY, a prescription support system that lists drugs by their generic name. The practice of generic prescription is also growing in other EU countries: in the Netherlands it is estimated to have reached 42 per cent of all prescriptions, and in France generic prescription has increased in exchange for a higher physician's fee per patient visit (CNAMTS 2003b). Other UK initiatives, including the collection of prescription data and face-to-face consultation with prescription advisers, have been integral to prescription budget schemes that indirectly promote generics through financial incentives. However, it should be noted that measures to promote generic prescribing are not introduced singly and it is difficult to disentangle their individual impact. Moreover, there is limited evidence on the impact of different measures, with the exception perhaps of prescribing budget schemes.

The concept of prescription budget schemes, as discussed in Chapter 10, and their impact on the use of generics is not exclusive to the UK, but is also found in Germany, Ireland and some regions of Italy. However, the evidence from the UK points to a clear link between profit incentives given to a selected group of physicians called GP-fundholders during the 1990s and the increased prescription of generic medicines (see Chapter 10). Evidence from a number of studies of the GP-fundholding scheme points to increased cost-awareness in this group of physicians compared with general practitioners (GPs) who were given indicative (non-cash-limited) prescription budgets, seen in an increase in generic prescription, the use of prescription data and the application of generic name formularies (Walley *et al.* 1995; Gosden and Torgerson 1997). A similar result was observed in Germany, where cash-limited prescription budgets were also set, but collectively for all physicians in a district, with a penalty for exceeding the budget. In the first year following the implementation of drug budgets in Germany, there was a 30 per cent decrease in prescriptions as well as a decrease in average prescription cost, largely associated with an increase in generic prescription (Busse and Howorth 1999). Both Germany and the UK replaced the cash-limited prescription budgets with indicative amounts, which are also used in Ireland (Molony 2002).

Role of the pharmacist and incentives

Since pharmacists are responsible for the dispensing of prescriptions, they can also play an important role in increasing the use of generic medicines. Generics are mainly promoted through generic substitution, although pharmacists in most EU countries can only select the multi-sourced drug if the prescription is written using the generic name (with the exception of Denmark, Finland, France, the Netherlands, Norway and Spain, as shown in Table 14.2). Where generic substitution is allowed, physicians and/or patients are generally reserved the right to refuse substitution; however, measures aimed at physicians (Denmark and Finland) and/or at patients, such as reference pricing, have been used to discourage this practice. In Denmark, pharmacists and patients generally tend to be more satisfied with the introduction of generic substitution schemes than physicians (Andersen *et al.* 2000; Rubak *et al.* 2000a,b).

Financial incentives have been used to motivate pharmacists to dispense less expensive generic medicines in several EU countries (see Chapter 11). Selection of a least-cost generic equivalent by pharmacists is encouraged through the use of preferential margins on generic products (Spain, France, the Netherlands, Norway). Financial incentives to motivate generic substitution in Denmark operate through fixed dispensing budgets. In the UK, when prescriptions are written using the generic name of the molecule, pharmacists have the incentive to select its least expensive version, as they are able to retain a proportion of the difference between the wholesale and the reimbursement price. A discount recovery scale or 'claw back' also operates to recover some of this excess profit for the government.[2] As discussed in Chapter 11, a number of countries have margins that are a percentage of product price (Austria, Belgium, Denmark, Finland, Germany, Greece, Italy, Portugal); these payment methods can make selecting cheaper medicines appear against the self-interests of pharmacists. The payment approach in Germany, combined with the reference price scheme, led

Table 14.2 Pharmacist incentives to promote generics in the EU

Method	Country
Generic substitution	Denmark, Finland, France, Norway, Spain
Multi-sourced product selection only if prescription written using the generic name	Italy, Germany, Luxembourg, Portugal, Netherlands, Sweden, UK
Margins that encourage generic dispensing	France, Netherlands, Norway, Spain, UK
Dispensing budgets	Denmark

to an artificial price floor (Mrazek 2001), as there was no incentive for decreases below the reimbursement limit; a new scheme has subsequently been introduced called the 'downward price coil', which attempts to overcome this problem (see below).

Patients

Financial incentives have also been used to influence the consumer demand for generics. When a payment equal to any excess in the price of a drug above the maximum reimbursement price (the reference price) is applied, patients have an incentive to request that a product priced at or below the reimbursement limit be prescribed or dispensed where selection of a multi-sourced drug is permitted. Evidence indicates that consumers responded to these additional out-of-pocket payments and consequently switched to alternatives available at the reference price, as in Germany for example (Zweifel and Crivelli 1996). However, as manufacturers eventually lowered the prices of their products to the reference price, these additional out-of-pocket costs were generally short-lived (Kanavos and Reinhardt 2003; see also Chapter 6). Although there is no explicit application of differential co-payments in Denmark, pharmacists must inform patients of price differences between original brands and generics. Pharmacists in Sweden are required to dispense the least expensive generic equivalent, and patients wanting a more expensive version must pay the full price differential. Ensuring that patients use generic medicines is certainly not only about financial incentives but also about gaining acceptance of the practice and confidence in the medicines. In Spain, generic medicine education programmes were an important component of increasing the use of generic medicines (Casado Buendia *et al.* 2002; Vallès *et al.* 2002).

The value of generics: price regulation and competition

Whether and how prices in the off-patent pharmaceutical sector are regulated varies among EU countries; this affects the difference in price between originator and generic products, which is estimated at 10–50 per cent, depending on the country. There are two common approaches to regulating generic drug prices in the EU. The first is to limit the generic price to X per cent less than that of a 'reasonably priced' originator product, or to make it equal to that of the cheapest generic equivalent on the market (Austria, Belgium, Finland, Greece, Italy and Portugal). The second common approach is to apply a reference price scheme that targets the off-patent drug market. Although, as discussed in Chapter 6, many of these schemes have been successful in having product prices converge at the reference price level, few have been able to motivate decreases below the reference price. This problem led Germany to supplement its reference price scheme with what is referred to as the *aut idem* regulation, or the downward price coil, which requires a pharmacist to select a lower cost generic equivalent if the price of the prescribed drug is above a defined comparative average price level, in an attempt to move the average price[3] downwards. The initial response by some companies was to launch dummy products to maintain an artificially high price level. German pharmacists still lack the financial incentive to select a least cost generic, as their margin remains higher, in general, for more expensive products.

By contrast, in the UK competition between unbranded generics can lead to discounts such that the actual reimbursement price falls below the maximum list price defined by the Statutory Maximum Price Scheme. However, the reimbursement price cannot exceed the maximum price. The reimbursement price for community pharmacists and dispensing doctors, known as the 'drug tariff', is frequently recalculated according to a basket of manufacturers' and wholesalers' actual supply prices. As pharmacists can retain a higher margin for dispensing an equivalent multi-sourced drug priced below the maximum price, competition drives prices downward. This approach has resulted in cost-savings to the government estimated at €474 million (Department of Health 2002b). The number of suppliers in the market (Mrazek 2001) and the extent of undisclosed discounts from wholesalers to pharmacists (Oxera 2001) continue to pose challenges in the UK.

Evidence from the US off-patent pharmaceutical market

Prescription drug spending in the USA, as in many EU countries, is among the fastest growing components of national health care spending, accounting for over US$131 billion in 2000 (Levit *et al.* 2002). Sales of generic drugs were approximately US$9 billion in 2002 and, as Figure 14.1 shows, accounted for nearly half of all prescriptions dispensed by volume but only around 7 per cent by value (Pharmaceutical Research and Manufacturers of America 2002). The high volume use of competitively priced generics in the USA has primarily followed legislative and market developments that included the repeal of anti-substitution laws in the late 1970s, the enactment of the Hatch-Waxman Act of 1984[4] and the expansion of managed care, particularly since the early 1990s.

Legislative and market developments

States have played an active part in defining the competitive role of generic drugs. During the 1970s and early 1980s, some states adopted laws allowing pharmacists to dispense a generic drug even when a brand name drug was specified on the prescription, as long as the physician had not indicated that the prescription should be 'dispensed as written'. By 1984, all states had enacted generic substitution laws. In addition, 12 states enacted laws making generic substitution at pharmacies mandatory. The purpose of these laws was to encourage substitution of generic for branded drugs, maintain quality of care and save consumers' money (Levy 1999). Before the abolition of anti-substitution laws in the late 1970s, there was little off-patent competition except in the antibiotic market, where substitution occurred between broad- and medium-spectrum antibiotics (Schwartzman 1976). Consequently, original brands were generally found to have maintained their prices while retaining market shares of not less than 92.4 per cent in drugstores and not less than 81.8 per cent in hospitals in the off-patent period (Statman 1981). However, these laws have had an increasingly important effect on the use of generic drugs, particularly when combined with active promotion of generics in managed care.

As in the EU, generic drugs are approved for marketing under a shorter regulatory review process than originator products. The current regulatory process governing market entry by generic drugs dates to the enactment of the Hatch-Waxman Act of 1984,[5] which stipulated that generic versions of previously approved drugs no longer had to undergo lengthy New Drug Applications (NDA) but could be approved on the basis of an Abbreviated New Drug Application (ANDA), demonstrating bioequivalence to an original branded drug. Furthermore, the Hatch-Waxman Act made it possible for the market approval process for generic equivalents to occur before the expiration of the patent on the original brand, which is better known as the Roche-Bolar early working provision (see above). Thus, Hatch-Waxman reduced both the entry requirements and the time to entry for generics.

The Act also contains a provision that grants a 180-day period of market exclusivity for the first generic manufacturer to file for an ANDA and successfully challenge the validity of a patent (paragraph IV certification). This provision, on its face, is a competition-enhancing policy. However, the Act also states that originator firms whose patents are challenged must be notified of the challenge and have the right to file a patent infringement claim, automatically resulting in a 30-month stay on any FDA (Food and Drug Administration) action approving the generic product. This creates incentives for original branded manufacturers to file infringement claims even when their claims are not strong. It also creates incentives and legal opportunities for rivals to communicate and enter into agreements that share profits between originator and generic manufacturers. The evidence suggests that firms respond to these incentives. A study by the US Federal Trade Commission (2002) found that in 72 per cent of 104 cases where a paragraph IV certification was claimed (75 applications), a patent infringement action was filed by the originator drug manufacturer. Among the 53 cases that were resolved, eight were decided in favour of the original branded manufacturer and 22 cases were found for the generic producer. The Federal Trade Commission has also settled several cases where the patent holder paid the generic entrant not to launch a generic product, effectively precluding other generics from entering the market as the exclusivity right cannot be transferred even if the first entrant does not market its product. Concern that these loopholes have delayed generic competition led to proposed legislative changes (Bill #S.54) put before Congress in 2003.

Managed care also drove cost-containment measures during the 1990s promoting the increased use of generics (Department of Health and Human Services 2000). As managed care has become a common feature of health insurance arrangements, attention has been directed to managing prescription drug utilization and costs. Pharmacy benefit managers administer formularies, create incentives for adherence to them, and engage in drug utilization review in an effort to make pharmaceutical prescription and distribution more cost-effective.

A key element in formulary management to realize cost savings by pharmacy benefit managers and other managed care organizations is to adopt measures that encourage the use of lower priced generic products in place of originator drugs (Levy 1999).

Pharmacy benefit managers commonly use so-called interchange programmes aimed at substituting lower priced drugs (Lipton *et al.* 1999). Interchange programmes come in two types: those aimed at generic substitution and those targeting therapeutic interchange among original branded products. The generic substitution programmes are more common and more widely accepted. All pharmacy benefit managers offer their clients generic substitution programmes that include: higher dispensing fees for generic products (an incentive for pharmacists to exercise the discretion permitted by state laws), establishing performance targets (rates of generic dispensing) for network pharmacies, and reminders to pharmacists. Another widespread practice is the multi-tier formulary, where generics are located in the lowest co-payment tier and original branded counterparts are in higher tiers. About 60 per cent of privately insured people are covered under a three-tiered formulary (Pharmaceutical Research and Manufacturers of America 2002). This approach relies on consumer-based incentives to promote generic substitution. By 1997, 82.5 per cent of health maintenance organizations had imposed an additional charge for choosing the original drug (Hoechst Marion Roussel 1998). As the gap between the price of original brands and generic equivalents increases, so do patients' preferences for generic drugs to non-formulary original brands at higher co-payment rates (Levit *et al.* 1995).

Generic competition

Economic research in the USA has shown that when generic manufacturers enter the market, they price their products well below their original branded counterparts and, as competition from other generic manufacturers increases, prices are driven down to a fraction of the original branded price at the time of generic launch.[6] A study by the US Congress Office of Technology Assessment (1993) showed that the average generic price was 25 per cent lower than the originator's price at the time of entry and fell to about 20 per cent of that price as generic entry continued. Several studies have shown that as the number of generic competitors increases, prices of generic products decrease: the Congressional Budget Office (1998) found that the retail prices of generic drugs facing competition from 16 to 20 firms were about two-thirds that of generics facing between one and five competitors; Caves *et al.* (1991) reported that generic prices fell to 34 per cent of the originator drug's price as the number of generic competitors went from 1 to 10; and Frank and Salkever (1997) showed that for each generic entrant after the first, prices fell by between 5 and 7 per cent. The increased generic competition has also been shown to rapidly erode the market share of the originator. The Congressional Budget Office study (1998) showed that within a year of entry, the generic products captured roughly 44 per cent of prescriptions dispensed by pharmacies and, for 34 drugs in the sample, up to 65 per cent of sales after 2 years on the market. Grabowski and Vernon (1992), in a study of 11 drugs losing patent protection between 1989 and 1992, found that on average generics had sales accounting for 50 per cent of prescriptions for the molecule one year after entry. More recent experiences with the cardiovascular drugs Cardizem CD and Dilacor show even more rapid erosion of the originator drug's market share: unpublished data on Cardizem CD indicates that it had lost 66 per cent of its market share to generic competitors 12 months following entry;[7] similarly, the antidepressant Prozac lost approximately 80 per cent of its sales to generic competitors within two months of entry.[8]

The implication of this research is that when generic products are permitted to enter markets for prescription drugs, a substantial segment of consumers avail themselves of the lower price generic products, enabling them to realize significant savings relative to the pre-generic entry period. This reflects a high level of substitutability in demand. Moreover, these shifts in market share and price all take place in the presence of potential therapeutic competition.

Comparative policy implications

The UK and France have achieved significantly different levels of generic consumption. Here, we briefly compare the policies introduced in the two countries to stimulate generic prescribing (Table 14.3). The development of a generic drug market in France was slowed in part because of already low prices of originator drugs; more importantly, however, generics had not been legally defined and designated for reimbursement until 1997. Until 1999, pharmacists retained a lower margin for dispensing a less expensive medicine as they were paid according to a digressive sliding scale. Financial incentives for both physicians and pharmacists in the UK have been an important part of developing the generic drug market. Although pharmacists in France have had the right to substitute drugs from a defined list, nevertheless physicians in both countries still retain an important role in the process: in France this means a physician not blocking substitution, while in the UK the use of generics is entirely dependent on the physician prescribing by the generic name. Quite unlike the USA, neither the UK nor France had targeted incentives to patients in the use of generics, although media campaigns in France facilitated wider patient acceptance of generic substitution. France agreed in 2002 to pay physicians higher fees on outpatient visits in exchange for their allowing generic substitution more often unless this was medically unjustified. These policy developments in France, and particularly the agreement with physicians, were an important part of the growth in the use of generics: rates of generic substitution increased from 18 per cent by volume of what can be substituted in 2000 (AFSSAPS 2002) to 48.2 per cent by 2002 (CNAMTS 2003a). However, as shown in Table 14.1, generics account for only 8.4 per cent by volume of all reimbursed medicines, compared with 52 per cent in the UK. These numbers in France are expected to increase following the implementation of a reference price scheme covering off-patent drugs in late 2003.

Certainly, market interventions and incentives that make the demand side (physicians, pharmacists and patients) more price sensitive are important for

Table 14.3 Key policies to promote generics in France and the UK

Policy	France	UK
Generic name prescribing	Offered physicians higher fees in exchange for increased generic prescribing but rejected by physician unions	Long taught in medical schools and widely encouraged as a key part of the generic medicine strategy; generic prescribing rates are approaching 80 per cent of all prescriptions written
Generic substitution	Introduced in 1998, allowing pharmacists to substitute from a defined list of products unless opposed by the physician; the opposition by the latter has decreased	Not allowed but if the prescription is written using the generic name of the drug the pharmacist can select the lowest cost generic equivalent
Pharmacist financial incentives	Pharmacists receive the same margin for the generic as they would for the originator	Pharmacists are paid a flat fee per medicine dispensed plus the list price of the drug; therefore, if they are able to purchase the drug below the list price, they are able to retain a higher margin, although the government does apply a discount recovery scale
Physician financial incentives	Increased physician fees for out-patient visits in exchange for physicians not blocking generic substitution	GPs have individual indicative budgets but previously when some GPs had cash-limited prescribing budgets they were found to have higher rates of generic name prescribing
Price regulation	Up to 2003, generics had to be priced 30 per cent below the price of the originator; however, a reference price scheme for off-patent drugs introduced in late 2003	The market price used to be the list price such that levels of supply and competition between wholesalers would determine actual price in the UK; however, after some gaming of the price system by wholesalers was uncovered, the government introduced a maximum price scheme

promoting generic medicines. Whether or not prescription budgets can or should be applied depends on incentives already in place, such as those inherent in the payment method of physicians, or on other mechanisms such as guidelines, formularies or monitoring of prescription data. The acceptance of generic substitution by pharmacists or the dispensing of lower-priced medicines is dependent on positive financial remuneration. When considering the generalizability of a differential co-payment approach in EU countries, it is important to keep in mind the values on which the health care systems are founded, especially equity (see also Chapter 13).

Regulation or market intervention is necessary to some extent in the off-patent pharmaceutical market. Without market interventions correcting for demand-side imperfections, even the market in the USA may not have achieved a high-volume use of generics with a lower price than the originator product. Whether generics are also price competitive depends not only on demand-side conditions (whether demand for individual products is price sensitive), but also on market factors. The adoption in the USA of drug product selection laws in the late 1970s and the lowering of market approval requirements of generic equivalents through the Hatch-Waxman Act in 1984 in many ways deregulated the off-patent market, and competition followed, albeit not fully until the demand-side initiatives associated with the spread of managed care really took hold.

Whether or not a given country should apply approaches adopted in other EU countries or the USA depends on a number of factors, for example the objectives of policy makers, the institutional and financial context of the health care system, and the role and ethics of health care professionals. It will also depend on the relative importance of the proprietary versus generic drug industries in the country from perspectives of both macroeconomics and supply availability. Measures may also raise politically sensitive issues such as the role of the pharmacist in the product selection decision, the ethics of financial incentive in prescribing and dispensing, and issues of equity in targeting the patient through differential user charges (Mrazek and Mossialos 2000). These are issues that should be discussed by policy makers, the industry, health professionals and the public as generics begin to play a wider role in pharmaceutical policies.

Notes

1 Estimates of the size of the generics markets in Sweden and Ireland were upwards of 33 per cent and 20 per cent by volume, respectively, by the mid-1990s (National Economic Research Associates 1998).

2 The government introduced a statutory maximum price scheme for generic medicines supplied to the NHS for primary care in August 2000 in an attempt to correct previous problems with the Drug Tariff Scheme, which made it possible for suppliers to game the system to achieve a higher list price (Department of Health 2000; Oxera 2001).

3 The price line is the average of the three least expensive generic equivalents plus one-third of the difference between the average of the three least expensive and the three most expensive products in the category.

4 Also known as the Drug Price Competition and Patent Term Restoration Act.

5 The language of the Act specifically states that its purposes are 'to make available more low cost generic drugs . . .'.

6 Examples of studies arriving at results reflected in this paragraph include: Caves *et al.* (1991), Grabowski and Vernon (1992), Treppel and Neugeboren (1994), Frank and Salkever (1997), Congressional Budget Office (1998), Suh *et al.* (2000) and Mrazek (2001).

7 Data obtained from Scott Levin, Inc.

8 Press release from Eli Lilly, 3 October 2001 (available from http://newsroom.lilly.com/news/story.cfm?id=856). Also, tabulations of sales data from Scott Levin, Inc.

References

Agence Française de Sécurité Sanitaire des Produits de Santé (2002) *Analyse des ventes de médicaments aux officines et aux hôpitaux en France 1988–2000*. Paris: AFSSAPS (available from http://agmed.sante.gouv.fr/pdf/5/ventmed.pdf) (accessed 20 July 2003).

Andersen, M.L., Laursen, K., Schaumann, M. *et al.* (2000) How do patients evaluate the newly introduced system of substituting prescriptions?, *Ugeskrift for laeger*, 162(45): 6066–9.

Atkinson, T.J. (2002) *European Generic Drug Markets Growth to 2007*. London: Urch Publishing.

Busse, R. and Howorth, C. (1999) Cost-containment in Germany 1977–97, in E. Mossialos and J. LeGrand (eds) *Health Care and Cost Containment in the European Union*. Aldershot: Ashgate.

Caisse nationale d'assurance maladie des travailleurs salariés (2003a) *Quelques aspects significatifs de la consommation de médicaments en France*. Paris: CNAMTS.

Caisse nationale d'assurance maladie des travailleurs salariés (2003b) *Des tendances de fond aux mouvements de court terme. Point de conjoncture No. 12*. Paris: CNAMTS.

Casado Buendia, S., Sagardui Villamor, J.K. and Lacalle Rodriguez-Labajo, M. (2002) The substitution of generic for brand medicines in family medical clinics, *Aten Primaria*, 30(6): 343–7.

Caves, R.E., Whinston, M.E. and Hurwitz, M.A. (1991) Patent expiration, entry and competition in the United States pharmaceutical industry: an exploratory analysis. *Brookings Papers on Economic Activity: Microeconomics 1991*. Washington, DC: Brookings Institute.

Congressional Budget Office (1998) *How increased competition from generic drugs has affected prices and returns in the pharmaceutical industry*. Washington, DC: CBO.

Delporte, J.P. (2002) Generic drugs, *Revue médicale de Liège*, 57(1): 13–22.

Department of Health (2000) *The Government's Response to the Health Select Committee's First Report on the Cost and Availability of Generic Drugs to the NHS*. London: HMSO.

Department of Health (2002a) *Prescriptions Dispensed in the Community, Statistics for 1991 to 2001: England*. London: HMSO.

Department of Health (2002b) *Roll Forward for the United Kingdom Wide Maximum Price Scheme for Generic Medicines in NHS Primary Care*. London: Department of Health (available from http://www.doh.gov.uk/generics/genericspressrelease2002.htm) (accessed 10 July 2003).

Department of Health and Human Services (2000) *Prescription Drug Coverage, Spending, Utilization and Prices*. Washington, DC: DHHS (available from http://aspe.hhs.gov/health/reports/drugstudy).

European Generic Medicines Association (2003) *G10 Workshop Identifies Key Measures to Stimulate Generics* (available from http://www.egagenerics.com) (accessed 14 May 2003).

Foundation for Pharmaceutical Statistics (2002) *Facts and Figures 2002*. The Hague: SFK.

Frank, R.G. and Salkever, D.S. (1997) Generic entry and the pricing of pharmaceuticals, *Journal of Economics and Management Strategy*, 6(1): 75–90.

Gosden, T. and Torgerson, D.J. (1997) The effect of fundholding on prescribing and referral costs: a review of the evidence, *Health Policy*, 40(20): 103–14.

Grabowski, H. and Vernon, J. (1992) Brand loyalty and price competition in pharmaceuticals after the 1984 Drug Act, *Journal of Law and Economics*, 35(2): 331–50.

Hellstrom, J. and Rudholm, N. (2003) *Uncertainty in the Generic Versus Brand Name Prescription Decision*. Umeå: Umeå University, Department of Economics.

High Level Group on Innovation and Provision of Medicines (2002) *Recommendations for*

Action. Brussels: European Commission (available from http://pharmacos.eudra.org) (accessed 14 May 2003).

Hoechst Marion Roussel (1998) *Managed Care Digest Series: HMO-PPO/Medicare-Medicaid Digest*. Kansas City, MO: HMR.

Kanavos, P. and Reinhardt, U. (2003) Reference pricing for drugs: is it compatible with United States health care?, *Health Affairs*, 22(3): 16–30.

Levit, K.R., Lazenby, H.C., Braden, B.R. *et al.* (1995) *National Health Expenditures*. Baltimore, MD: HCFA.

Levit, K., Smith, C., Cowan, C., Lazenby, H. and Martin, A. (2002) Inflation spurs health spending in 2002, *Health Affairs*, 21(1): 172–81.

Levy, R. (1999) *The Pharmaceutical Industry: A Discussion of Competitive and Antitrust Issues in an Environment of Change*. Washington, DC: Federal Trade Commission, Bureau of Economics.

Lipton, H.L., Kreling, D.H., Collins, T. and Hertz, K.C. (1999) Pharmacy benefit management companies: dimensions of performance, *Annual Review of Public Health*, 20: 361–401.

Molony, S. (2002) Generic drugs switch to cut soaring costs, *Irish Independent*, 29 October.

Mrazek, M. (2001) The impact of differing regulatory frameworks on post-patent pharmaceutical markets in the United Kingdom, United States and Germany 1990 to 1997. PhD thesis, London School of Economics and Political Science.

Mrazek, M. and Mossialos, E. (2000) Increasing demand while decreasing costs of generic medicines, *Lancet*, 356: 1784–5.

National Economic Research Associates (1998) *Policy Relating to Generic Medicines in the OECD: Final Report for the European Commission (III/E/3)*. London: NERA.

Office of Technology Assessment (1993) *Pharmaceutical R&D Costs, Risks and Rewards*. Washington, DC: US Government Printing Office.

Oxera (2001) *Fundamental Review of the Generic Drug Market* (available from http://www.doh.gov.uk/generics/oxerareport.htm) (accessed 9 October 2002).

Peterson, K.U. (2000) Original brands and generic preparations, *Medizinische Klinik*, 95(1): 26–30.

Pharmaceutical Research and Manufacturers of America (2002) *Pharmaceutical Industry Profile 2002*. Washington, DC: PhRMA.

Roche Products Inc. v. *Bolar Pharmaceuticals Co.* 733 F.2d 858 (Fed. Cir. 1984), cert. Denied, 469 United States 856 (1984).

Rubak, S.L., Andersen, M.L., Mainz, J., Olesgaard, P. and Lauritzen, T. (2000a) How do practitioners evaluate the newly introduced system of substituting prescriptions?, *Ugeskrift for laeger*, 162(45): 6070–3.

Rubak, S.L., Andersen, M.L., Mainz, J. *et al.* (2000b) How do pharmacists evaluate the newly introduced system of substituting prescriptions?, *Ugeskrift for laeger*, 162(45): 6074–7.

Schwartzman, D. (1976) *Innovation in the Pharmaceutical Industry*. Baltimore, MD: Johns Hopkins University Press.

Statman, M. (1981) The effect of patent expiration on the market position of drugs, in R.B. Helms (ed.) *Drugs and Health: Economic Issues and Policy Objectives*. Washington, DC: American Enterprise Institute for Public Policy Research.

Suh, D.C., Manning, W.G., Jr., Schondelmeyer, S. and Hadsall, R.S. (2000) Effect of multiple-source entry on price competition after patent expiration in the pharmaceutical industry, *Health Service Research*, 35(2): 529–47.

Treppel, J.I. and Neugeboren, E.A. (1994) Generic drug industry overview: statistical analysis and view point, *Kidder Peabody Industry Report*. New York: Kidder, Peabody & Co.

US Federal Trade Commission (2002) *Generic Drug Entry Prior to Patent Expiration*. Washington, DC: FTA.

Vallès, J.A., Barreiro, M., Cereza, G. *et al.* (2002) Acetación de los fármacos genericós en equipos de atención primaria: efecto de una intervención educativa y de los precios de referencia, *Gaceta Sanitaria*, 16(6): 505–10.

Walley, T., Wilson, R. and Bligh, J. (1995) Current prescribing in primary care in the United Kingdom: effects of the indicative prescribing scheme and GP fund-holding, *Pharmacoeconomics*, 7(4): 320–31.

Zweifel, P. and Crivelli, L. (1996) Price regulation of drugs: lessons from Germany, *Journal of Regulatory Economics*, 10: 257–73.

fifteen

The over-the-counter pharmaceutical market

Christine M. Bond, with Maria Pia Orru, Jean Marc Leder and Marcel Bouvy

This chapter summarizes the regulatory status of over-the-counter pharmaceuticals, and considers aspects of their distribution and use, including the market environment, safety and appropriateness of treatment.

Medicines classification and the over-the-counter market

In general, in all European countries, medicines are distributed/supplied according to their market regulatory status. This status is designed to ensure that the public benefit from the therapeutic actions of the drug while minimizing the chances of inappropriate use and of harm.

This is exemplified by the classifications of medicines currently existing in Europe. In the UK, these are known as POM (prescription-only medicine), P (pharmacy-supervised sale) and GSL (general sales list). The POM medicines are primarily only available to the public when recommended/endorsed by a medical practitioner. They may not all be reimbursable under an individual country's health service; for example, until recently, in Italy only 75 per cent of these prescription drugs were reimbursed. Dental practitioners also have limited prescribing rights. In some countries such as the UK and the Netherlands, this system is under review with legislation currently being prepared to allow nurses and other health care professionals, such as pharmacists, wider prescribing rights. This relaxation of earlier restrictions on supply is more advanced in the UK than in many other European countries. It should also be noted that in some countries, such as the Netherlands, as in the USA, there are also only two categories of medicines – the equivalent of POM and GSL – and in Australia and New Zealand there are four – there is an extra category of P medicines which can only be sold directly by the pharmacist and which require the pharmacist to ascertain additional information.

The over-the-counter (OTC) market includes the P and GSL categories, and also herbal and homeopathic medicines, which are discussed in more detail in Chapter 18, and which are currently not regulated under the same system. There can be major distinctions between the P and GSL categories. In the UK, France and many other countries, medicines in the P category can only be sold 'under the supervision' of a pharmacist, from registered pharmacy premises, whereas the GSL products can be sold both from pharmacies, without the supervision requirement, and from any retail outlet. This is not necessarily the case in all European countries. For example in Italy, the same three broad categories of medicines exist as prescription-only, SOP (senza obbligo di prescrizione) and PDB (prodotto da banco), commonly known as OTC. However, both the SOP and PDB medicines are only available through pharmacies and sold by the pharmacist; the difference is that the PDB medicines can be advertised directly to the public, and displayed in areas for customer self-selection, if the pharmacist so wishes. A similar position exists in France and some other European countries. In the Netherlands, however, there are only POM and OTC. Pharmacies focus on POM medicines and have a minority role in the sale of OTCs, 75 per cent of which are sold from *drogisten* (chemists), which also sell toothpaste and body care products.

In the UK, the pharmacy supervision requirement has been interpreted in its strictest sense with a requirement for the pharmacist to be both present and aware of all such sales. The exact interpretation of these stringent requirements are under review by the Royal Pharmaceutical Society of Great Britain. There are indications that, reflecting other professions, supervision may come to be understood as 'knowing that appropriate systems are in place'. This would necessitate the explicit use of protocols and audit trails, but permit easier access to these medicines.

In the UK, any new medicine seeking a licence is classified as a POM. After two years the classification automatically defaults to P unless there is a specific application to retain the POM status. In practice, the POM status is normally retained and subsequent moves to reclassify a product require a lengthy consultative process to demonstrate safety and the benefit of making the medicine more widely available (Medicines and Healthcare Products Regulatory Agency 2002). A similar process would also apply for medicines seeking further reclassification to GSL status.

Across Europe and the Western world, there have been moves generally to place more medicines into the OTC classes. The reasons for this are four-fold: to remove the drug distribution costs from government to individual consumer; to empower the public and encourage responsibility for self-medication; to widen access (Brass 2001); and to extend the life and market of products nearing the end of their patents. Again the extent to which these are applicable to an individual country will vary; for example, in Italy there is a greater emphasis on the need for professional input into all self-medication. To some extent, the transfer of costs from government to consumer is already achieved through a well-established, two-tier prescription system, whereby approximately 25 per cent of the products are not reimbursable.

In many countries, the moves to increase the range of OTC drugs have been generally supported by the pharmaceutical profession, as they have extended the armamentarium of drugs available to the pharmacist when giving advice on the management of symptoms of minor illness and self-limiting conditions. This traditional role is of increasing importance to the profession at a time when the technical aspects of dispensing have become relatively routine, and there is little call for the compounding skills required in earlier decades, although there is increased cognitive input, related to pharmaceutical care and medicines management that interface with both the patient and the prescriber. However, in the Netherlands, where OTC drugs are not primarily distributed through pharmacies, there has been less support for the deregulation process, reflecting the fact that the 'chemist' shops, rather than pharmacies, manage the bulk of supply.

The medical profession has also been shown to support the deregulation process in principle (Sivho *et al.* 1999), although some caveats have been expressed.

One of the early European moves to streamline the process of wider access was enshrined in a European Directive (European Community 1992), later revised (European Parliament and Council 2001), which declared that no medicine should remain a POM unless it met one of the following criteria:

- there is direct or indirect danger to health if the medicine is used without medical supervision (for example, the adverse drug reaction profile needs a doctor to assess risk–benefit; or misdiagnosis might lead to the patient being put at risk);
- the medicine is frequently used incorrectly, leading to direct or indirect danger to health (e.g. products liable to misuse);
- the activity of the drug or the side-effects require further investigation; or
- the drug is parenterally administered.

In 1989, Denmark was among the first of the Northern European countries to deregulate a large number of medicines, including cimetidine (Edwards 1992). Since then, other European countries, including Finland, have also rapidly increased the pace at which medicines are being reclassified. In the period January 1990 to December 1994, 50 products were switched, 19 of them in the preceding year. Products such as HRTs, haemorrhoid treatments, antihistamines, NSAIDs and vaginal imidazoles were involved. In contrast, changes have occurred much more slowly in other countries, notably those previously in the Eastern bloc. For example, in Slovakia it is perceived that the Slovak people need more education in self-medication before the Slovak regulations should be allowed to catch up with the legislation of the European Commission.

In the past 18 years in the UK, more than 50 products have been reclassified from POM to P and many further deregulated to GSL. A list of these is given in Table 15.1. There are well-publicized proposals to further extend this list into new therapeutic areas for chronic conditions, such as hypertension and lifestyle, including contraception (*OTC Bulletin* 2002). It may also be appropriate to prioritize some of the 'lifestyle' drugs (see Chapter 17) for deregulation.

While all European countries have a similar regulatory system in place, there are differences between countries as to the current classification for individual drug entities. For example, of the UK list shown in Table 15.1, 20 products are not yet available in the Netherlands. Similarly in the treatment of hay fever/

Table 15.1 List of medicines deregulated in the UK, 1983–1999

Date	Ingredient/product	Date	Ingredient/product
1983	ibuprofen	1994	diclofenac (topical)
	loperamide		felbinac (topical)
1984	terfenadine		piroxicam (topical)
1985	hydrocortisone 1% (topical)		flunisolide (nasal spray)
1986	miconazole		ranitidine
1988	ibuprofen (sustained release and		minoxidil (topical)
	topical)		Adcortyl in Orabase
1989	astemizole		Anusol Plus HC ointment
	mebendazole		Anusol Plus HC suppositories
	dextromethorphan	1995	hydroxyzine
1991	nicotine 2 mg gum		pyrantel
1992	hyoscine N-butyl bromide		fluconazole
	nicotine patches		ketoconazole (topical)
	vaginal imidazoles		Proctocream HC
	hydrocortisone with crotamiton		Iodosorb
	(topical)		Budesonide (nasal)
	carbenoxolone	1996	azelastine
	paracetamol and dihydrocodeine		nizatidine
1993	loratidine		hydrocortisone/lignocaine
	acyclovir (topical)		mebeverine
	acrivastine	1997	clotrimazole/hydrocortisone
	cetirizine	1998	domperidone
	ketoprofen (topical)		miconazole/hydrocortisone
	cimetidine		levocabastine
	famotidine		nedocromil sodium
	beclomethasone dipropionate		ketoconazole 2% (topical)
	(nasal)	1999	nystatin/hydrocortisone
	mebendazole (multiple dose)		aspirin 75 mg
	pseudoephedrine (sustained release)		isosorbide mononitrate
	sodium cromoglycate (ophthalmic)		
	tioconazole (vaginal)		
	nicotine 4 mg gum		
	hydrocortisone (oral pellet)		
	aluminium chloride hexahydrate		
	(topical)		

Source: Royal Pharmaceutical Society of Great Britain (2002). .

rhinitis, first- and second-generation antihistamines, cromoglycates and nasal corticosteroids are available as P medicines in the UK, whereas in some other European countries, such as France and Italy, only the first-generation antihistamines are available without a prescription. Further examples of these differences are shown in Table 15.2. Across these countries, and the illustrative 20 products, a range of three to six products is still only available by prescription, but there is no national pattern to this.

It is unlikely that there will be total agreement across Europe in drug classification in the near future, although recent changes may make more congruity

Table 15.2 Differences in regulatory status of different drugs across Europe

Ingredient	Austria	France	Germany	Italy	Netherlands	Sweden	Switzerland	UK
Analgesics, anti-inflammatory agents and antipyretics								
Acetyl salicylic acid	NPr	NPr	NPr	NPr	NPr	NPr	NPr	NPr
Diclofenac	NPr	NPr	NPr	NPr	NPr	Rx	NPr	Rx
Etofenamate (topical)	NPr	—	NPr	NPr	—	—	NPr	NPr
Ibuprofen (oral)	NPr	NPr	NPr	NPr	NPr	NPr	NPr	NPr
Ibuprofen (topical)	NPr	NPr	NPr	NPr	NPr	—	NPr	NPr
Ketoprofen	NPr	NPr	NPr	NPr	NPr	Rx	Rx	NPr
Naproxen	Rx	—	Rx	NPr	—	Rx	Rx	Rx
Paracetamol	NPr	NPr	NPr	NPr	NPr	NPr	NPr	NPr
Piroxicam (topical)	NPr	Rx	NPr	NPr	NPr	Rx	NPr	NPr
Antifungal agents								
Clotrimazole (topical)	NPr	NPr	NPr	NPr	NPr	NPr	NPr	NPr
Clotrimazole (vaginal)	Rx	NPr	NPr	Rx	Rx	NPr	Rx	NPr
Econazole	NPr	NPr	NPr	NPr	NPr	NPr	NPr	NPr
Isoconazole (topical)	NPr	NPr	NPr	Rx	—	—	Rx	NPr
Ketoconazole (topical)	NPr	NPr	NPr	NPr	Rx	NPr	NPr	NPr
Nystatin	Rx	Rx	NPr	Rx	Rx	Rx	Rx	Rx
H$_2$ antagonists								
Cimetidine	Rx	NPr	Rx	NPr	NPr	Rx	Rx	NPr
Famotidine	Rx	NPr	Rx	Rx	NPr	NPr	NPr	NPr
Ranitidine	NPr	NPr	Rx	Rx	NPr	NPr	NPr	NPr
Smoking cessation aids								
Nicotine (gum)	NPr	NPr	NPr	NPr	NPr	NPr	NPr	NPr
Nicotine (patch)	NPr	Rx	NPr	NPr	NPr	NPr	NPr	NPr

Note: Rx = available only with a doctor's prescription; NPr = without a doctor's prescription.
Source: Based on AESGP (2002) and Wilkes (1998).

easier. There are now procedures for mutual recognition, which 'enables manu-facturers to seek simultaneous marketing authorisation in two or more member states known as the Concerned Member States (CSM) providing they have an existing marketing authorisation for that drug in at least one member State, known as the reference member state (RMS)' (Abraham and Lewis 1999). Some of the differences of individual classification may also be historical and it is believed that some currently available GSL prescriptions would not have that status if they were assessed against today's criteria; for example, aspirin may be associated with severe adverse events, such as gastrointestinal bleeding or abuse/overuse as in analgesic-dependent headache.

Finally, it should be noted in this introductory section that medicines are constantly monitored even when fully deregulated. This is discussed in more detail below but it may mean that medicines may be reclassified back to a status with more control should concern arise about safety.

Market structure and competition

The OTC market is growing year on year. Self-medication products were estimated to account for 18 per cent by value of the total global pharmaceutical market in 2001 (*OTC Bulletin*-IMS Health Self-medication 2002). The proportion varies from country to country but is increasing in all areas worldwide. The Far East is the fastest growing market (*OTC Bulletin*-IMS Health Self-medication 2002). In North America, the proportion of OTC products is highest and accounted for 30 per cent of the global market in 1997, with Europe second highest at 27 per cent. It can thus be seen that there are global differences in patterns of self-medication, and these are also evident within Europe (AESGP 2002) (Figure 15.1).

One of the characteristics of the OTC market compared with the prescription specialities is that products can be advertised directly to the public. Such advertisements are subject to strict control but nevertheless can use emotive language, which may imply benefits beyond those stated. A US study of OTC advertisements in 1994 concluded that they lacked the information necessary for consumers to make informed choices, due to inaccuracies and insufficient information on side-effects (Sansgiry *et al.* 1999). A further survey of 167 adverts in top circulation women's magazines, some of which are also widely read in the UK, such as *Good Housekeeping*, demonstrated that adverts to the public are predominantly based on claims for performance of drug content and do not include information on price or research evidence (Rallapalli and Smith 1994). Thus, purchasing decisions are made on a different basis from the more, although not totally, objective decision making of a third-party prescriber. The data to support evidence of benefit is also unlikely to be demanded in the same way by the lay consumer as by the prescriber, and there is less external pressure, such as might come from governments, for cost-effective decision making. The reasons for this are two-fold. First, most decisions will be individual and occur in isolation and therefore differences between high and low cost options will be minimized. Secondly, market forces will be operating, under which a single consumer may feel able to opt for a higher cost purchase and be prepared to gamble that the more expensive preparation will have marginal benefit.

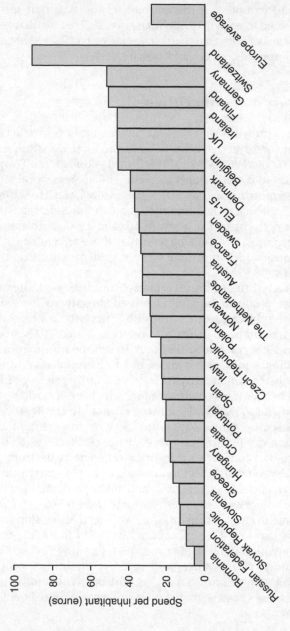

Figure 15.1 Self-medication spent per head of population across Europe in 2001.
Source: AESGP (2002).

The role of pharmacist

The pharmaceutical profession, and community pharmacists in particular, have a central supply role in the OTC market, although the extent of this is limited by the prevailing national legislation and custom and practice. Reflecting this, pharmacists in the Netherlands are less involved in the sale of OTCs than their counterparts elsewhere because of the intermediate category of retail outlets, the *drogisten*, which are not staffed by pharmacists, and in the UK where many GSL medicines are available outwith the pharmacy network, and only P medicines require pharmacy input. In this section, we consider the medicines for which the OTC licence requires that sales should be made 'under the supervision' of a pharmacist. The debate around the term 'supervision' has already been referred to and should be borne in mind when reading this section.

In most countries, for P medicines the pharmacist has a responsibility to ensure that preparations are sold appropriately. This is not dissimilar to the role of the doctor when prescribing a medicine, and many of the principles outlined in Chapter 8 on good prescribing practice could be applied in the OTC prescribing situation. In essence, therefore, the pharmacist should, as far as possible, ensure that medicines are sold for the indications for which the preparation has an OTC licence (which may not be the same as those for the prescribed use), that potential for drug interactions are assessed and avoided if relevant, and that patients with contraindications are not sold the drug. So, for example, the non-steroidal analgesic ibuprofen should not be sold to individuals with a history of peptic ulcer disease or a known sensitivity to aspirin, and patients with asthma should be warned that they may experience a worsening of their condition, in which case the drug should be stopped. This avoids the most common side-effects of NSAIDs which include gastric bleeding and exacerbations of asthma. Another example would be the OTC sale of vaginal imidazoles, which have few if any known adverse side-effects. However, with this particular preparation the concern would be to be confident of an accurate diagnosis and not to treat a condition other than vaginal candidiasis, for which the imidazole would be ineffective. This would be of particular concern if delay in diagnosing and treating the actual condition led to poorer prognosis (e.g. chlamydia, bacterial vaginosis). One of the problems with this set of diseases is that there are no definite presenting symptoms, and diagnosis can only be confirmed microbiologically. Novel ways of making such testing possible in the OTC context may be on the horizon with self-diagnostic kits emerging on the market in general (Anonymous 2000a), the use of self-administered tampons to detect sexually transmitted diseases (Wiesenfeld *et al.* 2001) and with a theoretical possibility of developing one for the diagnosis of candidiasis.

Thus the role of the pharmacist is to ensure compliance with the OTC licence at the point of sale, either through direct involvement at the point of sale or through supervising non-pharmacy staff involved in the transaction.

One of the difficulties for the pharmacist and his or her staff in carrying out their responsibilities is that the purchaser may be unaware of them, be resistant to answering the questions asked of them and of any attempt to refuse sale. This is particularly difficult if a GP has perhaps recommended an OTC purchase on the basis of financial economies for both the patient and government, yet for an indication for which the product does not have an OTC licence. For example, for hydrocortisone 1% cream, the OTC licence precludes use on the face, yet it is known that customers often wish to buy it for this purpose either because of prior use or because of a medical suggestion. The risk for the pharmacist in allowing such a sale, apart from violating the regulatory framework, would be one of liability. Should an individual subsequently suffer an adverse event, the pharmacist would be deemed liable, whereas if it had been sold within the OTC licence the manufacturer would be liable. This is the theoretical position but it has yet to be tested in case law.

As an increasing number of preparations originally deregulated to pharmacy sale are further deregulated to unlimited retail availability, and pack sizes are increased, this may further influence the customer's belief that the product is safe and undermines the pharmacist's attempt to contain sales with the OTC licence. In the Netherlands, it is now possible to buy 50-tablet packs of ibuprofen 400 mg, while a few years ago only 20 tablets of 200 mg were available.

Product selection

Product selection in the OTC market has traditionally been based on experience of benefit and safety as reported by customers. Under the current systematic approach to grading levels of evidence, this would be rated as lower than the current lowest level of 4 (US Department of Health and Human Services 1993), which refers to evidence obtained from expert committee reports or opinions and/or the clinical experience of respected authorities. Until the relatively recent increase in the armamentarium of OTC products, the actual benefit of most OTC products was unproven scientifically and much of the efficacy is often considered to be due to the placebo effect and time. However, drugs recently deregulated from previous prescription use are newer generation products that themselves had to go through extensive marketing applications to gain their original POM licence, and for which there is a body of evidence. Thus, for these newer products there is often sufficient information to generate evidence-based guidelines for use (Watson *et al.* 2001). The benefits of this are that patients are more likely to receive clinically effective treatments, which should be coherent with prescribing strategies for the same therapeutic area.

Appropriateness of product selection may be addressed by the use of evidence-based guidelines, but as in medical practice the extent to which such guidelines are used and their effect on patient outcome unclear. An early study on dyspepsia guidelines (Bond and Grimshaw 1994), designed to support appropriate H_2 blocker use, indicated that community pharmacists found the guidelines easy to use and of benefit to their practice (Bond 2000). They requested more guidelines for other therapeutic products, some of which were produced (Matheson and Bond 1995; Porteous *et al.* 1997, 1998).

The most effective way of disseminating such guidelines and their effect on behaviour and knowledge were explored in a later study addressing the appropriate use of vaginal imidazoles for symptoms of vaginal thrush (Watson *et al.* 2002). This study showed that there was no statistically significant difference between three routes of guideline dissemination (standard continuing education using workshops and didactic seminars, mailed printed material, or individual outreach visits to community pharmacists). Moreover, the relatively small proportion of appropriate sales (as measured by role-playing actions) despite good product knowledge demonstrated that OTC supply is a complex multifactorial combination of cognitive and affective skills, and is often mediated via a non-pharmacist. It may be appropriate to consider standard theoretical models, such as human error theory or the theory of planned behaviour, to design more relevant educational interventions to improve practice.

As discussed in Chapter 9, the doctor–patient relationship is changing, and this is no less true for the pharmacist–patient relationship. There is an increasing focus on the customer/patient in an OTC transaction and there is also greater patient influence on product choice that will be affected by previous use, lay advice and advertisement. Choice is also affected by advice from professionals such as GPs, nurses and pharmacists (Sinclair *et al.* 2000). Furthermore, products that are deregulated to a wider variety of retail outlets are available purely for self-selection and there is often little, if any, professional input in such selection. The GSL status reflects informed opinion that the product is safe to be used in this way, but it ignores the effect that such 'labelling' has on public perceptions. A recent Scottish study showed that there appeared to be differences in the public's perceptions of the safety and efficacy of products obtained on prescription from pharmacies compared with those from other outlets (Porteous *et al.* 2002).

In an increasingly European market and one in which consistency of practice is the ideal, a 'European' guideline for a particular condition should be the way forward. A first example of this is the ARIA guideline for the management of rhinitis in the pharmacy (ARIA 2003; Anonymous 2003). This innovative guideline (see Figure 15.2) has been produced by a multidisciplinary group (general practitioners, pharmacists, consultants) from seven countries that is applicable to all European countries and North America, despite variations in the availability of OTC treatments. For example, in the UK, first- and second-generation antihistamines, cromoglycates and nasal corticosteroids are available over the counter, whereas in France only the first-generation sedating antihistamines are available. Nonetheless, the guideline can be used in both these settings. It also incorporates physician management of disease, encouraging consistency across the pharmacist–self-care/medical interface.

In addition to supporting evidence-based management of rhinitis, the ARIA guideline is designed to detect undiagnosed or poorly controlled asthma. Rhinitis is a common co-morbidity of the potentially more serious asthma and thus the guideline should have benefit if it also improves the long-term management of this condition.

Economic impact

Early health economics research on newly deregulated products such as hydrocortisone and loperamide demonstrated significant government savings in drug-associated costs. For example, it was estimated using cost–benefit analyses that the deregulation of loperamide saved the UK government £4.2million in

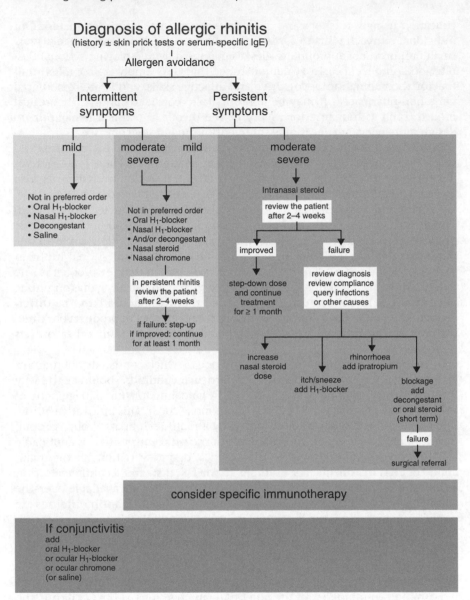

Figure 15.2 Stepwise approach for the treatment of allergic rhinitis according to the ARIA guideline. Reproduced with permission from ARIA (2003).

1987 and that of hydrocortisone £2 million (Ryan and Yule 1990). Similar studies in Sweden estimated a yearly saving of US$400 million for the national drug budget because of the deregulation of 16 different products (Carlsten *et al.* 1996). While such calculations are interesting, they may not always take into account the total effect of deregulation on the distribution and supply of a product. For example, if a product is for an acute condition, and requires a single treatment, such as topical aciclovir for the treatment of cold sores (herpes simplex), inspection of UK prescribing data for such a product shows that after deregulation prescriptions for this product fell sharply and remained low, thus saving the government significant amounts (Bond 1995). In contrast, such a fall was not recorded when the anti-ulcer drugs, the H_2 blockers such as cimetidine, famotidine and later ranitidine were deregulated. It is postulated that the reason for this is that OTC use of the product widened the target population and that different people purchased the product for dyspepsia – people who would have previously purchased a simple antacid from the pharmacist subsequently bought the more effective OTC product. Once an individual has experienced the better relief obtained from the H_2 blocker, but also the increased cost, it would be appear that long-term use is translated into increased prescription use. This is also seen with long-term antihistamine use (H. Sinclair, personal communication).

The mechanism of payment for prescription drugs will also inextricably affect the relative sales volume after deregulation. At the moment, OTC drugs in the Netherlands are only reimbursed on prescription when they are used chronically (e.g. paracetamol for arthrosis). These regulations can have unexpected effects. When topical aciclovir for cold sores became OTC, prescription drug sales remained the same until the drug was not reimbursed anymore. The original OTC availability just led to an increase in total sales unlike the UK situation described above.

Similarly in the Netherlands when ibuprofen 400 mg was deregulated, there was an increase in prescriptions for ibuprofen 600 mg, and when cetirizine and loratadine were deregulated, and were only reimbursed when used chronically, the newer prescription-only antihistamines were prescribed more (Bouvy and Egberts 2000).

Theoretical modelling of the deregulation process using standard economic theory of consumer surplus indicates that, in the UK, for those patients for whom the acquisition cost of the drug is cheaper over the counter than obtaining it on prescription (including direct and indirect costs in both cases), OTC purchase is financially beneficial for both patient and government (Ryan and Bond 1996). Again, this will vary from country to country depending on the extent to which patients contribute to the costs of their prescription medicines, and the OTC price (Shih *et al.* 2002).

Equity issues

It is clear from the above that those patients normally eligible for free prescriptions would be frequently disadvantaged by widespread policies to restrict distribution of particular products to OTC sale. In the UK, this was implemented in 1985 with the introduction of a blacklist for products of limited therapeutic value, such as multivitamins and those for which prescribing was not recommended (e.g. benzodiazepines). Subsequent supply of these drugs was therefore either through OTC purchase or private prescription. Thus in a single government action, drug costs were potentially reduced and prescribing quality was improved. However, there are obvious limitations on the range of drugs to which such a policy can be applied.

Interesting work has shown that many people who could self-medicate are unwilling to do so for financial reasons (Schafheutle *et al.* 1996; Payne *et al.* 1998; Hassell *et al.* 1999). This leads to unnecessary use of the medical consultation and means that, in effect, doctors are making social decisions when prescribing drugs. In a move to overcome this, recent projects in the UK have developed mechanisms for the direct supply of a list of drugs from community pharmacies, within the NHS, for those patients normally eligible for free supply (Whittington *et al.* 2001). Sometimes such schemes may reflect specific local need and other local examples include treatments for head lice (Anonymous 2001), smoking cessation (Anonymous 2002) and emergency contraception (Anonymous 2000b).

Side-effects and pharmacovigilance

By definition, drugs and their individual products that are made more widely available are deemed by the licensing authorities to be safe for use by a wider population. Side-effects and adverse events from drugs may be potentially predictable based on pharmacological principles, or idiosyncratic, and therefore unexpected. Such unexpected events, which may be rare but fatal, are often only identified after widespread and extensive use and may be due to the direct effects of the drug, or of an interaction with another drug or food product.

Thus, one of the first products to be deregulated in 1984, terfenadine (an early second-generation non-sedating antihistamine), was associated with a number of fatal events in wider non-prescription use. When taken by patients with cardiac or hepatic disease, in overdose or with drugs with which it interacted (e.g. ketoconazole) or certain foodstuffs such as grapefruit juice, it could produce serious or even fatal cardiac arrhythmias (Committee for Safety of Medicines and Medicines Control Agency 1992; Anonymous 1997). Subsequent to this association being recognized, the product was restored to prescription-only use and has since become unavailable in the UK, although it is still available on prescription elsewhere, such as in the Netherlands. It is likely that there were not many reports of actual arrhythmias due to the high detection of interactions by pharmacies and the high compliance of patients to one single pharmacy.

Another example of an adverse event arising from an OTC product was that related to the herbal preparation St John's Wort (*Hypericum perforatum*). St John's Wort is an inducer of various drug-metabolizing enzymes, resulting in reduced blood concentrations of some commonly prescribed drugs, including warfarin, cyclosporin, oral contraceptives, digoxin and theophylline. There are also interactions with selective serotonin reuptake inhibitors. As St John's Wort is a herbal preparation and, therefore, in the UK does not need a medicinal licence, there are limited regulatory mechanisms to protect the public. In addition, many people, both professionals and the public, do not recognize that herbal medicines and low doses of prescribed medicines are 'medicines', and do not consider them in their decision making. Awareness of the problem, particularly among pharmacists and doctors, has been raised through official letters from the Committee on Safety of Medicines (2000). A more recent example of concern over a herbal product is kava-kava (Breckenridge 2002).

Some side-effects may be predictable, such as the increased risk of gastro-intestinal bleeding from the use of NSAIDs. Thus ibuprofen, while deemed safe enough to be freely available from all retail outlets, may still be the cause of morbidity and potential mortality. In a Scottish study (Sinclair *et al.* 2000, 2001a), a cohort of 555 purchasers of ibuprofen was followed up over 26 weeks. There were indications that over a third of OTC purchasers used the product for chronic conditions (present for more than 13 weeks), over a quarter used it long term (more than 8 weeks) and 8 per cent took it above the recommended OTC dose. In the same study, 4 per cent of ibuprofen users had an active or past history of stomach or peptic ulcer, and 7 per cent had an active or past history of asthma. The important earlier positive findings that at OTC doses ibuprofen was as safe with respect to gastrointestinal events as other OTC analgesics such as paracetamol and aspirin (Moore *et al.* 1999), must therefore be questioned. The results of Sinclair *et al.* (2001b) illustrate the need to carry out studies in the real world when patients exceed recommended doses, or use drugs for prolonged periods, sometimes in combination with contraindicated conditions or products.

The examples given above illustrate the need to be alert to the potential for 'safe' OTC drugs to cause unexpected problems, either when used on their own or in combination with other prescribed products. Formal mechanisms should be in place to support this. At the current time, systems of pharmacovigilance include spontaneous reporting and signal generation in various databases fol-lowed by event monitoring (Mann and Andrews 1998) and post-marketing sur-veillance studies. Hypothesis-based case-control and cohort studies (Strom 1989) may also be used.

In the UK, the spontaneous reporting system is known as the yellow card system. It applies to events suspected of being associated with drug use – and the drug may be either an OTC or a prescribed drug. Professionals allowed to report such events include doctors, pharmacists and, most recently, nurses. However, it is widely recognized that the reporting of such events greatly underestimates the true number (Jarernsiripornkul *et al.* 2002), thus diluting the potential of the system to identify all events, or to identify them as early as possible. It is also likely that the under-reporting of OTC drug-related events is even higher than for prescription drugs because of the perception of safety on the part of both users and professionals, and also the need for the link between a new symptom and drug use to be made. This is difficult if the drug was originally supplied outwith a professional network, and even if symptoms experienced were severe enough to trigger a medical visit, it is unlikely that the doctor would remember to ask about OTC medicine use (Sinclair *et al.* 2001a), or that the patient when asked about drug usage would remember or even consider the role of OTC drugs.

Event monitoring is widely used in the prescription drug market and signifi-cant adverse events and associations have been identified in this way. It depends on a potential adverse event being suspected through signal generation, and then retrospectively identifying and following up people who have been pre-scribed the drug. However, because of the current lack of documentation of OTC use, it would be difficult to replicate such a system for OTC drugs.

Surveillance and dedicated exercises are therefore probably the most effective way of monitoring the safety of OTC drugs and the Scottish study described above did identify an increased reporting of gastrointestinal and dermatological symptoms in long-term users of ibuprofen, compared to those who purchased the drug for short-term use or 'stock'. However, rare events will only be identified through surveillance of a large number of users. The resources required for such an exercise would be significant. Advantages for the industry are unclear given the commercial implications of any adverse findings and there is still a general complacency about the safety of this product group despite calls for this to be addressed (Clark *et al.* 2001). All of the above systems should be integrated with, but not lost within, the systems for prescribed medicines already mentioned in Chapter 8.

Monitoring

At the moment, with rare exceptions, routine OTC product supply is undocumented, and therefore contact tracing would be on a self-report basis, as is the case for the recall of food products. This lack of documentation has important implications for both quality and safety, which are discussed in more detail below.

Product quality

Initial product quality at the point of manufacture is governed by standard quality assurance procedures for both content and stability. All products will have identifiable batch numbers and production codes, which will allow easy recognition in the event of a subsequent recall. In the UK, product quality and recall are managed through a system of drug alerts coordinated by the Committee on Safety of Medicines. Product-related problems such as inaccurate labelling (e.g. a paediatric product label on the adult product) or loss of potency, or contamination with particulate matter, are notified through this system for P products and traced as far as the retail supplier through the community pharmacy network. Products already supplied to the public cannot be traced routinely and are therefore lost to the system, although communication of the alert through the media should prompt individual customers to return products purchased to their pharmacist for checking against the drug recall.

However, products that are available through general retail outlets are dispersed through a large retail network making recall unrealistic. The media and local authority retail controls remain the only options.

Appropriate use

A lack of record keeping of product users and the reasons for the use is also problematic for monitoring both appropriateness of original supply and ongoing use with respect to clinical effectiveness and avoidance of adverse events. Likewise, as highlighted under the section on pharmacovigilance above, subsequent medical consultation for either the same or separate conditions cannot be informed by access to a comprehensive data set of information, including all previous treatment.

In the UK, a centrally maintained single electronic health record is much discussed. In such a system, each patient would have a single record to which all care – hospital, general practice, pharmacy – would be recorded (written) and to which all professionals involved in the care of the patient (e.g. medics, nurses, pharmacists, allied health care professionals) operating in either primary or secondary care settings would have agreed appropriate levels of access. A Scottish study has explored the acceptability of such a system to patients, general practitioners and pharmacists with respect to the two-way transmission of data between pharmacists and general practitioners. Assuming that concerns regarding data security and patient confidentiality are addressed, there was general support for such a system (Porteous *et al.* 2003). The system would certainly provide a mechanism for integrating OTC medicine use into overall patient management and address many of the concerns raised in this chapter.

Conclusion

The OTC market is expanding in terms of value, volume and range of products. This trend is common across all European countries, despite differences of detail in the exact products available and the regulations governing their distribution, supply and use. There are many advantages associated with this move, for patients, governments, professionals and the industry. There are, however, also common areas of concern. These are associated with equity of access, appropriate use and detection of adverse events. Issues of equity are more the realm of national policy makers. Because of the differences in health care systems *per se* across the different countries, and the implications of switching for patterns of use in access to medicines, it may be premature to recommend a centralized policy in switching from prescription to OTC status. The current system, whereby the principles of switching are agreed Europe-wide, but only applied nationally as part of a wider health care strategy, is therefore appropriate. However, ongoing appropriate and safe use in the wider population is of general concern and remains to be fully addressed across Europe. At the moment, the lack of systematic record keeping associated with the supply of these products, and the numbers of separate databases even within a single nation, are factors which limit the full potential of OTC drugs in contributing to health care. A single electronic patient health record, with different levels of read and write access according to stakeholder perspective, and issues of security and confidentiality addressed, would allow OTC drug use to be taken into account during history taking, used as an option for management, and for ongoing follow-up of benefit and risk. In addition, patients and professionals should be educated about appropriate use of self-medication to reduce unnecessary health care consultations, and to ensure symptoms requiring professional input are managed accordingly. It is essential that systems to integrate OTC medicine use into the core health care system of each country are developed to maximize the cost-effective contribution of the OTC group of drugs to the health of the European population.

References

Abraham, J. and Lewis, G. (1999) Harmonising and competing for medicines regulation: how healthy are the European Union's systems of drug approval?, *Social Science and Medicine*, 48: 1655–67.

Anonymous (1997) Terfenadine switches back to POM, *The Pharmaceutical Journal*, 259: 316.

Anonymous (2000a) Diabetes self-testing kit, *The Pharmaceutical Journal*, 265: 944.

Anonymous (2000b) Third pharmacy-based EHC pilot about to start in Derbyshire, *The Pharmaceutical Journal*, 264: 712.

Anonymous (2001) Pharmacy-based head lice management, *The Pharmaceutical Journal*, 267: 317.

Anonymous (2002) Pharmacists in Scotland target low income pregnant women who smoke, *The Pharmaceutical Journal*, 269: 182.

Anonymous (2003) International guideline on pharmacy management of hay fever, *The Pharmaceutical Journal*, 270: 428.

ARIA (2003) *The Management of Rhinitis in the Pharmacy: Pocketbook 2003* (available from www.whiar.com).

Association Européenne des Spécialités Pharmaceutiques Grand Public (AESGP) (2002) *OTC in Europe: Facts and Figures*. Brussels: AESGP.

Bond, C.M. (1995) Prescribing in community pharmacy: barriers and opportunities. PhD thesis, University of Aberdeen.

Bond, C.M. (2000) Reclassification of medicines: clinical aspects, in C.M. Bond (ed.) *Evidence Based Pharmacy*. London: Pharmaceutical Press.

Bond, C.M. and Grimshaw, J.M. (1994) Clinical guidelines for the treatment of dyspepsia in community pharmacies, *The Pharmaceutical Journal*, 252: 228–9.

Bouvy, M.L. and Egberts, T.C. (2000) Consequences of a change in reimbursement status on prescription patterns, *European Journal of Clinical Pharmacology*, 56(6–7): 511–12.

Brass, E.P. (2001) Changing the status of drugs from prescription to over-the-counter availability, *New England Journal of Medicine*, 345(11): 810–16.

Breckenridge, A. (2002) *CSM Advice on Liver Toxicity Associated with Kava-Kava and Proposed Regulatory Action by the Government Committee on Safety of Medicines* (CEM/CMO/2002/10). London: Department of Health.

Carlsten, A., Wennberg, M. and Bergendal, L.J. (1996) The influence of Rx-to-OTC changes on drug sales: experiences from Sweden 1980–1994, *Clinical Pharmaceutical Therapy*, 21(6): 423–30.

Clark, D., Layton, D. and Shakir, S. (2001) Monitoring the safety of over the counter drugs, *British Medical Journal*, 323: 706–7.

Committee for Safety of Medicines and Medicines Control Agency (1992) Astemizole and terfenadine. *Current Problems in Pharmacovigilance*. London: Committee on Safety of Medicines.

Committee on Safety of Medicines (2000) Reminder: St John's wort (*Hypericum perforatum*) interactions, in *Current Problems in Pharmacovigilance*. London: Committee on Safety of Medicines.

Edwards, C. (1992) Liberalising medicines supply, *International Journal of Pharmaceutical Practice*, 1(4): 186.

European Community (1992) Directive for medicines classification, 92/26/EEC of 31 March 1992 concerning the classification for the supply of medicinal products for human use, *Official Journal of the European Communities*, L113, 30.04.1992.

European Parliament and Council of the European Communities (2001) Directive 2001/83/EEC of 6 November 2001 on the Community code relating to medicinal products for human use.

Hassell, K., Noyce, P. and Rogers, A. (1999) A review of factors that influence the use of community pharmacy as a primary health care resource, *International Journal of Pharmaceutical Practice*, 7: 51–9.

Jarernsiripornkul, N., Krska, J., Capps, P.A.G. and Richards, R.M.E. (2002) Patient reporting of potential adverse drug reactions: a methodological study, *British Journal of Clinical Pharmacology*, 53: 318–25.

Mann, R. and Andrews, E. (1998) *Pharmacovigilance Handbook 1998*. Weimar, TX: Chipsbooks.

Matheson, C. and Bond, C.M. (1995) Lower gastrointestinal symptoms, *The Pharmaceutical Journal*, 253: 656–8.

Medicines and Healthcare Products Regulatory Agency (2002) *Changing the Legal Classification in the United Kingdom of a Medicine for Human Use*. London: MHRA.

Moore, N., van Ganse, E., Le Parc, J.-M. *et al.* (1999) The PAIN study: paracetamol, aspirin and ibuprofen new tolerability study, *Clinical Drug Investment*, 18: 89–98.

OTC Bulletin, (2002) *The Third Age of Switching*. Solihull, UK: OTC Publications.

OTC Bulletin-AESGP (2002) *Europe's Self-medication Market 1997* (available from www.otc-bulletin.com).

Payne, K., Ryan-Woolley, B. and Noyce, P. (1998) Role of consumer attributes in predicting the uptake of medicines deregulation and National Health Service prescribing in the United Kingdom, *International Journal of Pharmaceutical Practice*, 6: 150–8.

Porteous, T., Bond, C.M., Duthie, I. and Matheson, C. (1997) Guidelines for the treatment of hayfever and other allergic conditions of the upper respiratory tract, *The Pharmaceutical Journal*, 259: 62–5.

Porteous, T., Bond, C.M., Duthie, I. and Matheson, C. (1998) Guidelines for the treatment of self limiting upper respiratory tract ailments, *The Pharmaceutical Journal*, 260: 134–9.

Porteous, T., Bond, C.M., Sinclair, H. and Hannaford, P. (2002) *Non-prescribed Analgesics: How and Why are They Used?* Report to Chief Scientist Office. London: HMSO.

Porteous, T., Bond, C., Hannaford, P., Robertson, R. and Reiter, E. (2003) Electronic transfer of prescription related information: comparing the views of patients, GPs and pharmacists, *British Journal of General Practice*, 53: 204–9.

Rallapalli, K.C. and Smith, M.C. (1994) OTC drug advertising-information content, *Journal of Social Administrative Pharmacy*, 11(3): 139–47.

Royal Pharmaceutical Society of Great Britain (2002) *Bibliography: Prescription Only Medicines Reclassified to Pharmacy Only Medicines*. London: Pharmaceutical Press.

Ryan, M. and Bond, C.M. (1996) Using the economic theory of consumer surplus to estimate the benefits of dispensing doctors and prescribing pharmacists, *Journal of Social Administrative Pharmacy*, 13(4): 178–87.

Ryan, M. and Yule, B. (1990) Switching drugs from prescription-only to over-the-counter availability: economic benefits in the United Kingdom, *Health Policy*, 16: 233–9.

Sansgiry, S., Sharp, W.T. and Sansgiry, S.S. (1999) *Health Mark Q*, 17(2): 7–18. Department of Pharmacy Practice and Administrative Sciences, College of Pharmacy, Idaho State University.

Schafheutle, E., Cantrill, J., Nicolson, M. and Noyce, P. (1996) Insights into the choice between self medication and a doctor's prescription: a study of hay fever sufferers, *International Journal of Pharmaceutical Practice*, 4: 156–61.

Shih, Y.C., Prasad, M. and Luce, B.R. (2002) The effect on social welfare of a switch of second-generation antihistamines from prescription to over-the-counter status: a microeconomic analysis, *Clinical Therapy*, 24(4): 701–16.

Sihvo, S., Hemminki, E. and Ahonen, R. (1999) Physicians' attitudes toward reclassifying drugs as over-the-counter, *Medical Care*, 37(5): 518–25.

Sinclair, H.K., Bond, C.M. and Hannaford, P.C. (2000) Over the counter ibuprofen: how and why is it used?, *International Journal of Pharmaceutical Practice*, 8: 121–7.

Sinclair, H.K., Bond, C.M. and Hannaford, P.C. (2001a) Long term follow up studies of users of non-prescription medicines purchased from community pharmacies: some methodological issues, *Drug Safety*, 24(12): 929–39.

Sinclair, H., Lawton, S., Bond, C. *et al.* (2001b) *Report to Grampian Primary Care NHS Trust Research Committee*, July, Aberdeen.

Strom, B.L. (1989) Choosing among the available approaches for pharmacoepidemiologic studies, in B.L. Strom (ed.) *Pharmacoepidemiology*. New York: Churchill Livingstone.

US Department of Health and Human Services, Agency for Health Care Policy and Research (1993) *Acute Pain Management: Operative or Medical Procedures and Trauma*. Rockville, MD: AHCPR.

Watson, M.C., Grimshaw, J.M., Bond, C.M., Mollison, J. and Ludbrook, A. (2001) *Oral Versus Intra-vaginal Imidazole and Triazole Anti-fungal Treatment of Uncomplicated Vulvovaginal Candidiasis (Thrush): A Systematic Review*. Cochrane Library of Systematic Reviews.

Watson, M.C., Bond, C.M., Grimshaw, J.M. *et al.* (2002) Educational strategies to promote evidence-based community pharmacy practice: a cluster randomised controlled trial (RCT), *Family Practice*, 19: 529–36.

Whittington, Z., Cantrill, J., Hassell, K.J., Batres, F. and Noyce, P. (2001) Community pharmacy management of minor conditions – the 'care at the chemist' scheme, *The Pharmaceutical Journal*, 266: 425–8.

Wiesenfeld, H.C., Lowry, D.L.B., Phillips Heine, R. *et al.* (2001) Self collection of vaginal swabs for the detection of chlamydia, gonorrhea and trichomoniasis, *Sexually Transmitted Diseases*, 28: 321–5.

Wilkes, D. (1998) An international perspective on the OTC Market, *OTC Bulletin*, 9 December, 1998 (available from www.otc-bulletin.com).

chapter sixteen

The implications of pharmacogenetics and pharmacogenomics for drug development and health care

Munir Pirmohamed and Graham Lewis

Introduction

The completion of the first draft of the human genome project has raised enormous expectations, not only in terms of identifying genetic predisposition to disease, but also in improving drug therapy through the development and use of personalized medicines. This area of research, which is called pharmacogenetics or pharmacogenomics, is currently fashionable, and promises benefits for both the pharmaceutical industry and the patient. There are, however, many obstacles (technological, regulatory, social and ethical) that have to be overcome before (or if ever) the potential benefits are realized. The purpose of this chapter is to critically review this area, and the potential benefits that may accrue from it.

Definitions

Pharmacogenetics can be defined as the study of variability in drug response due to heredity. It is not a new term, having been coined by Vogel in 1957 (see Pirmohamed 2001). More recently, the term *pharmacogenomics* has also been introduced. The terms are often used interchangeably as there is no standard definition. However, for the purposes of this chapter, the term pharmacogenomics will be used in a wider sense to denote:

- all genes in the genome, and the variation within those genes, that may determine drug response; and
- the differential effects of different compounds on gene expression.

Therefore, pharmacogenomics, through examination of individual response profiles and elucidation of the differential effects of different compounds on gene expression, may ultimately lead to target identification, drug discovery and compound selection. Lindpaintner (2002) has suggested that pharmacogenetics should be used to refer to differences between patients, while pharmacogenomics should be used to refer to differences between compounds. This chapter mostly concentrates on pharmacogenetics, although where relevant we also discuss aspects that fall into the category of pharmacogenomics.

Current state of drug development and drug use

The whole process of drug development is extremely expensive. Industry-funded sources put the cost at approximately €500 million–800 million per marketed drug (Anonymous 2001; DiMasi 2002; DiMasi *et al.* 2003), although others suggest the figure is considerably lower (*Public Citizen* 2001; Henry and Lexchin 2002). It is time-consuming, with each drug taking approximately 10–15 years to reach the market after discovery of the compound (Anonymous 2001). In addition, there is a high attrition rate, with only one out of every 5000 chemical compounds considered to have a therapeutic potential being successfully developed for clinical use. The number of new applications submitted to regulatory agencies for approval has shown a decrease almost every year over the past five years. For example, the US Food and Drug Administration (FDA) approved only 15 new drugs in 2002, compared with a five-year annual average of 31. The trend is less noticeable in Europe, with the European Medicines Evaluation Agency (EMEA) approving 13 new products in 2002 compared with 14 in 2001 (five-year average 15.4) (Frantz and Smith 2003). Nonetheless, data provided by the industry-funded Centre for Medicines Research (Anderson *et al.* 2002) suggest there was a steady decline in the number of new active substances submitted to the major regulatory authorities from 1997 to 2001, as well as a decline in the number approved between 1999 and 2001. The incorporation of pharmacogenomics into the drug development process has the potential to improve target identification, accelerate the development process and reduce the attrition rate.

The problems for both pharmaceutical companies and health care systems do not stop after a drug has been marketed. It is becoming increasingly clear that there is marked variability in the way individuals respond to drugs, in terms of both efficacy and toxicity (Evans and Johnson 2001). For example, there is a 20-fold variation in the dose of warfarin required to achieve optimal anticoagulation across patients. Marked variability in efficacy has been demonstrated for compounds in almost every therapeutic class (Table 16.1). Adverse drug reactions are also a major problem (Pirmohamed and Park 2001): almost 4 per cent of the compounds that were originally licensed by the UK Medicines Control Agency were later withdrawn because of safety problems (Jefferys *et al.* 1998), which has

Table 16.1 Variable therapeutic responses to drugs for different conditions

Condition	Efficacy rate (%)
Alzheimer's disease	30
Asthma	60
Diabetes	57
Hepatitis C virus	47
Oncology	25
Osteoporosis	48
Rheumatoid arthritis	50
Schizophrenia	60

Source: Adapted from Physicians' Desk Reference (2000).

enormous financial implications for the industry and undermines public trust. Figures from EMEA show a similar picture, with 16 withdrawals from a total of 241 marketing authorizations since 1995 (EMEA 2003). Adverse drug reactions account for 5 per cent of all hospital admissions and increase the length of stay in hospital by two days at an increased cost of approximately US$2500 per patient (Pirmohamed et al. 1998). A meta-analysis in the USA suggested that adverse drug reactions killed over 100,000 patients in 1994, making them the fourth most common cause of death (Lazarou et al. 1998). A recent systematic review attempted to quantify the role of polymorphisms in drug-metabolizing enzyme genes in predisposing to adverse drug reactions (Phillips et al. 2001). Of the 27 drugs most frequently cited in adverse drug reaction studies, 59 per cent were metabolized by at least one enzyme with a variant allele associated with reduced activity, compared with 7–22 per cent of randomly selected drugs. This provides circumstantial evidence that dose alteration through a knowledge of the patient's genotype may have prevented some of these adverse reactions. However, it is important to note that the design of the study (relating published adverse drug reaction studies with review articles of drug-metabolizing enzyme gene polymorphisms) demonstrates an association and may not necessarily be causative. Furthermore, it does not take into account the fact that adverse drug reactions are likely to have more than one genetic predisposing factor.

It is difficult to calculate the likely cost savings in terms of reduced drug toxicity and/or improved efficacy because there are relatively few practical examples and little evidence based on actual clinical practice. Additionally, adverse reactions and efficacy are invariably the outcome of both genetic and non-genetic factors. Nonetheless, the potential benefits, in both health and economic terms, are considerable. However, therapeutic intervention based on individuals' genetic variation will not be applicable to all drugs and careful evaluation of cost-effectiveness will be needed on a case-by-case basis (Phillips et al. 2001; Veenstra et al. 2001).

The incorporation of pharmacogenetics into clinical practice, therefore, has the potential to improve efficacy and reduce toxicity, by allowing the choice of the right drug for the right patient in the right disease at the right dose. This also represents a culture change in clinical practice: currently the practice of evidence-based medicine is dependent on data from randomized controlled trials and meta-analyses, with the choice of appropriate treatment being dictated by an analysis of the whole population. Successful incorporation of pharmacogenetics will therefore lead to greater consideration of the individual rather than the whole population in the choice of drug. There are also many ethical issues that need to be considered, many of which are discussed in this chapter, and have also been addressed in the recent document from the Nuffield Council on Bioethics (2003).

Biological basis of pharmacogenetics and pharmacogenomics

Of the three billion base pairs in the human genome, 99.9 per cent are identical between different individuals. Variability that is observed in 0.1 per cent of the genome is thought to account for this variability in drug responses. Single nucleotide polymorphisms (SNPs) account for 90 per cent of the variability and are observed once every 500–1000 base pairs. The focus of pharmacogenetics has therefore largely been on SNPs, not only because they are the most common, but also because they are the most technically accessible class of genetic variant (Roses 2000). By definition, a SNP occurs in at least 1 per cent of the population, and those which have been mapped are freely available on the worldwide web (http://snp.cshl.org). Combinations of SNPs on the same DNA strand can be inherited together to form a haplotype. It has been suggested that the haplotype pattern may be more important in determining drug response and disease predisposition than individual SNPs. For this reason, there is currently an ongoing effort to map the haplotype structure of the human genome, which will also be freely available on the web. Looking further into the future, using whole genome scanning, it may be possible to correlate SNP and haplotype profiles in an unbiased fashion to drug response, but there is a need to develop cost-effective technologies to undertake this.

There have also been major advances in pharmacogenomic technologies, for example with microarrays (gene chips) and proteomics (the systematic study of protein expression within a whole organism). Drugs can have major effects on gene and protein expression, which may ultimately determine drug response. The ability to analyse changes in gene expression and protein profile on drug exposure in different tissues and in different patients, as well as the analysis and identification of disease categories, allied to the advances in bioinformatics, will provide us with unparalleled opportunities to identify new drug targets, novel candidate genes determining drug response, and allow the development of medicines targeted to individual disease sub-types. These technologies and developments, therefore, herald major potential changes for pharmaceutical companies, health care organizations and patients.

Pharmacogenomics, pharmacogenetics and the drug development process

Pharmacogenomics and pharmacogenetics may have a potentially beneficial effect on all aspects of the drug development process (Figure 16.1). These are considered in detail below.

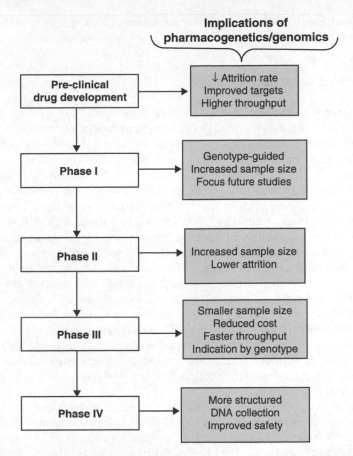

Figure 16.1   Possible implications of pharmacogenetics for drug development.

Target identification

Drugs currently on the market act on less than 450 of the estimated 10,000 targets in the human proteome (Norton 2001). Target diversity is also limited, with 75 of the top 100 drugs acting on four families of molecular targets; G-protein coupled receptors are the most common site of action. Proteomic and genomic technologies may increase the diversity of targets available for future medicinal products through:

- identification of novel proteins involved in disease processes;
- targeting of proteins with variant structure resulting from the presence of genetic polymorphisms;
- identification of mechanisms of action of currently used drugs and refinement of targeting to improve specificity of drug action;
- development of compounds with specific actions in disease sub-types; and
- increase specificity of drug action and thereby improvement in drug safety by reducing secondary targeting responsible for adverse effects.

It must be stressed, however, that these are theoretical possibilities and application on a large scale is eagerly awaited.

Pre-clinical drug development

Pharmacogenetics has already had an impact on this phase of drug development; arguably, this has been the major benefit to date of pharmacogenetics. It has been known for many years that individuals vary in their ability to metabolize certain drugs. The identification of the molecular defects underlying phenotypic variability has led to the development of *in vitro* screens. For example, a major advance has been the development of cell lines expressing drug-metabolizing enzymes, such as the cytochrome P450 enzymes. These are the most versatile group of biological catalysts known to exist in nature and are involved in the metabolism of many of the currently used drugs. This allows assessment of the interaction of a drug with a particular enzyme such as a P450 enzyme at an early stage of development, and the subsequent prediction of polymorphic metabolism in humans and the possibility of drug–drug interactions (Park and Pirmohamed 2001). The finding that a drug is a substrate for a polymorphically expressed drug-metabolizing enzyme often leads to abandonment of further development. However, if the drug is developed, it also provides an opportunity to draw the attention of prescribers to appropriate warnings in the Summary of Product Characteristics. As our knowledge increases, such screens may be extended to the protein targets on which drugs act, such as ion channels and receptors.

A further development in pharmacogenomics has been the use of gene expression profiling to predict toxicity; indeed, a large amount of money is being spent on developing databases of gene expression profiles with known toxicants in the hope that this will allow future candidate selection and reduce attrition rates later in the development process. Although this may help in certain situations, where the adverse effect depends on an idiosyncratic feature found only in a small proportion of patients, it is unlikely that the gene profiling patterns developed through animal studies will be of use in humans. It is also important to note that such screens will not be absolutely predictive, and therefore will not replace animal experimentation (Lindpaintner 2002). However, it is possible that these screens, because of their high throughput nature, will allow more focused animal experimentation, leading to a reduction in the total number of animals tested, and thereby savings in time and cost.

Phase I–III studies

These clinical studies, which provide the basis for regulatory approval, range from 'first in man' kinetic and tolerability studies (Phase I) in small numbers of healthy volunteers to the large randomized clinical trials designed to assess the efficacy of a compound (Phase III). The typical cost of a phase I study is US$7 million, but jumps to US$43 million for a Phase III study. Pharmacogenetics may lead to refinement of Phase I studies by focusing on individuals with known genotypes defined through pre-clinical testing (Brazell *et al.* 2002). An earlier identification of problems may lead to the compound being dropped during Phase I rather than in Phase III, with considerable savings in development costs. In Phase II, there may be further refinement of the pharmacogenetic determinants of drug response, which may provide information necessary for design of the Phase III studies. The net effect may be a reduction in sample size for Phase III studies, which may in turn result in more efficient and quicker drug development, and a net reduction in cost (Brazell *et al.* 2002). It must be stressed that although smaller numbers of patients will be required in phase III, there is a possibility that more individuals will need to be studied during Phases I and II to provide adequate power to identify the pharmacogenetic determinants of drug response. The net effect may be a more streamlined drug development process whereby potentially toxic or inefficacious compounds are screened out and abandoned at an earlier stage, while compounds that make it to Phase III studies are more likely to reach clinical use. However, the response of regulatory agencies to pharmacogenetics-based clinical trials remains unclear at this time, although they are increasingly supportive of the concept of personalized medicine.

Phase IV studies

Phase IV refers to the period after the drug is licensed; studies take several forms, ranging from hypothesis-generating spontaneous reporting to hypothesis-testing pharmacoepidemiological studies, and can continue for the whole period the drug is on the market. Historically, less effort has been expended on improving post-marketing surveillance than harmonization of marketing authorization procedures and the creation of a single market (Abraham and Lewis 2000). For both therapeutic and social reasons, existing pharmacovigilance systems may need to be considerably strengthened to 'fine tune' pharmacogenetics-based treatment regimes across different patient populations and encourage public acceptance.

Since Phase IV involves exposure of large numbers of patients to the drug, detection of rare adverse events usually occurs in this phase. Storage of DNA samples from patients treated with the drug in this phase may allow pharmacogenetic testing and identification of genetic predisposing factors, which will further allow an improvement in the risk–benefit ratio. This is perhaps best exemplified by abacavir hypersensitivity, where studies post-marketing have identified a major genetic predisposing factor in the MHC locus (Hetherington *et al.* 2002; Mallal *et al.* 2002). However, a note of caution needs to be added here: since detection of adverse events is a function of the power of the studies, any reduction in the total number of patients studied in Phase III may lead to the statistical need for larger, more structured Phase IV studies to identify rare and long-term toxicities. Prospective collection of DNA samples is a possibility in Phase IV (Roses 2000), but would be expensive. The cost of this may have to be borne by the pharmaceutical industry, but whether this may result in a more expensive product, and hence a shift in cost to health care, is unclear at present.

Phase IV also involves assessment of alternative uses of the drug; these studies may, in fact, be more streamlined given that pharmacogenetic determinants of efficacy will already have been identified prior to marketing.

Nature of pharmacogenetic tests

The aim of pharmacogenetic studies will be to provide a DNA-based test that allows determination of efficacy or toxicity with a high degree of sensitivity, specificity and accuracy before the patient takes the drug. However, it is important to appreciate that it is unlikely that such a test will be absolutely predictive, and will provide probabilistic information; for example, there is a 70 per cent chance of developing a severe adverse reaction with drug A. Furthermore, pharmacogenetic testing is unlikely to be dependent on one gene that determines efficacy or toxicity. It is more likely that the response to a drug, either efficacy or toxicity, will be dependent upon a number of genes, and these genes in combination may provide adequate sensitivity and specificity and therefore accuracy in determining drug response (Pirmohamed and Park 2001). The pharmacogenetic test may have been developed by the same company developing the drug, or in collaboration with a separate diagnostics or genomics company, and will require approval as part of the drug registration process. In other words, pharmacogenetic-based therapy is likely in some cases to take the form of a 'kit' comprising the drug plus diagnostic test. There may well be a proprietary-driven 'lock-in' with such an arrangement, with intellectual property rights surrounding not only the kit but the mechanism responsible for the genotype–drug interaction. This may have important cost implications for reimbursement decisions and health care budgets generally.

It is usually assumed that pharmacogenetics will proceed from observation that exposure to a drug generates a differential response, to identifying the predictive marker for that response, and then creating a diagnostic product that will then be co-marketed with the drug ('the right medicine for the right patient'). In contrast, others predict this process may well be reversed, with drug development based on diagnosis of new disease (sub)types, arising from improved knowledge of the molecular basis of diseases. Accordingly, the development and marketing of diagnostic tests becomes the 'driver', rather than such tests being seen as an 'add-on' to the drug development process, and maintenance of the conventional practice of treatment based on differential diagnosis (Lindpaintner 2002). Additionally, it appears that the same or similar genetic pathways may be active in more than one disease state. Therefore, a wide range of diagnostic products may be available in the future, some of which may have quite wide application, while others will be closely tied to a specific therapeutic product.

Any test developed after licensing, for example for an adverse reaction, will have to undergo a separate approval process, and a variation in licensing indications, the nature of which will depend on the accuracy of the test. The nature of the approval process for the pharmacogenetic test is unclear at present, but may well require a different set of standards that fall somewhere among a diagnostic device, a drug therapy and a clinical service. Responsibility for the regulation of genetic tests is in a state of flux. Although the FDA is responsible for regulating tests in the USA, in Europe this is not the responsibility of the EMEA, but this may well have to change for genotype-guided therapy. Presently, the regulation of *in vitro* tests in the European Union is the responsibility of member states, often through separate national device agencies, although some states have recently merged device regulation with the regulation of medicinal products.[1]

In Europe, the *In-Vitro* Diagnostic Medical Devices Directive regulates products used to examine substances derived from the human body, with the aim of achieving consistent interpretation and implementation across the EU. The Directive came into effect in June 2000, with a transition period until December 2003. There is pressure for harmonization of device regulation at the European level, although some states, such as the UK, remain opposed to this step. There are also efforts to achieve global harmonization across different regions, similar to that for medicinal products achieved through the International Conference on Harmonization.

Salvaging of drugs

Another possible benefit, and therefore a positive economic impact, of pharmacogenetics will be the possible salvaging of beneficial drugs – so-called 'drug rescue'. Many drugs have been withdrawn from the market because of an unacceptable frequency of adverse drug reactions occurring in a minority of patients. For example, as noted earlier, it is stated that 4 per cent of all drugs licensed by the Medicines Control Agency in the UK were withdrawn because of adverse drug reactions (Jefferys *et al.* 1998), and a similar percentage have been withdrawn by the EMEA after approval via the centralized procedure. The withdrawal was to protect the minority who developed the adverse drug reaction, at the expense of the majority who benefit from the drug without developing any adverse drug reactions. Thus, pharmacogenetic testing gives us a possibility of rescuing drugs that are beneficial in a large percentage of the population and avoiding their use in those who had adverse reactions. This is an important aspect to consider given the paucity of new drugs in the drug development pipeline at present.

There is conflicting evidence as to whether major pharmaceutical companies will wish to engage in this type of pharmacogenetics product because of the perceived risks involved. However, if large companies decide against developing such products, smaller 'niche' companies may well decide 'drug rescue' is financially worthwhile. Drug companies withdraw drugs at two stages, during clinical trials and after approval and introduction to the market. Media attention surrounding withdrawals tends to focus on 'blockbuster drugs' already on the market. However, the majority of withdrawals occur during clinical trials – that is, during the drug development process, rather than post-marketing – and this type of 'drug rescue' (i.e. reducing attrition) is perhaps likely to be most significant.

Economic impact of pharmacogenetics

The likely economic impact of pharmacogenetics upon the development of new medicines will depend on the disease being treated and whether other therapies are already available to treat that particular disease. Furthermore, the characteristics of the drug being developed, its therapeutic index and the characteristics of the pharmacogenetic test (its sensitivity, specificity and accuracy) will also act as determinants of the economic impact of a particular medicine. On the positive side, pharmacogenetics may allow more efficient and quicker drug development by reducing the number of patients that require drug exposure during Phase III of the development process. Since a large percentage of the expenditure of new drug development goes in the clinical phases and particularly in Phase III, reduction in the number of patients in Phase III should allow a corresponding reduction in drug development costs. Furthermore, the demonstration of a homogeneous therapeutic response with absence (or reduction) of adverse reactions may increase the likelihood of the drug passing through the licensing process. It will also reduce the chances of the drug being withdrawn from the market, since those individuals susceptible to developing adverse drug reactions, a major cause for drug withdrawal, should be excluded from drug exposure.

On the negative side, however, pharmacogenetic tests will almost certainly reduce the number of patients who are likely to receive the drug, as those with a different pharmacogenetic profile will be classed as non-responders. In other words, pharmacogenetics-based treatment is characterized by patient segmentation. This will therefore reduce the market uptake of the drug and, perhaps, will end the era of blockbuster drugs. Whether a drug is developed for a particular condition will depend on a complex set of scientific, regulatory and commercial factors. For example, there are likely to be differences *within* pharmaceutical companies as regards the (commercial) merits of pharmacogenetics-based drug development. It is also important to note that the reduction in the number of patients exposed during Phase III studies will necessitate careful post-marketing surveillance to ensure that serious idiosyncratic drug reactions are detected as early as possible after the drug goes onto the market, as discussed above.

Pharmacogenetics and regulatory issues

How regulatory agencies such as the FDA and the EMEA will deal with the whole area of pharmacogenetics in terms of clinical trials, licensing and labelling is not clear at present. As the predictive power of pharmacogenetic testing increases, labelling is likely to become more prescriptive (Robertson *et al.* 2002). Many of the guidelines in place for drug development do not encompass the new technologies, and thus new guidelines will have to be developed, an issue acknowledged by both the FDA and the EMEA. What is clear is that the FDA and, increasingly, the EMEA, are actively supporting the introduction of pharmacogenetics-based therapy (Lesko and Woodcock 2002), with regular meetings with industry and discussion of 'safe harbour' type arrangements to encourage joint discussion of the 'meaning' and interpretation of pharmacogenetics data.

Many drugs currently on the market contain information in their Summary of Product Characteristics (SPC) relating to polymorphic drug metabolism, for example when they are metabolized by CYP2D6, one of the cytochrome P450 metabolizing enzymes. In the future, when a drug has been shown to be efficacious in patients with a certain genotype, the indication in the SPC will have to reflect this. Therefore, the drug will be licensed not only for a particular condition, but will also be recommended for use in patients with certain genotypes. This is exemplified by the SPC for trastuzumab (Herceptin) in breast cancer. Any prescribing for patients without the particular genotype will therefore have to be considered to be outside the licensed indication. Labelling will also have to disclose recommended dosage based on stratified patient groups according to genotype profiles. Clearly, there are major issues here concerning how instructions for use will be encouraged or enforced (if, indeed, they should be enforced). Doctors currently have the right to prescribe 'off-label' and it is difficult to see why this would change. Indeed, regulatory agencies increasingly recognize off-label use for patient groups not included in the original approval or to extend indications. How regulatory agencies will ensure appropriate prescribing of medicines based on pharmacogenetic principles remains an outstanding question.

It is unlikely that pharmacogenetics testing will become part of regulatory requirements for all drugs. The need for pharmacogenetic testing for a particular drug will depend upon many factors, in particular on the genetic factors determining its disposition, pharmacodynamic characteristics and its therapeutic index. Therefore, a drug that has high efficacy in a large percentage of the population, shows little inter-individual variability in kinetics and dynamics and has a wide therapeutic index should not necessarily require pharmacogenetic testing, and indeed it would not be cost-effective to test every patient before drug prescription. By contrast, a drug that is efficacious in 30 per cent of the population and has a narrow therapeutic index, as is found with some antipsychotics at present, should arguably be subject to pharmacogenetic testing before prescription. Pre-clinical studies should be able to identify the routes of metabolism and disposition of any particular drug, and its mechanism of action. If any of these parameters are subject to genetic polymorphism that could theoretically or in practice effect the response to the drug, then pharmacogenetic testing should be encouraged. Therefore, in terms of drug development, constant dialogue between pharmaceutical companies and drug regulatory agencies will be important to ensure that the drug development process is as efficient as possible, but does not necessarily lead to cuts in standards.

Another issue to consider is that we may end up with some patients having an 'orphan genotype' – that is, a genotype that cannot be treated with currently available drugs because those patients have been classed as non-responders or as susceptible to particular adverse reactions. This, by definition, will represent a small proportion of the population, and may lead to pharmaceutical companies being reluctant to develop new medicines because of their potential unprofitability. In such cases, further regulatory measures may be needed so that these orphan genotypes are treated in the same way as orphan diseases are treated at present (Motl *et al.* 2003). This may provide financial incentives for the pharmaceutical industry to develop medicines for small patient populations with these orphan genotypes. Alternatively, as already mentioned, smaller genomics/drug development companies may enter such markets, in a similar way to the orphan drug market. Since many more medicines could fall into the category of 'orphan' products because of a reduced market, pharmaceutical companies might seek extension of orphan drug legislation to obtain development subsidies. On the other hand, treatments that are not commercially viable at present may well become viable with reduced clinical trial costs through pharmacogenetics. In other words, 'orphan patients' could stimulate new drug development. To qualify for orphan drug status in the USA, companies must demonstrate that there are less than 200,000 potential users of the drug, and similar legislation exists in the EU. However, defining the prospective patient population is often not straightforward, and hence is a potential source of conflict between regulators and industry. This has already been observed in the case of Herceptin, where orphan drug status was refused by the FDA.

Pharmacogenetics and the health service

The development of genotype-guided therapies will potentially result in a shift in costs of drug development from the pharmaceutical sector to the health care sector. For example, while the costs of drug development to the pharmaceutical industry up to licensing will be reduced through a more efficient streamlined drug development process, the use of the drug after licensing will incur the combined cost of the drug and the pharmacogenetic test. There is therefore a danger that new drugs developed with the aim of being prescribed to certain genotypes will prove to be too expensive for health care systems to introduce.

Where the costs of health care are met by a state-funded national health service, introduction will require careful assessment by governments to evaluate the cost- and clinical-effectiveness of genotype-guided therapy. In the UK, for example, this may well fall under the aegis of the National Institute for Clinical Excellence. Unless national guidance is given in these cases, individual health authorities may make different assessments, with the possibility that the utilization of genotype-guided therapies will be patchy, akin to 'postcode prescribing' that has been a major issue in the UK with expensive treatments such as the use of donepezil in Alzheimer's disease. There are also wider questions around whether Europe is willing to see the introduction of pharmacogenetics-based therapy in some member states and not others, particularly with the imminent expansion of the EU and the widely differing health care systems in the different member states. Similar considerations apply to private health care systems where insurer health management organizations paying for pharmacogenetic tests will require a rigorous evaluation of the cost- and clinical-effectiveness of genotype-guided therapies, in comparison to other therapies available to treat the same disease. There are also ethical and social issues around selective provision of such tests by health care systems of all types.

Given these considerations, there is a possibility that pharmacogenetics may exacerbate existing health inequalities, or initiate new ones. It may also lead to an even wider gulf in health care practices between the richer developed nations and poorer states, who cannot even afford the costs of drugs let alone the cost of pharmacogenetic testing. This has been acknowledged by the World Health Organization, which has strongly recommended that developing countries should not be deprived of potential health care gains afforded by genomic technologies (World Health Organization 2002).

The use of genotype-guided therapies requires that prescribers will have a level of knowledge sufficient to understand and interpret the rationale for prescribing for certain genotypes, but not for others (Robertson *et al.* 2002). This may be particularly important for primary care physicians, where the bulk of prescribing is performed. However, since most prescribers have only a limited knowledge of pharmacogenetics, training programmes will have to be put into place for existing prescribers and curricula altered to incorporate pharmacogenetics into undergraduate education (Gurwitz *et al.* 2003). Clearly, controversies currently arise in relation to all prescribing issues, and this is going to be no different with respect to pharmacogenetics. Each clinician will have their own opinion about the relative merits of different treatments available and the incorporation of pharmacogenetics into the clinical care of their patient. Clinician acceptance is presently an unknown factor. It is possible that this may be a significant barrier to introduction of widespread genotype-based therapy. Anecdotal evidence suggests that many physicians are unimpressed with the projected benefits within the context of general practice. However, it is important that such opinions are based on a good understanding of the issues involved. Where a doctor is not confident about treating a particular condition, he or she is likely to refer to a specialist, which is the current clinical practice. It is possible, therefore, that pharmacogenetics may be considered a specialty in its own right in the future, or as a sub-specialty of clinical pharmacology.

The nature of the pharmacogenetic test results fed back to the prescribing physician also needs to be considered. If most clinicians do not have the appropriate training and knowledge to interpret individual genotypes and thereby determine whether the patient would benefit from a particular drug, perhaps the information relayed to the clinician should indicate whether or not the patient should be prescribed the drug, and indicate the probability of the patient responding (efficaciously or adversely) to the drug. Depending on the predictive power of tests, clinicians may or may not be able to view such tests as a strict 'gatekeeper' on prescribing behaviour (Robertson *et al.* 2002). Based on this information, the clinician would be able to make an informed decision as to whether the patient should be prescribed the drug or whether they should get an alternative drug. But even with highly predictive tests, test information will need to be balanced against other clinical (and cost) considerations, and a modified rather than strict gatekeeper model may be most appropriate (Robertson *et al.* 2002). There may also be a role for pharmacists in interpreting genotypic information, as well as the provision of counselling and advice services (see below), with such services complementing the recent expansion of pharmacy practice. Not releasing individual genotypic information acts as another measure to enhance confidentiality and reduce any risks associated with secondary information contained within the test result.

There is also the question of test location. Will pharmacogenetic tests be conducted in doctors' surgeries – so-called 'point-of-care testing' – or by commercial laboratories, much like existing diagnostic tests? Current pharmacogenetic tests (such as that used to determine whether to prescribe Herceptin for breast cancer, and the hypersensitivity test prior to use of the HIV drug, abacavir) are conducted by specialist clinics. However, pharmacogenetic tests developed for other clinical situations, such as general practice, may in practice be less acceptable. Technologies for genetic point-of-care testing will eventually become available, but this will require considerable investment in infrastructure and training.

Whatever the test location, tests will need to be reproducible and reliable, and require validation, and clinicians will be faced with a range of quite complicated questions around which tests to conduct and how to interpret them (Manasco *et al.* 2002). Regulatory regimes for diagnostic tests are complex and vary across countries, and are also in a state of change. In the USA, for example, tests developed by commercial testing labs – so-called 'home-brew' tests – are exempt from regulations that apply to marketed tests, although the agency is expected to tighten controls in the future. In Europe, tests are governed by the *In Vitro Diagnostic Medical Devices Directive*, implemented in December 2003.

Pharmacogenetic testing can be viewed as part of the wider use of molecular diagnostics in health care systems. According to Hall *et al.* (2003), in state-funded systems the widespread introduction of molecular diagnostics in clinical practice has been hampered by a lack of funds for equipment and, more importantly, training for clinical and laboratory staff. Additionally, non-critical introduction will not necessarily lead to an improvement in clinical outcome if results do not affect clinical management, including ways of altering human behaviour as a method of disease prevention. As noted above, before introduction genotype-based tests should be subject to a detailed cost–benefit analysis that includes a realistic assessment of likely improvements in clinical outcome.

Pharmacogenetics and the patient

Currently, we prescribe on the basis of population data, which does not guarantee a benefit for the individual. Prescribing by genotype offers the patient the potential benefit that they will be given the right drug at the right dose, which will maximize efficacy and minimize toxicity. Pharmacogenetic tests may predict not only improvements in short-term measures, but also in long-term mortality. For example, in hypertension, treatment with thiazide diuretics preferentially leads to falls in blood pressure as well as in long-term measures such as myocardial infarction, cerebrovascular accidents and mortality in patients with certain adducin genotypes (Sciarrone *et al.* 2003). The possibility that we will be able to predict and prevent serious adverse reactions, which can be fatal, such as abacavir hypersensitivity (Hetherington *et al.* 2002; Mallal *et al.* 2002), will obviously be beneficial to patients.

Despite the potential benefits, there are other aspects of relevance to patients that have to be considered. First, given that these are going to be DNA-based tests, specific safeguards to maintain confidentiality will have to be put into place. Laboratories carrying out such testing will need to undergo an accreditation process to ensure safe and secure storage of both samples and information. However, if pharmacogenetic information leads to prescription of a particular drug, the mere fact that the patient is on the drug will betray their genotype, even without direct knowledge of the results of their genetic test.

There is a strong argument for pharmacogenetic testing to be accompanied by counselling so that any psychological impact of a non-optimal genotype is minimized, and the patient given information as to whether alternative therapies are available. This will have major cost implications in that significant resources will have to be found for training counsellors. It is important to note, however, that even for genetic tests for disease susceptibility, the psychological implications can vary enormously; for example, the implications of a test that indicates the possibility of Huntington's disease will be far greater than that which indicates susceptibility to haemachromatosis, because of the lower penetrance of the latter mutation. It has therefore been argued that by virtue of the fact that pharmacogenetic tests will provide probabilistic information, their psychological impact will be less than that of genetic tests used for Mendelian disorders. However, whether this will be the case in practice needs further study.

There is a possibility that secondary information may be conferred by the pharmacogenetic test (Buchanan *et al.* 2002), the most important of which will be susceptibility to a disease process, which may share some (but unlikely to share all) of the same genes determining drug response. However, this is also likely to provide probabilistic information, which in most cases will be less accurate than the primary purpose of the test – that is, to provide drug response data. Furthermore, it may be possible to minimize this secondary information to choose genetic markers more specific for drug response than for disease predisposition. Similar arguments will also apply in relation to other possible types of secondary information, including responses to other drug classes, or predisposition to addiction to cigarettes, alcohol or illicit drugs.

Pharmacogenetic tests may also have implications for family members. One issue that needs to be considered with all genetic tests is the possibility that non-paternity may be disclosed, particularly when other family members have been tested. The pharmacogenetic test may also indicate an increased predisposition to developing certain adverse effects. Where there are good data available, it may be necessary to undertake family screening, as is currently practised for probabilistic tests such as the Factor V Leiden mutation. However, the implications for individual family members may vary from none at all (for those who will never be exposed to the drug) to the same as those for the index individual.

There may be implications for the patient having a pharmacogenetic test in obtaining life insurance. Life insurance companies routinely use phenotypic information to decide on insurance information. It is perhaps naive to think that pharmacogenetic information will not be used in a similar manner eventually. It is likely therefore that in the future they will be given access to some information, but how this will affect insurance premiums and the ability to get insurance is difficult to predict. For example, an individual who has a high risk of developing a disease, but has a favourable response genotype, may actually have to pay lower premiums than an individual with a low risk of disease but with a genotype that indicates poor response to the drug. Overall, pharmacogenetic information is likely to be less controversial in most cases than genetic information predicting disease, with the possible exception of rare individuals who have a pharmacogenetic response profile that predicts non-response to any of the available drugs.

Nonetheless, one of the main challenges is addressing the ethical, privacy and social concerns affecting the willingness and acceptance of persons to be genotyped. For example, reportedly nearly one-third of women offered a genetic test for breast cancer at the US National Institutes of Health declined, due to concerns about potential health insurance discrimination. The question of who has access to an individual's genetic information generated by such tests is crucial (Park 2003).

If a particular medicine has been licensed on the basis that it is only prescribed to certain genotypes, and if a patient refuses the test, then the doctor does not have a legal duty to prescribe that particular medicine, and the patient should therefore not expect to receive that particular treatment. Obviously the patient has every right to expect some form of treatment (which is not dependent on pharmacogenetic testing). The clinician can prescribe a drug outside its licensing indication, but this will be an individual decision, and the legal implications of this will be different from that when the drug is prescribed within its licensed indications. Potentially there are also important legal and ethical implications arising when a doctor fails to offer a pharmacogenetic test when one exists. Health delivery systems of all types (state-funded, managed care organizations and health insurance companies) are likely to play a significant role in determining whether a pharmacogenetic test is required and/or reimbursed. Targeted treatment is likely to lead to fewer adverse drug reactions and/or improved efficacy in the targeted group, and hence reduce overall health costs. Where they exist, such tests may in fact be made compulsory by such organizations to reduce the potential for litigation in the advent of serious adverse events.

Some commentators have also raised concerns about genetic self-testing, such as via the internet, and some states have sought to investigate effective oversight of genetic tests supplied directly to the public (Human Genome Commission 2003).

Conclusions

Pharmacogenetics offers major potential benefits by allowing the use of the right drug at the right dose in the right patient. By virtue of this, it has many implications for all stakeholders, many of which are positive, although there are some negative implications as well, which will require consideration on a case-by-case basis. There has been a lot of hype about pharmacogenetics, which was particularly evident at the time of the first draft of human genome. The increasing realization of the complex technical, ethical and social issues that will be needed in making pharmacogenetics a reality has rapidly led to a dissipation in the hype, and has given way to a much more pessimistic outlook. This, we are sure, will be replaced by a more realistic outlook. It is likely that pharmacogenetics will play a major role in health care in the future, but it is unlikely to be important for all drugs, and will be of greatest benefit for drugs with a narrow therapeutic index.

Note

1   For example, the UK Medical Devices Agency merged with the Medicines Control Agency to form the Medicines and Healthcare Products Regulatory Agency (MHRA) in April 2003. Responsibility for medical devices in Sweden now resides with the Medical Products Agency (MPA); but in Germany it continues to reside with the Paul Erlich Institute.

References

Abraham, J. and Lewis, G. (2000) *Regulating Medicines in Europe: Competition, Expertise and Public Health*. London: Routledge.

Anderson, C., McAuslane, N. and Walker, S. (2002) The impact of the changing regulatory environment on review times, *R & D Briefing No. 35*, CMR International Institute for Regulatory Science (available from http://www.cmr.org/pdfs/r_d35.pdf) (accessed 15 March 2003).

Anonymous (2001) Tufts Centre for the Study of Drug Development pegs cost of a new prescription medicine at $802 million. *Press Release*. Tufts Centre for the Study of Drug Development, Tufts University, 30 November (available from http://www.tufts.edu/med/csdd/) (accessed 12 December 2002).

Brazell, C., Freeman, A. and Mosteller, M. (2002) Maximizing the value of medicines by including pharmacogenetic research in drug development and surveillance, *British Journal of Clinical Pharmacology*, 53: 224–31.

Buchanan, A., Califano, A., Kahn, J. *et al.* (2002) Pharmacogenetics: ethical issues and policy options, *Kennedy Institute Ethics Journal*, 12: 1–15.

DiMasi, J.A. (2002) The value of improving the productivity of the drug development process: faster times and better decisions, *Pharmacoeconomics*, 20(suppl. 3): 1–10.

DiMasi, J.A., Hansen, R.W. and Grabowski, H.G. (2003) The price of innovation: new estimates of drug development costs, *Journal of Health Economics*, 22: 151–85.

European Medicines Evaluation Agency (2003) *EMEA Centralised Procedures (Finalised)*. Annex 1 to CPMP Monthly Report (March), EMEA/CPMP/1358/03.

Evans, W. and Johnson, J.A. (2001) Pharmacogenomics: the inherited basis for interindividual differences in drug response, *Annual Review of Genomics and Human Genetics*, 2: 9–39.

Frantz, S. and Smith, A. (2003) New drug approvals for 2002, *Nature Reviews Drug Discovery*, 2: 95–6.

Gurwitz, D., Weizman, A. and Rehavi, M. (2003) Education: teaching pharmacogenomics to prepare future physicians and researchers for personalized medicine, *Trends in Pharmacological Sciences*, 24(3): 122–5.

Hall, A.G., Coulthard, S.A. and Irving, J.A.E. (2003) Molecular diagnostics: a healthcare perspective, *Expert Review of Molecular Diagnostics*, 3(1): 13–16.

Henry, D. and Lexchin, J. (2002) The pharmaceutical industry as a medicines provider, *Lancet*, 360: 1590–5.

Hetherington, S., Hughes, A.R., Mosteller, M. *et al.* (2002) Genetic variations in HLA-B region and hypersensitivity reactions to abacavir, *Lancet*, 359: 1121–2.

Human Genome Commission (2003) *Genes Direct: Ensuring the Effective Oversight of Genetic Tests Supplied Directly to the Public*. London: Human Genome Commission (available from http://www.hgc.gov.uk/genesdirect/#report).

Jefferys, D.B., Leakey, D., Lewis, J.A., Payne, S. and Rawlins, M.D. (1998) New active substances authorized in the United Kingdom between 1972 and 1994, *British Journal of Clinical Pharmacology*, 45: 151–6.

Lazarou, J., Pomeranz, B.H. and Corey, P.N. (1998) Incidence of adverse drug reactions in hospitalized patients: a meta-analysis of prospective studies, *Journal of the American Medical Association*, 279: 1200–5.

Lesko, L.J. and Woodcock, J. (2002) Pharmacogenomic-guided drug development: regulatory perspective, *The Pharmacogenomics Journal*, 2(1): 20–4.

Lindpaintner, K. (2002) Pharmacogenetics and the future of medical practice, *British Journal of Clinical Pharmacology*, 54: 221–30.

Mallal, S., Nolan, D., Witt, C. *et al.* (2002) Association between presence of HLA-B*5701, HLA-DR7, and HLA-DQ3 and hypersensitivity to HIV-1 reverse-transcriptase inhibitor abacavir, *Lancet*, 359: 727–32.

Manasco, P., Reiser, P., Renegar, G. and Mosteller, M. (2002) Pharmacogenetics and the genetic basis of adverse drug reactions, in R.D. Mann and E.B. Andrews (eds) *Pharmacovigilance*. Chichester: Wiley.

Motl, S., Miller, S.J. and Burns, P. (2003) Programs established by FDA to expedite patient access to medications, *American Journal of Health-System Pharmacy*, 60: 339–45.

Norton, R.M. (2001) Clinical pharmacogenomics: applications in pharmaceutical R&D, *Drug Discovery Today* 6: 180–5.

Nuffield Council on Bioethics (2003) *Pharmacogenetics: Ethical Issues* (available from http://www.nuffieldbioethics.org) (accessed 14 October 2003).

Park, B.K. and Pirmohamed, M. (2001) Toxicogenetics in drug development, *Toxicology Letters*, 120(1–3): 281–91.

Park, R. (2003) Growth of diagnostics in SNP detection market shows promise, *IVD Technology*, May (available from http://www.devicelink.com/ivdt/archive/03/05/004.html) (accessed 14 May 2003).

Phillips, K.A., Veenstra, D.L., Oren, E.E.O., Lee, J.K. and Sadee, W. (2001) Potential role of pharmacogenomics in reducing adverse drug reactions: a systematic review, *Journal of the American Medical Association*, 286(18): 2270–9.

Physicians' Desk Reference (2000) 54th edition. Montvale, NJ: Thomson Healthcare.

Pirmohamed, M. (2001) Pharmacogenetics and pharmacogenomics, *British Journal of Clinical Pharmacology*, 52(4): 345–7.

Pirmohamed, M. and Park, B.K. (2001) Genetic susceptibility to adverse drug reactions, *Trends in Pharmacological Sciences*, 22: 298–305.

Pirmohamed, M., Breckenridge, A.M., Kitteringham, N.R. and Park, B.K. (1998) Adverse drug reactions, *British Medical Journal*, 316: 1295–8.

Public Citizen (2001) *Rx R&D Myths: The Case Against the Drugs Industry 'Scare Card'*, Public Citizen (available from http://www.citizen.org/publications/release.cfm?ID=7065).

Robertson, J.A., Brody, B., Buchanan, A., Kahn, J. and McPherson, E. (2002) Pharmacogenetic challenges for the health care system, *Health Affairs*, 21(4): 155–67.

Roses, A.D. (2000) Pharmacogenetics and the practice of medicine, *Nature*, 405: 857–65.

Sciarrone, M.T., Stella, P., Barlassina, C. *et al.* (2003) ACE and alpha-adducin polymorphism as markers of individual response to diuretic therapy, *Hypertension*, 41: 398–403.

Veenstra, D.L., Higashi, M.K. and Phillips, K.A. (2001) Assessing the cost-effectiveness of pharmacogenomics, *American Association of Pharmaceutical Scientists*, 2(3): article 29 (available from http://www.pharmsci.org/).

World Health Organization, Advisory Committee on Health Research (2002) *Genomics and World Health*, Geneva: WHO.

chapter seventeen

Should we pay for lifestyle drugs?

Tom Walley

Introduction

Lifestyle drugs have attracted much attention, with concerns for the future funding of health services around the world if such therapies are included in the package of care provided and, more basically, about what are the limits of collective responsibility for health, and what are the limits of medical care. Examples of such drugs (Table 17.1) include orlistat for obesity and sildenafil for erectile dysfunction. The term 'lifestyle drugs' may trivialize serious medical conditions for which the drugs are indicated, but encapsulates concerns that the indications for these drugs might be regarded as issues of personal choice rather than illness.

Perception of what is illness and what is personal responsibility rather than health care depends on social and cultural norms (Reissman 1999; Gilbert et al 2000), and perhaps on whether one is a potential patient or a potential payer. 'Lifestyle' refers to how a medicine might be used rather than the medicine itself; for instance, most would agree that sildenafil for a healthy man unhappy with his sexual performance is a lifestyle use, but would think differently about the use of the same drug for a diabetic with neuropathy. An arbitrary working definition for this chapter might therefore be that a lifestyle drug is one that is used either for 'non-health' problems, or for problems that lie at the margins of health and well-being.

This definition is also problematic: a wider definition might include drugs that are used for health problems that might be caused by one's lifestyle, or might be better treated by altering one's lifestyle. This might include, for instance, lipid-lowering drugs (risk of cardiovascular disease might be better reduced by stopping smoking in many cases). The margins between these two definitions might not always be clear; for example, in regard to obesity, which at one level is a cosmetic problem but at another causes significant co-morbidity

Table 17.1 Examples of 'lifestyle' drugs

Indication	Examples	Comments
Erectile dysfunction	Sildenafil, phentolamine, apomorphine	NHS use of sildenafil defined for physical illness and for psychosexual disorders
Obesity	Orlistat, sibutramine	Obesity should be considered 'a serious medical issue rather than a perversity of current fashion' (Royal College of Physicians of London 1999)
Smoking cessation	Bupropion, nicotine replacement therapy (NRT)	Many NRTs currently blacklisted, but considerable stress on reducing smoking in many national health policies
Male pattern baldness	Minoxidil, finasteride	In the UK, the manufacturer of Propecia (finasteride) has requested that the drug be placed on the selected list of drugs not reimbursed by the NHS, alongside other drugs for the same indication
Prevention of skin ageing	Vitamin A creams	Efficacy uncertain, not available in the UK
Skin wrinkling	Botulinum toxin	Widely used in private dermatology and outside medicine
Contraception	Oral contraceptives	Well-established and accepted
Hormone replacement therapy	Testosterone in males (or females for libido)	Well-defined hormone deficiency states uncommon in males but advocated by some for wider use. Role in female libido uncertain
	Oestrogen replacement in women	For menopausal symptoms: until recently advocated with little evidence for cardiovascular disease prevention
Delaying menstruation	Norethisterone	Convenience
Dyspepsia	Proton pump inhibitors	Often used for minor indications and to avoid lifestyle changes
Patient convenience	Transdermal preparations; Modified – release preparations	Often expensive and rarely medically essential
Fungal toenail infections	Terbinafine	Unsightly toenails apparent depending on current fashions; rarely medically harmful
Depression, dysthymia, 'social dysfunction'	SSRI antidepressants	'Unhappiness' a medical condition? Potential serious adverse effects

Infertility treatments		Is having children a right or a lifestyle choice? With deliberate delays in fertility more socially desirable, infertility seems an increasing problem
Body-building	Anabolic steroids	Rarely indicated medically and potentially dangerous but widely available illicitly
Constitutional short stature in children	Growth hormone	Long-term efficacy uncertain
Patient convenience	Transdermal preparations; Modified – release preparations	Often expensive and rarely medically essential. Useful aid to compliance or concordance? Or a marketing attempt at product life extension?

and is a major public health concern. Many health services recognize this by health promotion or education campaigns; if they do, why should they not go on to actively treat these problems?

Definition of disease

Well-being and ill-health are difficult concepts to define, as their boundaries are not static but blurred and changing. For instance, studies have reported rates of self-perceived morbidity in the USA to be around 160 diseases per 100 people, but in India around 35 per 100. This is not new – throughout medical history, new diseases have 'appeared' and old ones 'disappeared', sometimes driven by the available treatment. In the 1960s, patients were often diagnosed as anxious and prescribed benzodiazepines. Today, with benzodiazepines less acceptable, such patients are more likely to be diagnosed as suffering from mild depression with anxiety, and prescribed an SSRI (selective serotonin reuptake inhibitor) antidepressant. So the technology has redefined the condition and perhaps even created it, if it has transformed the stresses of daily life into a medical condition.

Who should actually define when a problem or a risk factor becomes a disease – that is, is it worthy of medical attention? This was traditionally the domain of doctors, who have tended to define disease as disruption in physiological processes. But other stakeholders might legitimately claim this right: the first of these is the person who suffers from the problem. But are all problems (e.g. loneliness) illnesses? A different stakeholder might be the general public whose views may differ from that of the sufferer. Others might be third-party payers in many health services, who may define illness by what they are willing to pay for, rather than the other way round. A final stakeholder here might be the pharmaceutical industry, discussed in more detail below.

So when does a lifestyle issue become a disease? A lifestyle wish may become medicalized by doctors as a health problem when a biomedical cause (e.g. biochemical or genetic factor) or a treatment is found. Lifestyle issues may also be medicalized when associated with long-term public health concerns (e.g. obesity or smoking). Lifestyle wishes are then portrayed as amenable to health care – that is, medical intervention that can remove responsibility and/or control from the individual and/or society.

A second way might be by patient definition: the former WHO definition of health as a state of total physical, mental and social well-being, opens the question of whether health care should seek to meet all of these aims – should it embrace social as well as physical or mental well-being? This is often the demand in a consumerist society, where wishes become needs. One conceptualization of the problem (Stolk *et al.* 2002) distinguishes two types of utility gain: 'pain avoiding', which might be seen as the collective responsibility of the health service; and 'pleasure seeking', which is not a collective but rather a personal responsibility. 'Pleasure-seeking' treatments are those that people may want to raise themselves above some socially defined reference point for their health or functioning. 'Pain-avoiding' treatments are those that allow them to aspire to that social reference point. So if we expect the elderly to forego sexual activity, for instance (a social reference point), sildenafil is a lifestyle drug for them. For other groups of patients (e.g. younger diabetics with neuropathy), however, sexual activity might be seen as a basic need and within the social reference point, and so sildenafil is not a lifestyle therapy in such patients. In practice, this is how many governments have tackled these drugs – by refusing them for pure 'lifestyle use' but allowing them where they might be seen almost as 'compensatory' therapy.

Thirdly, the pharmaceutical industry can, in effect, create new 'diseases', defining these as those that can be treated by the company's products. Whether this is true or not is very contentious. For instance, recent discussion in relation to 'female sexual dysfunction', a possible indication for drugs such as sildenafil, ranged from those who decried the role of industry in sponsoring the definition of the condition that might cover as many as 43 per cent of women (Moynihan 2003) to those who argued that this condition deserved greater recognition and were less concerned about industry involvement (Basson *et al.* 2003).

The pharmaceutical market drives drug development by potential profitability rather than by public health needs. Lifestyle medicines are a growth area: increasing affluence in developed countries means more disposable income to spend on what might be seen as luxuries. Furthermore, the 'baby boomer' generation grows old, a generation more used to demanding benefits than accepting restrictions, and who already try to make ageing optional through cosmetic surgery: so why not do this via medicines? This generation may be less happy to accept that ageing causes a natural decline in many functions such as sexual activity. And who is to say that they are wrong? While such treatments may add what the patient perceives as quality rather than quantity to life, why should they not demand it as long as no-one else suffers as a result (Ebrahim 2002; Walley 2002)?

This view of a condition as a disease may be driven by advertising, which may seek to redefine the illness in the minds of doctors and of potential patients, converting wishes into health care problems and portraying health problems as primarily amenable to pharmaceutical treatment. Patients, similarly, may acquiesce in this: getting a tablet legitimizes the problem as medical, and it may be much easier to take a tablet than to change diet and lose weight. Though 'direct-to-consumer advertising' is currently proscribed in the European Union, companies are able to target patients indirectly through 'disease awareness' campaigns (e.g. Pfizer, makers of sildenafil, supporting impotence awareness), sponsorship of information materials and press releases. Companies might also sponsor patient advocacy groups for the same purpose (Moynihan *et al.* 2002).

This awareness raising may sometimes be highly appropriate. For example, one effect of the sildenafil controversy has been to reduce the taboo surrounding erectile dysfunction and to encourage people to seek help. Data from the UK suggest that the number of men presenting with erectile dysfunction increased from 80,000 to 257,000 per year between 1997 and 2000 (Wilson *et al.* 2002).

Costs and rationing

There are policy implications with lifestyle drugs, which may create a dichotomy between public and private interests. Those with public health benefits will probably be funded, as in the long run it may be most cost-effective. In most Western health services, lifestyle drugs are not purely a matter of personal choice, or of a debate about the extent of medicalization, but rather raise questions of whether such drugs should be paid for by a public health service (Mitrany 2001). With overstretched health care budgets almost universal, funding these drugs inevitably means limiting other forms of treatment for other patients. In theory at least, treating one patient's impotence threatens another patient's well-being.

This issue is therefore essentially one of rationing, and this is handled differently in different countries. The UK's centralized National Health Service (NHS) in practice has rarely made explicit central rationing decisions, depending instead on implicit rationing at local levels – a useful approach to diffuse responsibility and blame. In the case of sildenafil, however, there were dramatic predictions of the likely cost to the NHS of £1.25 billion per year (in fact, the cost rose from £29 million to £74 million) (Ashworth *et al.* 2002; Wilson *et al.* 2002), and central action was thought necessary. The Secretary of State for Health hoped that his Standing Medical Advisory Committee would provide a technical reason to avoid explicit rationing, but it responded that there was no medical justification for refusing sildenafil (to at least some patients) and that the issues were of affordability. He then said of sildenafil: 'Impotence is in itself neither life-threatening, nor does it cause physical pain, although it can in exceptional circumstances cause psychological distress. I do not consider it to be a priority for any additional NHS expenditure compared with, say . . . cancer, heart disease and mental health' (Beecham 1999).

This blurs the issues of what is legitimate medical use with questions of what the state is willing to spend or, given limited resources, how it prioritizes its services. In practice, the UK NHS already funds drugs and other treatments that are neither life-saving nor pain or disability reducing, but whose benefits to individuals and society mean they have become part of accepted medical practice. An example is oral contraceptives, which, in their early days, also gave rise to concerns of state-funded sexual licence (in some countries, such drugs could at one time only be supplied to married women and even today in some countries, e.g. Denmark, are only reimbursed for those under the age of 21). There are many other examples and to suggest that lifestyle enhancement is not a legitimate part of medical treatment is simply nonsense, although this is not the same as saying that the collective purse should fund it.

Despite the flawed logic, the statement above had general public and professional support. As a result, sildenafil is funded by the NHS for patients with a limited number of physical conditions (e.g. diabetic neuropathy) and for patients with defined psychosexual disorders. It is not clear how well such restrictions work. Even in countries with apparently tight systems of control, doctors notoriously lie to prescribe what they wish (McManus *et al.* 1998)!

In other European countries, there has generally been less discussion and introspection, and more proscription of such drugs from public funding (see Table 17.2). But in principle at least, the situation has often ended up not all that different from the UK – that is, general proscription but available for selected patients with more medically defined indications (Klein and Sturm 2002). In the Netherlands, sildenafil was initially approved by the insurers' organization but then excluded by ministerial order, a centralist approach not dissimilar to the UK. In Germany, the committee of the doctors and the sickness funds (Bundesausschuss der Artze und Krankenkassen) decided that sildenafil should not be made available, but this decision was partially overturned by the Federal Social court, which held that the Bundesausschuss did not have the right to ban it. The matter has not been resolved: the sickness funds provide limited funding for patients on a case-by-case basis and often after court

Table 17.2 Reimbursement status of some 'lifestyle' drugs across key European markets

	Sildenafil	Sibutramine	(Topical) minoxidil
France	X	X	X
Germany	X/S[a]	X	X
Spain	X	X	X
Italy	S	X	X
UK	S	G	X
Netherlands	X	X	X
Austria	S	S	S
Belgium	X	X	X
Sweden	S	X	X
Finland	S	S	X
Ireland	L	G	X
Denmark[b]	S	S	S

Note: X = not reimbursed; S = reimbursed only for special circumstances; L = reimbursed for limited amount; G = reimbursed as for other drugs.
[a] See text. [b] In Denmark, these drugs are not generally reimbursed but the patient can apply for individual reimbursement; this is seldom granted for minoxidil, but is granted to 10–15 persons a month for sibutramine, and about 100 per month for sildenafil.

decisions. The sickness funds have avoided seeking a definitive decision from the higher courts, lest it require more general funding and establish precedents for other areas.

In Sweden, sildenafil was at first included in the package of approved drugs but then relegated to a secondary category of drugs available only in special circumstances, as decided by the Ministry of Health on a case-by-case basis. In 2001, of the 3000 applications, less than 10 per cent were approved.

In the USA, health care providers have taken a range of views, with some refusing it, others providing limited supplies or introducing steep patient co-payments (Mitrany 2001; Klein and Sturm 2002). The role of co-payments are considered in Chapter 13, but it is worth repeating that at least some 'lifestyle' medicines may have an important role in public health (e.g. nicotine replacement therapy or treatments for obesity) and anything which reduces their utilization, such as co-payments or other forms of limitation, may have important adverse effects in the long term.

In all of these countries, there was successful containment of the costs of sildenafil to the state, broad medical and public support for the government approaches and a disparate patient group who might hesitate to identify themselves publicly. There was also a safety valve: sildenafil was easily available on private prescription or via the internet, and at a cost most could afford. This success contrasts with the difficulties governments have had in controlling other therapeutic areas, where there is a well-defined patient population with advocacy groups (e.g. multiple sclerosis and beta-interferon in the UK; Walley 2004).

Managing lifestyle drugs

Traditional drug regulation and licensing is intended to deal with the three hurdles of efficacy, safety and quality and not with issues such as the cost or cost-effectiveness of a new drug, or the need for the drug. In the UK, the National Institute of Clinical Excellence (NICE), created after the launch of sildenafil, addresses these other issues, distancing these difficult decisions from politicians. Health economics can play a role by defining measures of the quality of life and patient and citizen utilities, and the likely cost-effectiveness of achieving gains in utilities. This is useful in that it uses patient-defined quality of life to allow lifestyle drugs to be measured in the same terms as other more traditional treatments, at least in theory. The difficulties of using the Quality Adjusted Life Year (QALY) in this area have been well recognized (most recently in relation to a study of sildenafil; Freemantle 2000), but there is difficulty in finding an alternative. But health economics, like drug efficacy, only addresses a limited technical question – that is, cost-effectiveness compared with defined comparators. Interestingly, NICE does not consider affordability (i.e. the total cost to the health service); that is a political decision. Nor does NICE provide the funding for the medicines it approves, causing problems for local managers.

Decision-making principles

Can we establish principles in deciding whether a health service should fund an intervention, such as a lifestyle drug? The 'compensatory' principle is useful but requires definition of a social reference point. The Dunning Report (Stolk *et al.* 2002) in the Netherlands described four filters to be passed before a treatment should be considered for public funding; the first that it constituted necessary care, the second that it should be effective, the third efficient, and the fourth that it was more appropriately an issue of public and collective responsibility rather than individual responsibility.

How would this apply to a drug like sildenafil? The second and third questions are the easiest: there is ample clinical trial evidence that sildenafil is effective. For the third, efficiency, sildenafil is more cost-effective than papaverine-phentolamine (Stolk *et al.* 2000). The remaining two questions are much more difficult, since they are not technical but really depend on value judgements. The first question on 'necessary care' begs the definition of necessary and of disease as discussed already; in the case of sildenafil, it might be thought necessary for some (e.g. diabetic neuropathy) but inappropriate for others (e.g. young men wishing to enhance their sexual performance). The last question is also difficult; if we have a problem defining what disease is, how are we to define the limits of collective responsibility versus individual responsibility? Debates on these two points have undermined the operationalization of the Dunning principles in the Netherlands; for instance, attempts to stop reimbursement of oral contraceptives failed because of such disagreements and intense lobbying. So the technical issues are often the easiest to address, but do not aid us in the difficult political, ethical and social decisions. It is important not to confuse these two questions.

Solutions?

The ethical, clinical and financial arguments here are not independent, and do not have individual answers. In European health services, lifestyle medicines are not just matters of personal choice, but also of public concern. The ethical questions are around how far we should bow to consumer forces and industry, or whether we should take a more planned approach, and how to balance individual and public responsibility. The only solution to this would seem to be social and political debate (Lexchin 2001), but medicine has tended to be led on such issues rather than leading. The clinical debate is around how we ensure that patients are well-informed consumers, and how we minimize risk while preserving patient choice and autonomy.

Klein and Sturm (2002) identify a common theme running through the rationing of sildenafil across Europe and the USA – that it was better to avoid blanket proscription and allow instead a leaky bucket approach (i.e. availability within some defined parameters). By allowing doctors to determine medical need, it encourages medical cooperation and restores some of the medical authority that might otherwise be undermined by consumerism. Klein and Sturm suggest that the same principles could be applied to all lifestyle drugs.

Table 17.3 Scenarios for the future of the pharmaceutical market

Sobriety in sufficiency
A scenario involving a dramatic shift in social values resulting in a culture of restraint – people reject the consumer society and concentrate on essential, intrinsic values, and emphasize solidarity and collectivism

Risk-avoidance
This scenario is characterized by a general feeling of mistrust of technology and the practice of medicine becomes highly defensive and conservative

Technology on demand
This scenario is driven by technological optimism, both by professionals and by the public. Trust in medical technology is implicit

Free market unfettered
In this scenario, health care is dominated by market forces accompanied by high consumption, a focus on self-help, and demand for medical technology and health care services. The negative aspect of this scenario is the acceptance of inequality in society

Source: Leufkens *et al.* (1994).

This has an air of muddling through, but may be politically easier than a more rational planned approach. Supply-side changes would need to be balanced with demand-led work, requiring the management of expectations and, possibly, making patients more accountable for their own treatments (Smith 1999).

In fact, any call for restraint opposes the forces that are fuelling demand, such as modern medical technology, including the development and marketing of lifestyle drugs (Leufkens *et al.* 1994). The pharmaceutical industry should be a responsible partner in the debate about services and rationing, but perhaps it is unrealistic to expect the pharmaceutical industry to limit itself any more than the tobacco or the motor industries. At present, the pharmaceutical market is less to do with meeting health needs and more about the industry's growth requirements. The goals of health care policy are in danger of becoming subsidiary to those of the industry. A more sustainable approach would be for an informed debate (led by societal interests) about what constitutes need and how this can be translated into useful products – how stakeholders more than shareholders can shape the future of health care. This would re-evaluate and re-prioritize research and development activities in the long term, centred on an awareness of what health systems can and cannot afford. If this does not happen, the pace of medicalization and new technologies threatens to outstrip the capabilities of institutions and providers (both financially and organizationally) and may ultimately overwhelm societal control and central planning. Leufkens and colleagues (1994) described four broad scenarios for the future of pharmaceuticals (Table 17.3). These are not the only options and we currently see elements of all of these in the pharmaceutical market. Lifestyle drugs should prompt us to think carefully where we want the balance to lie between these extremes.

References

Ashworth, M., Clement, S. and Wright, M. (2002) Demand, appropriateness and prescribing of 'lifestyle drugs': a consultation survey in general practice, *Family Practice*, 19: 236–41.

Basson, R., Leiblum, S., Potts, A. *et al.* (2003) The making of a disease: female sexual dysfunction (letter), *British Medical Journal*, 326: 658.

Beecham, L. (1999) UK issues guidance on prescribing Viagra, *British Medical Journal*, 318: 279.

Ebrahim, S. (2002) Medicalisation of old age – to be encouraged, *British Medical Journal*, 324: 861–3.

Freemantle, N. (2000) Valuing the effects of sildenafil in erectile dysfunction, *British Medical Journal*, 320: 1156–7.

Gilbert, D., Walley, T. and New, B. (2000) Lifestyle medicines, *British Medical Journal*, 321: 1341–4.

Klein, R. and Sturm, H. (2002) Viagra: a success story for rationing?, *Health Affairs*, 21: 177–87.

Leufkens, H., Haaijer-Ruskamp, F., Bakker, A. and Dukes, G. (1994) Scenario analysis of the future of medicines, *British Medical Journal*, 309: 1137–40.

Lexchin, J. (2001) Lifestyle drugs: issues for debate, *Canadian Medical Association Journal*, 164(10): 1449–51.

McManus, P., Marley, J., Birkett, D.J. and Lindner, J. (1998) Compliance with restrictions on the subsidized use of proton pump inhibitors in Australia, *British Journal of Clinical Pharmacology*, 46: 409–11.

Mitrany, D. (2001) Lifestyle drugs: determining their value and who should pay, *Pharmacoeconomics*, 19: 441–8.

Moynihan, R. (2003) The making of a disease: female sexual dysfunction, *British Medical Journal*, 326: 45–7.

Moynihan, R., Health, I. and Henry, D. (2002) Selling sickness: the pharmaceutical industry and disease mongering, *British Medical Journal*, 324: 886–91.

Reissman, D. (1999) The pros and cons of covering lifestyle drugs, *Disease Management and Health Outcomes*, 6: 249–51.

Royal College of Physicians of London (1999) *Clinical Management of Overweight and Obese Patients – With Particular Reference to the Use of Drugs*. London: Royal College of Physicians of London.

Smith, R. (1999) The NHS: possibilities for the endgame, *British Medical Journal*, 318: 209–10.

Stolk, E.A., Busschbach, J.J., Caffa, M., Meuleman, E. and Rutten, F. (2000) Cost utility analysis of sildenafil compared with papaverine-phentolamine injections, *British Medical Journal*, 320: 1165.

Stolk, E.A., Brouwer, W.B. and Busschbach, J.J. (2002) Rationalising rationing: economic and other considerations in the debate about funding of Viagra, *Health Policy*, 59(1): 53–63.

Walley, T. (2002) Lifestyle medicines and the elderly, *Drugs and Aging*, 19: 163–8.

Walley, T. (2004) Prescribing of neuropsychotherapeutics in the UK: what has been the impact of NICE?, *CNS Drugs*, 18: 1–12.

Wilson, E.C., McKeen, E.S., Scuffham, P.A. *et al.* (2002) The cost to the United Kingdom National Health Service of managing erectile dysfunction: the impact of sildenafil and prescribing restrictions, *Pharmacoeconomics*, 20: 879–89.

eighteen

Alternative medicines in Europe

Edzard Ernst and Anna Dixon[1]

Introduction

The market for alternative medicines has a long and varied history in Europe. In recent years, growth in the demand for alternative medicines has led to an increased interest from policy makers in regulating the market. As the bulk of the sales are in the private market, with only a low level of public reimbursement, regulation has tended to focus on quality in the interests of consumer protection rather than price regulation. In this chapter, we present an overview of the market for alternative medicines in Europe and the current developments in the regulation of products. We first set out the main types of alternative medicine and their uses. We then go on to analyse the key market characteristics, in particular the utilization and the size of the commercial market, and the relative size of the over-the-counter and publicly financed market. Quality regulation has taken a number of forms, including product licensing at the European Union (EU) and national levels, and pharmacovigilance of products. We conclude by assessing the future direction of the market, including the implications of EU regulation.

Definitions and use of alternative medicines

The term 'alternative medicine' implies that these therapies are used as a substitute for conventional treatments. While this may be the case for some, the vast majority of consumers embrace both types of treatment (Murray and Shepherd 1993). The National Library of Medicine, whose keywords are utilized in the main electronic databases such as Medline, increasingly uses the term 'complementary therapies', which implies that the therapies are used alongside conventional treatments. Other terms that are often employed are natural, unconventional, unorthodox, irregular or integrative medicine; and the choice of terminology is often motivated by social and political factors (Jonas 2002). Comparative work in this area is complicated by the lack of clear translations for terminology (Dixon *et al.* 2003).

The Cochrane Collaboration defines complementary medicine as 'diagnosis, treatment and/or prevention which complements mainstream medicine by contributing to a common whole, by satisfying a demand not met by orthodoxy or by diversifying the conceptual frameworks of medicine' (Ernst *et al.* 1995). The Office of Alternative Medicine at the National Institutes of Health (USA) defined alternative medicine as 'A broad domain of healing resources that encompass all health systems, modalities and practices, and their accompanying theories and beliefs, other than those intrinsic to the politically dominant health system of a particular society or culture in a given historical period' (Kelner *et al.* 2000). For the purpose of this chapter, 'alternative medicine' refers only to the products used in the delivery of complementary and alternative medicine (CAM).

More than a hundred different therapies and associated products fall outside orthodox medicine and are therefore termed 'alternative'. However, some are more established than others (often depending on the country). A useful classification is between those that are frontier therapies (those that challenge conceptual and paradigmatic assumptions about biological and scientific reality), emerging therapies (those that involve common areas of interest for CAM and conventional medicine) and integrating therapies (those that may be considered conventional but overlap with CAM practices) (Jonas 2002). The main products are homoeopathic medicines, herbal medicines, essential oils and flower remedies. Apart from herbal medicines, these could all be classified as frontier therapies.

Homoeopathic medicine

Homoeopathy was founded by Samuel Hahnemann (1755–1843), based on the Law of Similars, the 'like cures like' principle. Homoeopathic medicines are produced through a process of serial dilution and vigorous shaking ('potentiation'). Homoeopaths believe that the dilutant retains a memory of the original substance ('the memory of water').

Homoeopathy is employed mainly for mental, infectious and rheumatological disorders (Colin 2000). According to a survey of professional organizations (Long *et al.* 2001), the four most important medical indications are respiratory problems, menstrual complaints/pre-menstrual syndrome, arthritis/rheumatic conditions and irritable bowel syndrome.

Herbal medicine/phytotherapy

Herbal medicine or phytotherapy uses various remedies derived from plants and plant extracts to treat disorders and maintain good health. It relies on the principles of pharmacology. Chinese herbal medicine has developed over thousands

---

Box 18.1   Selection of medicinal herbs and their uses

Aloe vera: used for a variety of skin conditions including psoriasis
Echinacea: supposed to promote the immune system and is used to prevent or treat colds
Garlic: used to lower blood pressure and cholesterol
Gingko: used to treat dementia and supposed to improve memory and mental concentration
Ginseng: believed to be a panacea
Kava: traditionally known for its relaxing and calming properties, it is used to treat anxiety, stress and tension
Feverfew: used to prevent migraines; also commonly used for arthritis and menstrual pain
Saw palmetto: widely used to treat benign prostate hyperplasia
St John's wort: widely used to treat mild to moderate depression
Valerian: used to reduce anxiety and insomnia

---

of years and is now popular in European societies. However, there are European traditions of herbal medicinal use too. The number of remedies derived from plants are too numerous to detail here. Some medicinal herbs and their uses are listed in Box 18.1 (Mar and Bent 1999; Rotblatt 1999).

A survey of UK herbal practitioners, who represent only a small proportion of herbal use in the UK, indicated that the most frequently treated conditions were pre-menstrual syndrome, irritable bowel syndrome, eczema and arthritis (Barnes and Ernst 1998).

Essential oils

Essential oils are used in a variety of products, including food, toiletries, conventional and aromatherapy oils. Aromatherapy accounts for only about 4 per cent of the entire production. Aromatherapy is the controlled use of plant essence for therapeutic purposes (Ernst *et al.* 2001). Plant essences are essential oils that are fragrant and highly volatile compounds generated by plants through photosynthesis. Essential oils can be applied directly to the skin through massage or a compress, added to baths, inhaled with steaming water or spread throughout a room with a diffuser. The oils are thought to have effects at the psychological, physiological and cellular levels. These effects can be relaxing or stimulating depending on the chemistry of the oil and also the previous associations of the individual with a particular scent (Ernst *et al.* 2001).

According to a survey of professional organizations (Long *et al.* 2001), the indications for aromatherapy span a wide spectrum, including anxiety and stress, arthritis, chronic fatigue, hormonal problems, cancer, multiple sclerosis, insomnia and depression.

Flower remedies

Flower remedies belong to a therapeutic system developed by Dr Edward Bach at the beginning of the twentieth century that uses specifically prepared plant infusions to balance physical and emotional disturbances (Ernst *et al.* 2001). Inspired by Hahnemann and Jung, Edward Bach developed his own system of medicine. According to Bach, all human disease and suffering are rooted in emotional imbalances. He identified 38 flower remedies that, he believed, could treat most illnesses. These were divided into seven therapeutic groups according to the following emotions: depression, fear, lack of interest in the present, loneliness, overconcern for the welfare of others, oversensitivity and uncertainty. Bach associated each of these emotions with flowers to be used as remedies (Ernst *et al.* 2001).

The remedies are produced by placing freshly picked sun-exposed flowers into spring water, into which brandy is added for preservation. The prescription of these remedies by specialized therapists is highly individualized and intuitive. According to Bach, the remedies work not through their pharmacological actions but through their 'energy'. Thus there are similarities with homoeopathy, even though many homoeopaths deny this. Flower remedies are used to treat the above-named emotional states and often also to treat (mostly chronic benign) medical conditions believed to be caused by such states.

Efficacy and effectiveness

Criticism of alternative medicines has tended to come from a narrow biomedical perspective, which argues that only scientifically proven evidence-based medicine is legitimate. Critics regard the lack of systematic proof of the efficacy of alternative medicines using 'scientific methods' (by which they mean randomized control trials) to be unacceptable (Angell and Kassirer 1998). Increasingly, the appropriate use of alternative medicines is supported by scientific evidence of their efficacy and effectiveness. This is partly influenced by the wider trend in evidence-based medicine (Ernst 2000; Ernst *et al.* 2001), but this trend is also due to the understanding among practitioners that any future integration with conventional medicine or the public reimbursement of alternative medicines will only occur if their efficacy is based on evidence (Mason *et al.* 2002). There has been significant debate among practitioners and professional CAM organizations about the appropriateness of scientific methods, in particular the double-blind randomized controlled trial (RCT), in the evaluation of alternative medicines. Opposition arises for a variety of reasons: for example, the belief that holistic or individualized treatments defy science; that RCTs eliminate the important effect of the therapeutic relationship and the placebo effect; that no account is taken of wider quality-of-life measures in the narrow clinical outcomes; and the fear that science might destroy the uniqueness or subtlety of alternative medicine (Ernst 2002a). Increasingly, proponents of CAM have become more open to the idea of scientifically testing the value of their treatments and are developing appropriate methods to establish an evidence base. Numerous trials of herbal and homoeopathic medicine have been published

Table 18.1 Systematic reviews of homoeopathy and herbal medicines

Remedy	Indication	Result[a]
Homoeopathy[b]		
any	any	(+/+/−/±/±/±/−/−)
any	post-operative ileus	±
any	delayed-onset muscle soreness	−
arnica	any	−/−
any	migraine prophylaxis	−
any	comparisons with conventional drugs	−
oscillococcinum	influenza prevention/treatment	+
any	asthma	−
any	any rheumatic conditions	+
any	osteoarthritis	−
Herbal medicines		
aloe vera	any	−
cranberry	urinary tract	±
echinacea	common cold	±
evening primrose	pre-menstrual syndrome	−
evening primrose	eczema	+
feverfew	migraine prevention	±
garlic	hypercholesterolaemia	±
ginger	nausea/vomiting	+
ginkgo biloba	intermittent claudication	+
ginkgo biloba	tinnitus	±
ginkgo biloba	dementia	+
ginkgo biloba	cerebral insufficiency	+
ginkgo biloba	macular degeneration	±
ginseng	any	±
hawthorn	congestive heart failure	+
horse chestnut	venous insufficiency	+
kava	anxiety	+
peppermint	irritable bowel syndrome	±
saw palmetto	benign prostate hyperplasia	+
St John's wort	depression	+
tea tree	skin infections	±
valerian	insomnia	±

[a] The number of plus or minus (±) signs reflects the number of systematic reviews. +, positive; −, negative; ±, inconclusive.
[b] Because of the nature of homoeopathic treatment, the remedy is often tailored to the individual and therefore systematic reviews have often looked at the effectiveness of 'any' homoeopathic remedy on a particular indication.
Note: Data based on Ernst (2001, 2002b)

and dozens of systematic reviews or meta-analyses have also become available (Cooke and Ernst 2000; Ernst 2001, 2002b) (see Table 18.1).

Such research obviously requires financial resources. Several initiatives in Britain, Germany and Switzerland have earmarked considerable sums for research into this area (Ernst 1999). In the UK, for example, the Department of

Health has launched a series of fellowships to increase research capacity in this area. Compared with the funds available for conventional medical research, these sums are still minute, but the trend appears to be for creating more support for this under-researched field. Compared with the pharmaceutical sector, commercial research and development (R&D) spending is also minute. Within the EU, only the German herbal industry is investing sizeable amounts into R&D (exact figures unavailable).

Utilization of alternative medicines

Numerous surveys have attempted to define the prevalence of use of alternative medicines in various European countries. Some are based on samples of the general population, while others focus on particular sub-populations such as children or specific disease groups. Higher prevalence rates are found among particular patient populations, for example patients with cancer or rheumatological conditions (Ernst and Cassileth 1998; Ernst 1998). However, most of the surveys do not distinguish between use of practitioners and self-care (which usually involves the purchase of an alternative medicine).

In the UK, where surveys covered both self-care and care provided by a practitioner, self-care life-time prevalence rates were much higher than practitioner-only usage – in the region of 40–50 per cent compared with 10–30 per cent (Thomas *et al.* 1991, 2001; Ernst and White 2000). Thomas *et al.* (2001) report that over 12 months (data relate to 1998), homoeopathic remedies accounted for 8.6 per cent of over-the-counter (OTC) transactions and herbal remedies 19.8 per cent. Another UK survey conducted in 1999 found an overall one-year prevalence of 20 per cent and suggested that herbal medicine was more popular than any other form of alternative medicine (Ernst and White 2000). Longitudinal data from Scotland show that, between 1993 and 1999, the use of herbal or homoeopathic medicines in the general population had increased from 4 to 6 per cent and from 7 to 10 per cent, respectively (Emslie *et al.* 2002). The herbal products most commonly utilized are garlic, ginseng, gingko, St John's wort and echinacea (Skinner and Rangasami 2002). According to one survey (Allensbacher Archiv 2002), there has been a continuous increase in the utilization of 'natural remedies' over the past three decades in Germany (Table 18.2). One-year prevalence increased from 30 per cent in 1970 to 56 per cent in 2002.

Table 18.2   Percentage of population reporting having used natural remedies in West Germany, 1970–2002

	1970	1980	1989	1997	2002
In the last 3 months	14	20	25	28	35
In the last 6 months	22	27	35	41	46
In the last 12 months (one-year prevalence)	30	33	44	52	56
Ever in their life (lifetime prevalence)	52	51	58	65	73

Source: Allensbacher Archiv (2002).

Table 18.3 Conditions and frequencies of treatment with herbal medicinal products in Germany

Condition	2002 (%)	1997 (%)	1970 (%)
Common cold	69	66	41
Flu	34	38	31
Digestive or intestinal complaints	24	25	24
Headache	24	25	13
Insomnia	27	25	13
Stomach ulcer/problems	26	24	21
Nervousness	·21	21	12
Circulatory disorders	19	17	15
Bronchitis	18	15	12
Skin diseases	14	12	8
Fatigue and exhaustion	15	12	8

Source: Allensbacher Archiv (2002).

Table 18.3 shows common conditions frequently treated with herbal medicinal products in Germany in 2002 (Allensbacher Archiv 2002). Data from Austria suggest that homoeopathy (12.1 per cent life-time prevalence) was the second most popular form of CAM after acupressure in 1988 (Haidinger and Gredler 1988). An epidemiological study of French workers showed that, in 1986, 2.7 per cent of that population used homoeopathic remedies; in 1996, this proportion had fallen slightly to 2.1 per cent. Also, women were about three times more likely than men to use homoeopathy (Lapeyre-Mestre *et al.* 1999). Finally, recent data from Sweden suggest that 31 per cent of the general population had used some form of CAM within the last 14 days and that vitamins/minerals and biological products were the most popular category (Nilsson *et al.* 2001).

Financing of alternative medicines

Much of the European alternative medicine market constitutes self-administered remedies bought over the counter in outlets ranging from pharmacies to direct sale companies. The total European OTC market for herbal remedies in 1991 was £1.5 billion (Fisher and Ward 1994) and in 1998 around £4.5 billion (Blumenthal *et al.* 1998). Licensed herbal medicines constitute more than half of the total complementary medicines market in the UK (estimated to amount to £38 million in 1996) (Mintel International Group 1997).[2] In Germany, herbal medicines made up a third of the total OTC market, equivalent to US$1.8 billion in 1997. In France, where figures currently comprise pharmacy sales only, total sales of herbal products reached US$1.1 billion in 1997, representing 28 per cent of the total OTC market. The annual growth rates in these markets have been in the range of 5 per cent (Fasihi 1996). Growth in the German herbals market, however, halted in 1997, mainly as a result of the delisting of products by German health insurance funds in an attempt to reduce their expenditures (Institute of Medical Statistics 1998).

The leading categories of herbal products in Germany were cough/cold and circulatory products. In France, circulatory products were a leading category (Institute of Medical Statistics 1998). The sales figures of aromatherapy oils have increased sharply during recent years. In the UK, retail sales of aromatherapy oils were £2.0 million in 1991 and £14.0 million in 1996 (Mintel International Group 1997). In other European countries, they have followed a similar trend.

Most OTC sales are paid for privately. Publicly funded alternative medicines account for a smaller market share but some countries with explicit positive lists of publicly funded drugs do include licensed natural remedies. In Germany, Social Code Book V states that medicines associated with 'special therapeutic approaches' (phytotherapy, homoeopathy and anthroposophy[3]) are reimbursable under social health insurance. However, a number of alternative medicines have been delisted in recent years by the Federal Committee of Physicians and Sickness Funds, which makes decisions on exclusions from the benefits catalogue, due to increasing concerns about cost-effectiveness (Dixon *et al.* 2003). As a result, from 1996 to 2000, sales of anthroposophic and homoeopathic remedies reimbursed by social health insurance decreased from €66.5 million to €49.9 million (Wissenschaftliches Institut der Ortskrankenkassen 2002). In 2002, three natural remedies were among the 100 most commonly prescribed pharmaceuticals, compared with eight in 1989 (Schwabe and Paffrath 2003). In the UK, doctors are able to prescribe homoeopathic remedies and estimates suggest that approximately 75,000 consultations per year by doctors yield a homoeopathic prescription (Swayne 1989). In addition to self-care, alternative medicines are dispensed and utilized by CAM practitioners and integrated as part of orthodox medical treatment (however, no figures on quantities prescribed are available).

Historical and cultural background

Trends in the utilization of alternative medicines and reimbursement policies vary substantially between countries. This is often a result of historical tradition rather than any objective measure of (cost) effectiveness. For example, hydrotherapy was widespread throughout Europe at the turn of the twentieth century. In England, hydrotherapy died out in all but a few spas, whereas in Germany and much of Central and Eastern Europe, spas and balneotherapy remained popular (Porter 1989; Lindemann 1999). Anthroposophic medicine is widespread in both Germany and the Netherlands but is only a minority therapy in the UK. On the other hand, aromatherapy is widespread in the UK but less popular in other countries. Table 18.4 shows the top therapies, as identified in major national reports on CAM, in Germany and the UK (Rosslenbroich *et al.* 1994; House of Lords Select Committee on Science and Technology 2000).

History may also explain the varying degree to which CAM products are included in, or excluded from, the publicly funded health care systems. For instance, when the British NHS was created in 1948, all alternative medicine except homoeopathy (which benefited from strong royal patronage) was not included. This is in stark contrast with Germany, where herbal medicine, for example, has had uninterrupted support from governments, doctors, lay practitioners and patients; in fact, during the Nazi era, it was even specifically

Table 18.4 Top CAM therapies in the UK and Germany at the
end of the twentieth century

UK	Germany
acupuncture	phytotherapy/herbal medicine
chiropractic	homoeopathy
herbal medicine/phytotherapy	anthroposophic medicine
homoeopathy	acupuncture
osteopathy	

Sources: Rosslenbroich *et al.* (1994), House of Lords Select Committee
on Science and Technology (2000).

promoted under the banner of 'New German Art of Healing' (*Neue Deutsche
Heilkunst*). Within the constraints of this chapter, it is not possible to provide
further detailed information on the historical tradition in European countries,
but several writers have provided fascinating studies (see Porter 1989; Jütte
1996; Schepers and Hermans 1999).

Regulation of alternative medicines

There are a number of options for the regulation of alternative medicines: (i)
that they be subject to the same regulatory requirements as other pharmaceutical products; (ii) that they be exempt from all regulatory requirements; (iii)
that there be partial exemptions from regulatory requirements (such as evidence
or registration and marketing authorization); or (iv) that there be separate
regulatory requirements for alternative medicines (World Health Organization
1998).

Where herbal medicines and related products are neither registered nor controlled by regulatory bodies, a special licensing system may be used to enable
health authorities to screen the constituents, demand proof of quality before
marketing, ensure correct and safe use, and also to oblige licence holders to
report suspected adverse reactions within a post-marketing surveillance system
(De Smet 1995).

Licensing

Herbal medicines can be licensed through identical procedures to conventional
medicines. By obtaining a pharmaceutical licence for an alternative medicine,
the product would have greater legitimacy and the producers may find it easier
to market or obtain public reimbursement of the product (World Health
Organization 1998, 2001). Several such licences exist in Germany, while in
other European countries herbal medicines have found it difficult to obtain
similar licences.

In addition, there are special licensing procedures for herbal medicines.

Regulatory evaluations of medicinal herbs have been laid down in more than 300 monographs in Germany, and in France more than 200 herbs have been listed as acceptable ingredients of phytomedicines (De Smet 1995). 'Special therapeutic approaches' (phytotherapy, homoeopathy and anthroposophic medicine) receive special protection in Germany with respect to licensing of products.

Products classified as 'special therapeutic approaches' account for a major share of the total medicines market, although the share has declined as a result of changes to licensing requirements. In 1988, for example, there were 70,000 phytopharmaceuticals, 24,000 homoeopathic drugs and 3000 anthroposophic drugs out of a total of 126,000 medicinal drugs available in Germany (Matthiessen *et al.* 1992). Between 1988 and 1993, 70,000 drugs that did not fulfil the licensing requirements were removed from the list; a substantial number of these were alternative medicines (Busse 2000).

The number of alternative medicines available on the German market is expected to decrease further by the end of 2004 when all drugs must have undergone re-licensing procedures.

European Union regulation

Homoeopathic medicines are regulated throughout the EU according to a specialized licensing system. As long as the medicine is highly dilute, no evidence of efficacy and safety is required and essentially only the quality of the product is regulated. In terms of registration and marketing authorization, anthroposophic medicinal products described in an official pharmacopoeia and prepared by a homoeopathic method are treated in the same way as homoeopathic medicinal products (Council of the European Union 2001).

The establishment of effective regulation for registration and quality assurance of herbal medicines was recognized as a priority by the World Health Organization (WHO) in their Traditional Medicine Strategy 2002–2005 (World Health Organization 2002a) and followed an earlier worldwide review of herbal medicine regulation (World Health Organization 1998). A new European Union directive on traditional herbal medicinal products, which is still under discussion, is likely to be implemented by 2004 (European Commission 2002). Under this proposal, a herbal product would only obtain a traditional use licence if the applicant demonstrates that the herbal medicine or a 'comparable product' has been in medicinal use in the EU for 30 years; up to 15 years of use outside the EU can be used to make up this 30-year period. The evidence required in the traditional use licensing process would be bibliographic or based on expert reports of traditional use, meaning that there is a very wide range of possible sources: authoritative literature, practical evidence of licensed/unlicensed products on the market to date, lists of herbal medicines accepted as traditional by member states, and testimony of recognized experts. Such evidence would be used as a substitute for the usual requirement for demonstrating efficacy; in particular, safety would be assessed on existing bibliographic data where possible. This represents a compromise between relying on the test of time and having to subject all herbal medicines to RCTs (Ernst *et al.* 1998).

Under the proposed new regulatory scheme, there would be a positive list, established at community level by the Committee for Herbal Medicinal Products. The primary purpose of having such a list is to remove the need for companies to provide evidence of traditional use and safety where this has already been established. Each herbal medicine on the list would have therapeutic indications, specified strength, route of administration and relevant safety information. Moreover, the quality of the product would have to be demonstrated (i.e. demonstrate good manufacturing practice) to obtain a manufacturer's licence or wholesale dealer's licence where appropriate. The labelling of traditional use herbal medicines would be the same as for conventional pharmaceutical products and would state that indications are not clinically proven. More details on this new directive can be found elsewhere (see Steinhoff 2002).

Developments in EU regulation of homoeopathic remedies and herbal medicines can be viewed as a means of promoting consumer safety in the sector and enabling the free movement of goods between member states. However, there is concern that the costs of meeting the proposed regulatory requirements may have a negative impact on smaller businesses, favouring the industrial manufacturers of products.

Aromatherapy oils and flower remedies presently are not regulated as medicines in Europe.

Pharmacovigilance

In a survey of leading pharmaceutical and herbal companies, as measured by revenue from pharmaceutical/herbal sales for the year ending December 1999 (Thompson Coon *et al.* 2003), the heads of research and development were asked: (i) whether herb–drug interactions are considered important and whether studies are conducted; (ii) whether funds are specifically allocated to research the topic; and (iii) if this were the case, how much of their annual research and development budget was allocated in the year 2000. Approximately 67 per cent (10 of 15 companies) conducted studies and only around 13 per cent (2 of 15) regularly allocated funds to such research, with only two herbal companies reporting that 5 per cent and 6 per cent of their annual R&D budget, respectively, was allocated to research into herbal drug interactions in 2000.

The Yellow Card Scheme in the UK, which is operated for the reporting of adverse drug reactions, explicitly covers the reporting of adverse reactions to herbal remedies. The Medicines and Healthcare Products Regulatory Agency and the Committee on Safety of Medicines request information on ingredients, source or supplier, and what the product was being used for. Once the new EU Directive on herbal products is implemented, provisions on pharmacovigilance will apply to herbal products and all member states will have to include them in reporting procedures for adverse drug reactions.

Professional regulation

As discussed above, the majority of alternative medicines are bought over the counter and utilized as part of self-care. However, a significant number of practitioners (both medical and non-medical) also utilize these alternative medicines as part of their therapeutic practice (such as homoeopaths, aromatherapists and herbalists). Clinical integration between doctors and practitioners of alternative and complementary therapies is becoming more common and is usually described as 'integrative' or 'integrated health care' (Cohen 2003). In some European countries, such as Austria, France, Belgium, Spain and Italy, the practice of these therapies by non-medical practitioners remains illegal. In others, such as Denmark, Finland, the Netherlands and Sweden, legislative reform has created a more permissive environment (Monckton 1998). Other countries, such as the UK, have historically had a more liberal legal environment in which the practice of these therapies by non-medically qualified practitioners has flourished. Only in a few countries are non-medical practitioners statutorily regulated. For example, in Germany the title of *Heilpraktiker* is conferred on those practitioners who have passed a public health exam but no specific training or qualifications are required to practise any of the above-mentioned therapies. In most countries, these therapists have formed voluntary self-regulating bodies (indeed, there are pan-European bodies such as the European Herbal Practitioners Association). Whether voluntary or statutorily regulated, professional groups usually set standards for training and professional conduct, and hold a register of qualified professionals (Stone 1996). Professional regulation is one means by which the administering/prescribing of alternative medicines can be controlled. However, there has been no attempt to restrict the prescribing of alternative medicines only to registered professionals (as is the case with allopathic medicines). Such a development would represent a radical shift given that currently the majority of alternative medicine sales are direct to consumers.

Conclusions

The demand for alternative medicine in the EU is significant and growing, the majority of it is financed directly by the consumer and is part of self-care. The accumulating evidence of the efficacy and effectiveness of alternative medicines is likely to challenge their exclusion from public financing systems. In the future, one might expect a growing tension between popular demands for alternative medicines and the need of insurers/governments to reduce public health expenditure overall. The process of integration of alternative medicine into orthodox medical practice is likely to continue, but the tension between orthodox medical doctors who traditionally prescribe (and dispense) allopathic medicines and those practitioners (and patients) who utilize alternative medicines will not dissipate rapidly.

These trends have implications for health policy makers, regulators and practitioners. Continued growth in the market for alternative medicines will require orthodox medicine to adapt if not to integrate. Ignoring alternative medicine consumption may result in unexpected interactions with orthodox treatment. Integration of practice is still a long way off in many countries, but steps may be needed to strengthen mutual understanding and facilitate dialogue and openness between practitioners and users of allopathic and alternative medicines.

The approach to the regulation of alternative medicines in Europe is highly variable. However, licensing of homoeopathic and herbal medicines is being strengthened at the EU level together with systems of pharmacovigilance. As alternative medical practitioners gain statutory recognition or further develop systems of voluntary self-regulation in certain member states, provisions may be needed to ensure that regulations are compatible and facilitate free movement of people.

There is a range of regulatory measures that countries can implement to ensure the quality, safety and availability of alternative medicines to consumers. The Executive Board of WHO recommends that countries implement policies and regulations on traditional and complementary and alternative medicine that: support the proper use of traditional medicine, and its integration into national health care systems; set up or expand and strengthen existing national drug-safety monitoring systems to monitor herbal medicines; and promote sound use of traditional medicine and complementary and alternative medicine by consumers and providers (World Health Organization 2002b). Some action in the EU is already beginning to implement these recommendations, but countries may need to do more both nationally and supranationally to facilitate the safe utilization of alternative medicines by consumers.

Notes

1 The authors are grateful to Dr Alyson Huntley and Dr Annette Riesberg for help with this chapter.
2 The UK data are likely to be a gross underestimate, since garlic, ginkgo and unlicensed herbal products were excluded from the analysis.
3 Anthroposophical medicine determines the nature of illness based on a system developed by Austrian scientist and philosopher, Rudolf Steiner (1861–1925). Anthroposophy is coined from the Greek words for 'man' and 'divine wisdom'. Influenced by Hindu and Buddhist beliefs, as well as his scientific training, Steiner believed that the body was not purely a physical entity and that health and well-being depended on treating every human being as unique. In particular, his principle of polarity attempts to link and harmonize both the upper and lower poles of the body. Good health then depends on a harmonious relationship between the physical, ethereal and astral bodies, and the ego. Practitioners are trained as medical doctors and may treat childhood infections, hay fever and asthma, anxiety, depression, cancer, musculoskeletal problems and fatigue (see http://www.holistic.com/holistic).

References

Allensbacher Archiv (2002) *Naturheilmittel 2002*. Allensbach: Allensbach Institut.

Angell, M. and Kassirer, J.P. (1998) Alternative medicine: the risks of untested and unregulated remedies, *New England Journal of Medicine*, 339(12): 839–41.

Barnes, J. and Ernst, E. (1998) Traditional herbalists' prescriptions for common clinical conditions: a survey of members of the UK National Institute of Medical Herbalists, *Phytotherapy Research*, 12: 369–71.

Blumenthal, M., Busse, W. and Goldberg, A. (eds) (1998) *The Complete German Commission E Monographs*. Boston, MA: American Botanical Council.

Busse, R. (2000) *Health Care Systems in Transition: Germany*. Copenhagen: European Observatory on Health Care Systems.

Cohen, M.H. (2003) *Future Medicine: Ethical Dilemmas, Regulatory Challenges and Therapeutic Pathways to Health Care and Healing in Human Transformation*. Ann Arbor, MI: University of Michigan Press.

Colin, P. (2000) An epidemiological study of a homeopathic practice, *Homeopathic Journal*, 89: 116–21.

Cooke, B. and Ernst, E. (2000) Aromatherapy: a systematic review, *British Journal of General Practice*, 50(455): 493–6.

Council of the European Union (2001) Directive on traditional herbal medicinal products, 2001/83/EC.

De Smet, P.A. (1995) Should herbal medicine-like products be licensed as medicines, *British Medical Journal*, 310: 1023–4.

Dixon, A., Riesberg, A., Weibrenner, S. *et al.* (2003) *Complementary and Alternative Medicine in the UK and Germany: A Synthesis of Research and Evidence on Supply and Demand*. London: Anglo German Foundation.

Emslie, M.J., Campbell, M.K. and Walker, K.A. (2002) Changes in public awareness of, attitudes to, and use of complementary therapy in North East Scotland: surveys in 1993 and 1999, *Complementary Therapies in Medicine*, 10(3): 148–53.

Ernst, E. (1998) Usage of complementary therapies in rheumatology: a systematic review, *Clinical Rheumatology*, 17: 301–5.

Ernst, E. (1999) Funding research into complementary medicine: the situation in Britain, *Complementary Therapies in Medicine*, 7(4): 250–3.

Ernst, E. (2000) *Assessing the Evidence Based for CAM. Complementary and Alternative Medicine: Challenge and Change*. Amsterdam: Harwood Academic.

Ernst, E. (2001) Herbal medicinal products: an overview of systematic reviews and meta-analyses, *Perfusion*, 14: 398–404.

Ernst, E. (2002a) A systematic review of systematic reviews of homeopathy, *British Journal of Clinical Pharmacology*, 54: 577–82.

Ernst, E. (2002b) What's the point of rigorous research on complementary/alternative medicine?, *Journal of the Royal Society of Medicine*, 95(4): 211–13.

Ernst, E. and Cassileth, B. (1998) The prevalence of complementary/alternative medicine in cancer: a systematic review, *Cancer*, 83: 777–82.

Ernst, E. and White, A. (2000) The BBC survey of complementary medicine use in the UK, *Complementary Therapies in Medicine*, 8(1): 32–6.

Ernst, E., Resch, K., Mills, S. *et al.* (1995) Complementary medicine – a definition, *British Journal of General Practice*, 45: 506.

Ernst, E., De Smet, P.A., Shaw, D. and Murray, V. (1998) Traditional remedies and the 'test of time', *European Journal of Clinical Pharmacology*, 54(2): 99–100.

Ernst, E., Pittler, M.H., Stevinson, C., White, A.R. and Eisenberg, D. (2001) *The Desktop Guide to Complementary and Alternative Medicine*. Edinburgh: Mosby.

European Commission (2002) Proposal for a Directive of the European Parliament and of the Council amending Directive 2001/83/EC as regards traditional herbal medicinal products COD 2002/0008, *Official Journal of the European Communities*, CI26E, 28.05.2002: 0236–0267.

Fasihi, A. (1996) *Complementary Medicine: Harnessing the Profit Potential*. London: FT Pharmaceuticals & Healthcare.

Fisher, P. and Ward, A. (1994) Medicine in Europe: complementary medicine in Europe, *British Medical Journal*, 309: 107–11.

Haidinger, G. and Gredler, B. (1988) Bekanntheitsgrad, Anwendungshäufigkeit und Erfolg alternativer Heilmethoden in Österreich – Ergebnisse einer Bevölkerungsbefragung, *Offtenliche Gesundheitswesen*, 50: 9–12.

House of Lords Select Committee on Science and Technology (2000) *Complementary and Alternative Medicine*. London: The Stationery Office.

Institute of Medical Statistics (1998) *Herbals in Europe*. Dusseldorf: IMS.

Jonas, W.B. (2002) Policy, the public, priorities in alternative medicine research, *Annals of the American Academy*, 583: 29–43.

Jütte, R. (1996) *Geschichte der Alternativen Medizin: von der Volksmedizin zu den unkonventionallen Therapien von heute*. Munich: Beck.

Kelner, M., Wellman, B., Pescosolido, B. and Saks, M. (eds) (2000) *Complementary and Alternative Medicine: Challenge and Change*. Amsterdam: Harwood Academic.

Lapeyre-Mestre, M., Chastan, E., Louis, A. and Montastruc, J.L. (1999) Drug consumption in workers in France: a comparative study at a 10-year interval (1996 versus 1986), *Journal of Clinical Epidemiology*, 52(5): 471–8.

Lindemann, M. (1999) *Medicine and Society in Early Modern Europe*. Cambridge: Cambridge University Press.

Long, L., Huntley, A. and Ernst, E. (2001) Which complementary and alternative therapies benefit which conditions? A survey of the opinions of 223 professional organizations, *Complementary Theropies in Medicine*, 9(3): 178–85.

Mar, C. and Bent, S. (1999) An evidence-based review of the 10 most commonly used herbs, *Western Journal of Medicine*, 171(3): 168–71.

Mason, S., Tovey, P. *et al.* (2002) Evaluating complementary medicine: methodological challenges of randomised controlled trials, *British Medical Journal*, 325: 832–4.

Matthiessen, P. F., Roßlenbroich, B. and Schmidt, S. (1992) *Unkonventionelle medizinische Richtungen*. Bremerhaven: Verlag für neue Wissenschaft.

Mintel International Group (1997) *Complementary Medicines*. London: Mintel International Group Ltd.

Monckton, J. (1998) *The Final Report of the European Commission Sponsored Cost Project on Unconventional Medicine*. Brussels: European Commission.

Murray, J. and Shepherd, S. (1993) Alternative or additional medicine? An exploratory study in general practice, *Social Science and Medicine*, 37(8): 983–8.

Nilsson, M., Trehn, G. and Asplund, K. (2001) Use of complementary and alternative medicine remedies in Sweden: A population-based longitudinal study within the northern Sweden MONICA Project. Multinational Monitoring of Trends and Determinants of Cardiovascular Disease, *Journal of Internal Medicine*, 250(3): 225–33.

Porter, R. (1989) *Health for Sale: Quackery in England, 1660–1850*. Manchester: Manchester University Press.

Rosslenbroich, B., Schmidt, S. and Matthiessen, P.F. (1994) Unconventional medicine in Germany: a report on the situation of research as basis for state research support, *Complementary Therapies in Medicine*, 2: 61–9.

Rotblatt, M.D. (1999) Cranberry, feverfew, horse chestnut, and kava, *Western Journal of Medicine*, 171(3): 195–8.

Schepers, R.M. and Hermans, H.E. (1999) The medical profession and alternative medicine in the Netherlands: its history and recent developments, *Social Science and Medicine*, 48(3): 343–51.

Schwabe, U. and Paffrath, D. (eds) (2003) *Arzneiverordnungsreport 2002*. Berlin: Springer-Verlag.

Skinner, C.M. and Rangasami, J. (2002) Preoperative use of herbal medicines: a patient survey, *British Journal of Anaesthesia*, 89(5): 792–5.

Steinhoff, B. (2002) Future perspectives for the regulation of traditional herbal medicinal products in Europe, *Phytomedicine*, 9: 572.

Stone, J. (1996) Regulating complementary medicine, *British Medical Journal*, 312: 1492–3.

Swayne, J.M. (1989) Survey of the use of homeopathic medicine in the UK health system, *Journal of the Royal College of Practitioners*, 39(329): 503–6.

Thomas, K. J., Carr, J., Westlake, L. and Williams, B.T. (1991) Use of non-orthodox and conventional health care in Great Britain, *British Medical Journal*, 302: 207–10.

Thomas, K. J., Nicholl, J.P. and Coleman, P. (2001) Use and expenditure on complementary medicine in England: a population based survey, *Complementary Therapies in Medicine*, 9(1): 2–11.

Thompson Coon, J., Pittler, M. and Ernst, E. (2003) Herb–drug interactions: survey of leading pharmaceutical/herbal companies, *Archives of Internal Medicine*, 163(11): 1371.

Wissenschaftliches Institut der Ortskrankenkassen (2002) *Statistiken des GKV Arzneimittelmarkts*. Bonn: WIdO.

World Health Organization, Programme on Traditional Medicine (1998) *Regulatory Situation of Herbal Medicines: A Worldwide Review*. Geneva: WHO.

World Health Organization (2001) *Legal Status of Traditional Medicine and Complementary/Alternative Medicine: A Worldwide Review*. Geneva: WHO.

World Health Organization (2002a) *Traditional Medicine: Report by the Secretariat*. Geneva: WHO.

World Health Organization (2002b) *WHO Traditional Medicine Strategy 2002–2005*. Geneva: WHO.

nineteen

The pharmaceutical sector and regulation in the countries of Central and Eastern Europe

Monique Mrazek, Kees de Jonchere,
Guenka Petrova and Elias Mossialos

Introduction

In this chapter, we examine the changing pharmaceutical sector in the countries of Central and Eastern Europe (CCEE) and the Baltic countries.[1] The reform process began in these countries in the early 1990s, when communist ideology and central planning gave way to democracy and market liberalization. The manufacture, procurement and distribution of pharmaceuticals was previously centralized and supply based on projections often did not accurately reflect need. Structural changes in the wider economy also influenced the need for health system reforms that have focused on the introduction of health insurance schemes and improving the efficiency of resource utilization. These political and economic changes, together with the drive towards accession to the European Union (EU), have liberalized the pharmaceutical sector; however, considerable re-regulation has been introduced to meet Western standards.

Despite the diversity across the CCEE, there are some common political, economic and health status patterns. Table 19.1 shows data on expenditures in health and pharmaceutical care across the CCEE. There have been some common patterns in gross domestic product (GDP), health care funding and life expectancy. In the Czech Republic, Hungary, Poland and Slovakia, all three indicators declined briefly in the early stages of the reforms but steadily recovered. The three indicators dipped in the Baltic countries during the mid-1990s, but rapidly improved. In Bulgaria and Romania, none of the three

Table 19.1 Expenditure on health care and pharmaceuticals in the CCEE, 2000

Country	Real GDP per capita (US$ PPP)[a]	Total expenditure on health (% GDP)[b]	Private expenditure on health (% total expenditure on health)[b]	Total pharmaceutical expenditure (% total health care expenditure)[a]	Total public pharmaceutical expenditure (% total pharmaceutical expenditure)[a]
Albania	3 506	3.4	37.9	25.0 (1999)[c]	—
Bosnia & Herzegovina	—	4.5	31.0	11.1 (1991)	—
Bulgaria	5 710	3.9	22.4	46.6[d]	72.0[d]
Croatia	8 091	8.6	15.4	16.8[e]	—
Czech Republic	13 991	7.2	8.6	25.2	80.6
Estonia	10 066	6.1	23.3	22.3	43.6
Hungary	12 416	6.8	24.3	33.2	56.5
Latvia	7 045	5.9	40.0	16.6 (1999)[f]	51.0[k]
Lithuania	7 106	6.0	27.6	30.0[g]	41.7[g]
Poland	9 051	6.0	30.3	8.9 (1998)[h]	—
Romania	6 423	2.9	36.2	20.0 (1998)	37.0 (1999)[m]
Slovakia	11 243	5.9	10.4	28.0 (1999)[j]	—
Slovenia	17 367	8.6	21.1	19.6	71.7
Former Yugoslav Republic of Macedonia	5 086	6.0	15.5	13.5	70.0
Serbia & Montenegro	—	5.6	49.0	11.9	65.0[n]

Sources: [a]World Health Organization (2002a), [b]World Health Organization (2002b), [c]Nuri (2002), [d]Benisheva (2002), [e]Croatian Ministry of Health (personal communication, 2002; *note:* prescription drugs only); [f]Karaskevica and Tragakes (2001); [g]Cerniauskas and Murauskiene (2000; note: public pharmaceuticals expenditure accounts for the outpatient drug market only), [h]Karski and Koronkiewicz (1999), [j]Hlavacka and Skackova (2000), [k]Behmane (2003), [m]Government of Romania (2000), [n]McCormick (2001).

indicators showed much improvement until the late-1990s (Mossialos *et al.* 2003). Armed conflict and social unrest in the early and mid-1990s slowed reform and development in Albania, Bosnia-Herzegovina, Croatia, the Former Yugoslav Republic of Macedonia (FYROM) and Serbia-Montenegro. Private expenditures and informal payments represent a sizeable proportion of all health care spending in many of these countries (Ensor and Duran-Moreno 2001) with some notable exceptions, such as the Czech Republic, where physician salaries have risen above the rate of inflation for average salaries (Mossialos *et al.* 2003). As Table 19.1 shows, pharmaceuticals represent a significant component of total health expenditures in the CCEE, due in part to the increased use of higher priced imports. Furthermore, total pharmaceutical expenditures may be underestimated, as it is difficult to obtain accurate data on out-of-pocket expenditures.

Life expectancy for both sexes across the CCEE remains below the EU average of 78.5 years (World Health Organization 2002a). There is also a notably higher incidence of cardiovascular disease, violent injuries, cancers and infectious diseases in the CCEE than in Western Europe, influenced by lifestyle choices, social circumstances and environmental conditions (European Communities and the World Health Organization 2002; World Health Organization 2002b). The opening up of markets to previously unavailable therapies has had a direct impact on the treatment of certain conditions; for instance, new chemotherapeutic drugs have led to higher cure rates for cancers in the CCEE (Levi *et al.* 2001; Mossialos *et al.* 2003) and better control of hypertension in the Czech Republic and Hungary (Euroaspire I and II Group 2001). Yet with high levels of out-of-pocket expenditures for pharmaceuticals, equity of access is a problem, particularly for the more vulnerable social groups (McKee and Jacobsen 2000).

In this chapter, we examine some of the key changes in the pharmaceutical markets of the CCEE in the last decade, particularly the impact of market reforms and the subsequent re-regulation driven by the desire for EU accession. For the pharmaceutical sector, the systemic changes of the 1990s meant, above all, privatization of the once centralized and government-owned drug manufacturing and distribution networks. Quantities of imported pharmaceuticals, particularly from Western Europe, have grown dramatically. Re-regulation of the sector has included market authorization, patent legislation, manufacturing standards, licensing requirements, as well as drug pricing and reimbursement. As this is a diverse region with ever changing developments, we do not attempt to provide a comprehensive country-level analysis, but aim to summarize some common approaches to reform, as well as their limitations and implications for policy development. Moreover, given the limited sources of information available and the common-theme approach adopted here, some generalizations are inevitable.

Market reforms in the pharmaceutical sector

Market reforms in the pharmaceutical sector of the CCEE included both privatization of manufacturing and drug distribution, and a liberalization and opening of the markets to more Western imports. While the centrally planned government drug manufacturing and distribution of the past did, for the most part, deliver and pay for basic medicines, there were often difficulties in estimating the need for and producing sufficient quantities of required drugs. Furthermore, the development of new drugs and the uptake of foreign medicines was not common. Some CCEE countries had successful pharmaceutical sectors, which have remained strong as predominantly generic manufacturers (see Box 19.1). These changes did not occur in all the countries at the same time and in Bosnia-Herzogovina, FYROM and Serbia-Montenegro, public pharmacies operating alongside an increasing number of private pharmacies maintain a role in the dispensing of prescriptions reimbursed through the health insurance system.

State-owned manufacturing across the region has for the most part been sold to both domestic and foreign interests. Although local preference clauses protect domestic firms in tenders in some countries, tax incentives in other countries have been used to attract foreign investment. The penetration of foreign products was generally quite rapid and dramatic: the consumption of domestic pharmaceuticals in the Slovak Republic decreased from 80 per cent in 1989 to 17.6 per cent by 1999 (Hlavacka and Skackova 2000); in Bulgaria, the market share of domestics decreased from 90 per cent in 1987 to 60 per cent in 1997 (Hinkov *et al.* 1999). More than 50 per cent of the market in most of the CCEE is sourced abroad and there has been a shift towards the use of branded medicines

---

Box 19.1 Pharmaceutical production capabilities in Slovenia and Croatia

The pharmaceutical sectors in Slovenia and Croatia are important for their respective national economies. The Slovenian market is led by three predominantly generic manufacturers: Krka, Lek and Bayer Pharma. All three export a significant amount of their annual production throughout the CCEE and countries of the Former Soviet Union (FSU) but also to the EU, Asia and Africa. Both Krka and Lek pursue developing 'value added generics' such as existing treatments using novel delivery systems. Lek has also formed a strategic partnership with Sanofi-Synthelabo to market and sell its products in the CCEE. Bayer Pharma was German drug manufacturer Bayer AG's entry into the Slovenian market in 1971.

The pharmaceutical market in Croatia is dominated by domestic producers Pliva and Belupo. These two companies produce active ingredients as well as finished products. One major success of Pliva was the licensing of its antibiotic azithromycin to Pfizer in 1986, which helped Pliva to generate significant revenues. This company also benefits from exports to the CCEE, Western Europe, Russia, North and South America and other markets. Belupo predominantly manufactures generic pharmaceuticals, as well as those licensed from foreign drug companies. Nevertheless, imported pharmaceuticals, particularly from Slovenia, account for a growing percentage of the domestic market in Croatia.

(both originator and branded generics). The penetration of imports benefited from the perception that they were generally superior to locally manufactured drugs (Nuri and Healy 1999) and the marketing strategies of suppliers. Drug distribution (wholesalers and pharmacies) was also widely privatized with a significant change in the structure of the market. In Poland, there was only one wholesaler until 1990, but by the end of the decade the number of wholesalers had increased to over 1000. The number of pharmacies in Poland increased from 3500 state-owned and 60 private pharmacies in 1989 to 6315 private and 533 state-owned pharmacies by 1996 (Tacis 1999). It is not clear, however, whether these changes improved access to, and the quality of, the services provided. Nor is it clear whether there is a continuing need for public pharmacies in markets where the number of private pharmacies is increasing and safety regulations are better enforced. Improved transparency and inspection to mitigate corruption, ensuring safe and affordable medicines, remains a key issue in both public and private distribution channels for a number of countries of Central and Eastern Europe.

One important consequence of the rapid shift to imported drugs was the subsequent escalation in pharmaceutical expenditures. For example, in Slovenia, the average cost of a prescription drug increased by 70 per cent between 1990 and 1999 (Albrent *et al.* 2002). Currency fluctuations, tariffs, import duties, taxes and preferential treatment of domestic products often added to the price burden of imports. The escalation in pharmaceutical expenditures added to the pressures on public health care budgets, which in most countries were also burdened by wider economic constraints. In Romania, for example, real public expenditure on drugs approximately doubled between 1993 and 1995 (Chellaraj *et al.* 1997). In Hungary, in 1990, there were 1300 drugs available, all government subsidized; by 2002, there were 10,577 drugs available, 3867 of them subsidized (Gulacsi *et al.* 2002). The rapid increase in the number of products available on the market put pressure not only on public financing but also on the ability of the system and health professionals to keep informed of the new medicines coming onto the market, often relying solely on information provided by the suppliers (Kiivet *et al.* 1998). Consequently, the cost of pharmaceuticals was shifted onto households as reimbursements were lowered and products were delisted or excluded from reimbursement. This has meant that many patients cannot afford to buy necessary medicines (Karaskevica and Tragakes 2001). In Hungary, the average family expenditure on pharmaceuticals was estimated to have increased ten-fold during the 1990s (Gaal *et al.* 1999).

Development of pharmaceutical policies

To regulate public sector pharmaceutical costs, drug reimbursement and pricing approaches similar to those in Western Europe have been widely adopted in the CCEE. Public drug reimbursement in most of the countries is based on reimbursement lists or essential drugs lists with sub-categories of: full, partial or no reimbursement (Czech Republic, Poland, Slovakia); partial coverage according to disease severity (Hungary, Latvia, Slovenia); type of patient (Hungary, Poland); or type of drug (Poland, Romania). Some countries have applied a combined approach. Certain countries have had more than one positive list depending on disease or social group (Lithuania), a list for partially reimbursed drugs (Poland, Slovenia) and/or a negative list (Hungary, Poland, Slovenia). Hungary and the Czech Republic set conditions for reimbursement that include designating certain medicines to be prescribed by particular specialists only. Most countries maintain an inherited concern with protecting certain vulnerable social groups (Bulgaria, Estonia, Hungary, Lithuania, Poland, Slovenia) or those suffering from particular serious or chronic diseases (Bulgaria, Estonia, Hungary, Latvia, Lithuania, Poland, Romania, Slovenia). Often the criteria for full reimbursement have become more stringent. For example, in Lithuania revised criteria for full reimbursement were introduced in 2002 to cover diseases (cancer, tuberculosis, schizophrenia) that if untreated could cause death or disability in a short time or pose other dangers to society. Although the inclusion criteria for reimbursement lists vary from country to country, common requirements include safety, efficacy and cost considerations. Supplementary voluntary insurance is available in Slovenia to cover prescription charges.

The prices of reimbursed drugs have been regulated by a number of mechanisms, including price negotiation (Hungary, Poland, Latvia, Lithuania), international price comparisons (Bulgaria, Czech Republic, Estonia, Hungary, Latvia, Lithuania, Poland, Romania, Slovenia), setting the ex-manufacturer's price (Bulgaria, Romania, Slovakia, Bulgaria, Lithuania), economic evaluation (Estonia, Latvia, Lithuania) and reference pricing (Czech Republic, Estonia, Hungary, Lithuania, Poland, Romania, Slovakia). As in Western Europe, the approaches are multiple, ever changing and complex. Public sector procurement practice remains a critical issue, especially when considering the uptake and expansion of the statutory health insurance system. Some countries require tender of drug supplies for hospitals or certain medicines on a national level, while in others the tender may be separate for each hospital. However, often procurement criteria and the transparency of the process remain problem areas. In general, both wholesaler and pharmacist margins are regulated, but are usually high compared with those in the EU.

An interesting development has been the collaborative approach to the pharmaceutical sector by the Baltic countries. All three have small markets, predominantly supplied by imports: 2001 consumption per capita was US$73 in Lithuania, US$70 in Estonia and US$55 in Latvia (Behmane 2003). In addition, they faced the common problem of medicines marketed at EU prices despite the fact that their GDP per capita was six to seven times less than the EU average. Consequently, in 1993 the Baltic countries signed an agreement on the mutual recognition of the registrations of pharmaceutical products, followed by a 1995 cooperation agreement in the fields of medicine, health care and health insurance that led to the establishment of the Baltic Coordinating Committee on Pharmaceuticals. Since January 2003, the countries have used common guidelines on the cost minimization, cost-effectiveness and cost utility analysis of pharmaceuticals (http://www.zca.gov.lv).

Following the pattern in Western Europe, CCEE countries have predominantly focused on drug reimbursement and pricing, paying much less attention to the demand side of the market (physicians and pharmacists) and the promotion of rational drug use. Anecdotal evidence and unpublished surveys suggest prescription rates in the CCEE are high, reflecting patient expectations and the marketing practices of the pharmaceutical industry. A survey at a Croatian teaching hospital found that only 46 per cent of prescriptions could be deemed rational (Cicin-Sain and Francetic 1994). The lack of policies for the rational use of antibiotics is critical given the rise in antibiotic resistance. Furthermore, higher incidences of penicillin-resistant pneumococci, ampicillin-resistant *Haemophilus influenzae* and methicillin-resistant *Staphylococcus aureus* have been reported in the CCEE than in Western Europe (Krcmery and Gould 1999). The availability of prescription-only medicines without a prescription in parts of the Balkans and problems of unregistered drugs highlight the need for improved pharmacy practices and inspection.

Although many countries have acknowledged problems with prescription rates, policies promoting the rational use of medicines have been limited and often directed at the use of lists and standard treatment guidelines (Petrova 2002). Most health insurance funds in the region do collect prescription data but few feed this information back to physicians as a way of improving rational prescribing. Bulgaria, Estonia, Poland, Romania and Slovakia have introduced national formularies and prescription guidelines, and Lithuania has disease treatment algorithms, but there is little positive or negative incentive to follow these guidelines. The Czech Republic and Latvia have introduced prescription budgets with penalties for over-spending to increase cost-awareness and the prescription of generics, but the impact of these is not yet clear.

The possibility for generic substitution remains limited in much of the CCEE. For example, pharmacists may substitute with the physician's consent in Poland, if the original brand is not available in the Czech Republic and unless a brand is specified in Hungary. Reference price schemes and requirements that pharmacists dispense the least-cost multi-sourced product encourage the use of unbranded generics in Estonia and Romania. However, branded generics predominate in the region and concepts such as generic prescription and substitution still need to be further developed with physicians and pharmacists, and payment for the latter adjusted to be consistent with such objectives (see Chapter 14).

Patients in the CCEE generally have high out-of-pocket expenditures on pharmaceuticals. Where public reimbursement of medicines is in place, patients have to pay some portion of the reimbursement price although there are certain exemptions or lower out-of-pocket payments in most countries for the elderly, children and those with certain medical conditions or from particular income groups. Also, countries with reference pricing introduce an additional payment for those patients having a product dispensed that falls above the reference price.

EU accession

The EU accession process has had an important influence on the candidate countries, as well as other countries in the region, in redefining pharmaceutical sector regulations. Of the ten CCEE applying for accession, the Commission closed negotiations with eight – the Czech Republic, Estonia, Hungary, Latvia,

Lithuania, Poland, the Slovak Republic and Slovenia – in December 2002, with accession in May 2004. In the pharmaceutical sector, accession means the implementation of the *acquis communautaire*, entailing the adoption of EU pharmaceutical legislation and Commission decisions relating to the protection of public health and completing the single market (see Chapter 3).

Several collaborative initiatives have helped countries to update their regulations in preparation for accession. Since 1997, ten CCEE countries engaged in the Collaboration Agreement of Drug Regulatory Authorities in EU Associated Countries (CADREAC), with multiple aims: implementation of EU standards and obligations; involvement in EU activities before official admission; introduction of mutual recognition procedures and activities; development of common strategies for accession; and improvement of information exchanges among the regulatory authorities of EU associated countries. In addition, the EU established the Pan European Regulatory Forum in 1999 as a technical support project with the accession countries in order to implement the *acquis communautaire* and prepare for EU membership.

The implementation of the *acquis communautaire* has meant a number of regulatory reforms and developments for the pharmaceutical sector in the candidate countries. All countries are in the process of upgrading the drugs on their markets to make sure that all are in line with EU requirements. Drugs that may have been voluntarily withdrawn for safety reasons from the EU may not have been withdrawn in the CCEE because such information from manufacturers may not have been forthcoming and pharmacovigilance capacity was limited (Freemantle *et al.* 2001). This meant that several older products produced domestically or imported from other CCEE or FSU countries disappeared from the market and wider imports of Western original brands and generics. One major challenge to domestic manufacturers in these countries was the cost of restructuring to implement the EU GMP requirements. The adoption of the EU Transparency Directive (89/105) on drug pricing and reimbursement (see Chapter 3) and the implementation of the *acquis* posed challenges to the regulatory regimes, including fees for certain types of products, priority evaluation and lack of patent protection.

Reforms of intellectual property regimes are also part of the accession process. Patent protection was generally provided on processes during the communist era but product patents were only introduced more recently. Since products already on the market or in the pipeline at the time of this introduction were not eligible for product patent protection, full harmonization of EU patent rights will not occur until 2011–2019, depending on the country and product. There is, however, an agreement that parallel trade cannot occur because of these intellectual property differentials. Nor should it be assumed that parallel imports will move from the new EU member states to the existing (older) member states as drug prices in the former are in some cases higher than in the latter. In fact, trade may move in the other direction as the new member states seek ways to lower their pharmaceutical expenditures. Furthermore, the candidate countries have implemented data exclusivity periods and Supplementary Protection Certificates[2] (all products with market authorizations of 1 January 2000 or later must qualify).

Policy challenges

The health care and pharmaceutical markets of the CCEE countries have shifted from the centralized planning and control of the communist era to decentralization and market liberalization. Privatization of pharmaceutical manufacturing and distribution has opened the market to foreign companies. The penetration of imports has been an important source of drug supply, as well as of the observed cost increases. Some evidence suggests that where affordable the imports may have contributed to better health status, but the rapid price rise has increased the burden on the public purse and – of greater concern – on individual households. Higher prices are also driven by non-transparent markets where corruption, mark-ups along the distribution chain, as well as import duties and taxes can add to the burden facing health care payers and patients.

Continued attention to effective pharmaceutical policy measures is required to improve access, particularly considering the effect of wider economic constraints on public health care spending. Drug procurement based on competitive tender should be fair and transparent. Careful examination of current price regulatory mechanisms should be undertaken to ensure that they operate with clear and transparent criteria. It is also important not to overlook the size of the distribution and retail margins. Distribution chain incentives should be introduced to foster a more competitive market. For example, competitive retail margins that encourage discounting and the dispensing of the cheapest multi-sourced drug, as discussed in Chapters 11 and 14, could be considered. Collaborative approaches such as that in the Baltics or among accession countries, as stimulated by the EU and World Health Organization, could also assist countries facing similar challenges.

Despite pressures to reduce budgets, careful attention should be given to the impact of changes in reimbursement and their impact on access to the needed medicines, particularly by the most vulnerable patients. Attention should be given in particular to cost-effective and affordable medicines. At the same time, the prescription and dispensing of these medicines calls for an integrated policy approach with the incentives for physicians' and pharmacists' involvement. Government assistance may be necessary for manufacturers to meet EU standards.

In most of these countries, the pharmaceutical sector has gone through deregulation and re-regulation. Whereas for the accession countries regulatory systems – and their implementation – have been largely brought in line with EU requirements, regulation in Albania, Bosnia-Herzegovina, Croatia, FYROM, and Serbia and Montenegro remains more problematic; legislation has greatly improved, but enforcement remains a problem.

Professional education programmes for both physicians and pharmacists need to keep pace with policy developments and new drug introductions. Rational prescription should be promoted in both basic and continuing professional education programmes (Petrova 2001). Initiatives should be further supported through the dissemination of relevant, reliable and timely drug information. The development and implementation of prescription guidelines will require sustainable support and approaches. Longer-term investments in further strengthening prescription data monitoring systems and dissemination strategies should be considered as part of any strategic changes. Consideration could be given to payment incentives for health professionals that ensure rational prescription and dispensing.

Although several challenges remain, much progress has been made in reforming the health care and pharmaceutical sectors in these countries. The demands of the next decade, however, do not pose less of a challenge, particularly for the new countries of the EU. Accession to the EU will demand full compliance to standard requirements for where protectionism or practices involving corruption will be subject to greater scrutiny. Sourcing of medicines in the coming years will continue to be an issue (and with it the affordability of pharmaceutical supply), and EU accession will have an important impact both in terms of parallel trade – in all directions – and the restructuring of pharmaceutical manufacturing and trade.

Notes

1   The three Baltic countries are Estonia, Latvia and Lithuania. For the remainder of the chapter, the term CCEE includes the Baltic countries.
2   A supplementary protection certificate (SPC) can take effect for a maximum of 5 years after expiry of the original patent term and is capable of extending the exclusivity for a particular medicinal product to a maximum of 15 years.

References

Albrent, T., Cesen, M., Hindle, D. *et al.* (2002) *Health Care Systems in Transition: Slovenia.* Copenhagen: European Observatory on Health Care Systems.

Behmane, D. (2003) Baltic collaboration on pharmaceuticals. Communication to the *Baltic Conference on Medicines*, Riga, 28 March (available from http://www.zca.gov.lv/eng/konference.htm) (accessed 19 March 2003).

Benisheva, T. (2002) *National Drug Policy in Bulgaria. National Conference on National Drug Policy*, Sofia, 26 September 2002 (available from www.mh.government.bg).

Cerniauskas, G. and Murauskiene, L. (2000) *Health Care Systems in Transition: Lithuania.* Copenhagen: European Observatory on Health Care Systems.

Chellaraj, G., Adeyi, O., Preker, A.S. and Goldstein, E. (1997) Trends in health status, services and finance: the transition in Central and Eastern Europe, Vol. II, *World Bank Technical Papers*, No. 348.

Cicin-Sain, A. and Francetic, I. (1994) Analysis of justifications for prescribing drugs which must be obtained abroad, *Lijecnicki vjesnic*, 116(9–10): 258–63 (in Serbo-Croat).

Ensor, T. and Duran-Moreno, A. (2001) Corruption as a challenge to effective regulation in the health sector, in R. Saltman, R. Busse and E. Mossialos (eds) *Regulating Entrepreneurial Behaviour in European Health Care Systems*. Buckingham: Open University Press.

Euroaspire I and II Group (2001) Clinical reality of coronary prevention guidelines: a comparison of EUROASPIRE I and II in nine countries, *Lancet*, 357: 995–1001.

European Communities and the World Health Organization (2002) *Health Status Overview for Countries of Central and Eastern Europe that are Candidates for Accession to the European Union* (available from http://www.who.dk/Document/E76888.pdf) (accessed 22 May 2002).

Freemantle, N., Behmane, D. and de Joncheere, K. (2001) Pricing and reimbursement of pharmaceuticals in the Baltic States, *Lancet*, 358: 260.

Gaal, P., Rekassy, B. and Healy, J. (1999) *Health Care Systems in Transition: Hungary.* Copenhagen: European Observatory on Health Care Systems.

Government of Romania (2000) Ministry of Health and National Health Insurance Fund Budget, *Romanian Government Newspaper*, No. 1, Bucharest.

Gulacsi, L., David, T. and Dozsa, Cs. (2002) Pricing and reimbursement of drugs and medical devices in Hungary, *European Journal of Health Economics*, 4: 1–8.

Hinkov, H., Koulaksuzov, S., Semerdjiev, I. and Healy, J. (1999) *Health Care Systems in Transition: Bulgaria.* Copenhagen: European Observatory on Health Care Systems.

Hlavacka, S. and Skackova, D. (2000) *Health Care Systems in Transition: Slovakia.* Copenhagen: European Observatory on Health Care Systems.

Karaskevica, J. and Tragakes, E. (2001) *Health Care Systems in Transition: Latvia.* Copenhagen: European Observatory on Health Care Systems.

Karski, J.B. and Koronkiewicz, A. (1999) *Health Care Systems in Transition: Poland.* Copenhagen: European Observatory on Health Care Systems.

Kiivet, R.A., Bergman, U., Rootslane, L., Rago, L. and Sjoqvist, F. (1998) Drug use in Estonia in 1994–1995: a follow-up from 1989 and comparison with two Nordic countries, *European Journal of Clinical Pharmacology*, 54(2): 119–24.

Krcmery, V. and Gould, I.M. (1999) Antibiotic policies in Central/Eastern Europe (CEE) after 1990, *Journal of Hospital Infection*, 43 (suppl.): S269–S274.

Levi, F., La Vecchia, C., Boyle, P., Lucchini, F. and Negri, E. (2001) Western and eastern European trends in testicular cancer mortality, *Lancet*, 357: 1853–4.

McCormick, K. (2001) Terms of reference for a restricted service tender for provision of support to the pharmaceutical industry in Serbia. Unpublished report, European Agency for Reconstruction, July.

McKee, M. and Jacobsen, E. (2000) Public health in Europe, *Lancet*, 356: 665–70.

Mossialos, E., McKee, M. and MacLehose, L. (2003) *Health and Health Care in the EU Accession Countries.* Brussels: European Commission.

Nuri, B. (2002) *Health Care Systems in Transition: Albania.* Copenhagen: European Observatory on Health Care Systems.

Nuri, B. and Healy, J. (1999) *Health Care Systems in Transition: Albania.* Copenhagen: European Observatory on Health Care Systems.

Petrova, G.I. (2001) Monitoring of national drug policies: regional comparison between Bulgaria, Romania, Macedonia, Bosnia Herzegovina, *Central European Journal of Public Health*, 9(4): 205–13.

Petrova, G.I. (2002) Prescription patterns analysis: variations among Bulgaria, Romania, Macedonia and Bosnia Herzegovina, *Central European Journal of Public Health*, 10(3): 100–3.

Tacis (1999) *The Country Profile of Poland: Diagnosis and Elaboration of a Strategy for the Development of the Pharmaceutical Industry.* Kiev: CII Group GbR (available from http://www.pharma-tacis.kiev.ua/index.html).

World Health Organization (2002a) *Health for All Database.* Copenhagen: WHO (available from http://www.who.dk/hfadb).

World Health Organization (2002b) *World Health Report.* Geneva: WHO.

twenty

Access to pharmaceuticals and regulation in the Commonwealth of Independent States

Monique Mrazek and Armin Fidler[1]

Introduction

The pharmaceutical sectors in the countries of the Commonwealth of Independent States (CIS) have undergone considerable change since independence in the early 1990s. Following independence, economic conditions across the CIS deteriorated, particularly after the Russian currency crisis in 1998; in 2000, the combined gross domestic product (GDP) of the region was 63 per cent of that in 1990 and one in five people were estimated to be living on less than US$2.15 a day[2] (World Bank 2002a). These economic conditions have meant less money flowing into once universal public health care services. As shown in Table 20.1, total expenditure on health as a percentage of GDP remains low in most CIS countries and public expenditure on health is very low in some. During the 1990s, many CIS countries experienced a decline in real GDP together with decreasing public expenditures on health care, resulting in households bearing an increasing amount of their health care expenditures, including pharmaceuticals, out-of-pocket (Falkingham 2002). Official statistics and measures of informal payments are unlikely to fully account for out-of-pocket spending on medicines given a sizeable trade in unregistered drugs (Sargaldakova *et al.* 2000) and informal distribution networks. Furthermore, a simultaneous deterioration in health status, due in part to an increase in communicable diseases, environmental pollution, economic-related stress and high levels of alcohol consumption and smoking, has increased the need for health care and pharmaceuticals (Shkolnikov *et al.*

Table 20.1 Expenditure on health care and pharmaceuticals in the CIS, 2000

Region	Country	Total expenditure on health (% GDP)[a]	Private expenditure on health (% total expenditure on health)[a]	Total pharmaceutical expenditure (% total health care expenditure)[b]
Eastern European	Belarus	5.7	17.2	25.8
	Republic of Moldova	3.5	17.6	11.1
	Russian Federation	5.3	27.5	—
	Ukraine	4.1	29.9	11.6
Caucasus	Armenia	7.5	57.7	—
	Azerbaijan	2.1	51.1	16.5
	Georgia	7.1	89.5	45.6
Central Asian	Kazakhstan	3.7	26.8	2.8
	Kyrgyz Republic	6.0	38.3	14.3
	Tajikistan	2.5	19.2	15.7 (1998)[c]
	Turkmenistan	5.4	15.1	18.0 (1997)[d]
	Uzbekistan	3.7	22.5	11.4

Source: [a]World Health Organization (2002a), [b]World Health Organization (2002b), [c]Rahminov *et al.* (2000), [d]Mamedkuliev *et al.* (2000).

2001; Savas *et al.* 2002). Further concern is raised by rapidly rising rates of HIV/AIDS in the region.

For the pharmaceutical sector, the break-up of the Soviet Union led to the dissolution of the centralized pharmaceutical supply, regulation and distribution systems. The immediate effect of the breakdown in this network was a severe shortage of drugs across the CIS because pharmaceutical manufacturing capacity had not been evenly distributed across the Soviet Union. Consequently, for many countries imports of pharmaceuticals increased rapidly, as did the costs of the pharmaceutical supply chain (Sargaldakova *et al.* 2000; Business Credit Co. 2001). The break-up also meant a lack of self-sufficiency in the supply of vaccines, leading to an increased import of these, but the high cost of doing so resulted in lower rates of immunization and subsequent disease outbreaks (measles, whooping cough).

The framework shown in Figure 20.1 incorporates the expenditure equation (expenditure = price × volume), an essential component of the regulatory framework, as well as concepts of the drug supply management framework developed by the World Health Organization and Management Science for Health (MSH) (Quick *et al.* 1997). For the countries of the CIS, the areas of drug management that surround the expenditure equation remain problematic. However, all are essential components of an integrated national drug policy. Within a context of significant social and economic changes in the CIS, this chapter examines the experiences, problems and potential options regarding key issues of access to medicines and regulation of pharmaceutical markets along several lines: availability of supply and product quality; coverage, procurement and pricing; and prescription and distribution.

Availability of supply and product quality

The dissolution of the Soviet Union severely affected the drug production and distribution system in CIS countries. It is important to note that there were

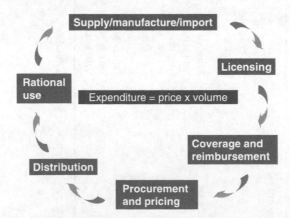

Figure 20.1 Framework for pharmaceutical policy development in transition economies. Adapted from Quick *et al.* (1997).

often problems with the quality and availability of supply during the Soviet era because central planning poorly anticipated demand, and the range of medicines did not keep pace with the introduction of medicines elsewhere. The collapse of the distribution network and a lack of pharmaceutical manufacturing capacity in many countries resulted in medicine shortages and an increase in imported raw and finished pharmaceuticals, followed by a rapid escalation of local drug prices, as in Belarus (Karnitski 1997) and Uzbekistan (Ilkhamov and Jakubowski 2001). The perception that imported products were of a higher quality than domestics, as well as the influence of direct-to-consumer advertising, also drove the shift to the former and from cheaper generics to brands. Imports have been estimated to account for 60–90 per cent of the local market in most CIS countries. Traditional Eastern European sources of cheaper generics also shrank as many of these manufacturers were privatized. After the Russian currency crisis in 1998, and the subsequent devaluation of some regional CIS currencies, imports of drugs decreased because they had become very expensive, as in Kazakhstan (US Commercial Service 2001), and subsequently supplies shifted away from western European sources to low price suppliers and counterfeit drugs of questionable quality (Tacis 1999b).

Developing local pharmaceutical manufacturing capacity has not been a viable solution to supply problems for several CIS countries. Establishing manufacturing or upgrading existing capacity involves high fixed costs, a stable supply of raw materials and utilities (i.e. gas, electricity), as well as technical and regulatory expertise. Despite these economic constraints, several CIS countries have developed domestic manufacturing capacity either through joint ventures with foreign investors (Tajikistan: Rahminov *et al.* 2000; Georgia: Gamkrelidze *et al.* 2002) or through tax advantages, preferential real estate purchases, customs exemptions and other incentives (Kazakhstan: Tacis 1999a). Nevertheless, it may be difficult to attract investment from foreign firms because of non-transparent customs regulations and registration procedures, as well as concerns about political and economic stability, a lack of human resource capacity and corruption. Of those CIS countries with manufacturing facilities, few meet Good Manufacturing Practice (GMP) standards[3] and upgrading to do so can be very costly (Tacis 1999b). By 2005, Russian-defined GMP standards are to be mandatory for all firms manufacturing drugs in that country; it is important to note that these standards are less stringent than the GMP standards defined by WHO or those of the European Union.

Of particular concern is the quality of supplies in CIS markets, where it is not uncommon to see expired or unregistered 'black market' drugs being sold. In 2001, these products represented 36 per cent of the total in Georgia (Lotuashvili 2001) and 10–12 per cent in Russia (Startseva 2002) of the market by value but these estimates may be low. To combat counterfeiting, the multinational pharmaceutical industry has lobbied for wider patent protection and enforcement (AIPM and CIPR 2002). Armenia, Georgia, the Kyrgz Republic and Moldova, as members of the World Trade Organization, have adopted the patent standards of the Trade Related Aspects of Intellectual Property Rights (TRIPS) Agreement; however, concerns have been raised about the implementation of the TRIPS requirements in poor countries and the impact this may have on drug prices (World Health Organization 2001).

The problem of drug quality and the availability of unregistered drugs is also due to poor regulatory monitoring and enforcement of legislation. In the Soviet Union, product registration and quality control were undertaken by Moscow and therefore the equivalent institutions across the CIS are newly established bodies with limited financial and human capacity. Many of these countries are trying to bring their national drug legislation and market authorization process in line with European Union and internationally accepted standards. The lack of enforcement is blamed on the absence of a single authority that is effective in enforcing existing laws and preventing or dealing with corruption (Tacis 1999a). The situation is often further complicated by an ineffective judicial system in some countries (Tacis 1999b) and limited financial resources to pay staff adequately. The concerns over product quality and safety extend to where drugs are sold; it is not uncommon for drugs to be traded in unlicensed pharmacies, kiosks, bazaars or other forms of informal distribution, and prescription requirements for dispensing a particular drug are often overlooked.

Drug coverage, procurement and pricing

As mentioned previously, the burden of pharmaceutical financing has shifted to a greater extent from the state onto households since the dissolution of the Soviet Union. It is estimated that over 89 per cent of pharmaceuticals in Kazakhstan in 1999 (Tacis 1999a), between 50 and 90 per cent in Uzbekistan in 2001 (World Bank 2002b) and almost 80 per cent in Armenia in 2000 (Hovhannisyan et al. 2001) were purchased out-of-pocket through both formal and informal charges.[4] This is a significant shift away from the full government pharmaceutical coverage of inpatient medicines and free or highly subsidized outpatient prescriptions of the Soviet Union; subsequently, there has been an impact on access to medicines. Table 20.2 shows that a high percentage of the population in Tajikistan and the Kyrgz Republic did not obtain the required medicines because of price. The burden of paying for medicines out-of-pocket is greater for low-income groups and those living in rural areas than for those with higher incomes or those living in urban centres (Sari and Langenbrunner 2001).

Government coverage of pharmaceuticals in the CIS varies but is generally based around the Essential Drugs List (EDL), a concept developed and widely promoted by the WHO.[5] Most countries in the CIS have adopted an EDL as a starting point for their drug policy strategy; however, the size of the list and the

Table 20.2 Reasons for not obtaining required drugs in the Kyrgz Republic and Tajikistan

Reason	Kyrgz Republic (1996) (%)	Tajikistan (1999) (%)
Too expensive	73	84
Not in stock/could not find	9	7
Other	18	9

Source: Falkingham (2002).

products included vary among countries. A study by Jafarov and Laing (2002), comparing the WHO 1999 EDL to those of Uzbekistan, Kazakhstan, the Kyrgz Republic and Tajikistan, found that although the countries' lists contained 40–80 per cent of the items on the WHO list, they also included a number of drugs of unproven efficacy. The large number of branded generic drugs on both the Kazak and Tajik EDLs were of concern for the development of generic drug policies. Furthermore, the promotion of generic drugs often meets resistance over their quality, as they are often manufactured locally.

Shortfalls in public health care budgets have meant a reduction in eligibility for public drug coverage and the drugs covered (Tacis 1999a). Although in practice inpatient drugs are to be covered through public funds, often inpatients have had to pay the cost of their drugs out-of-pocket in a number of countries, including Russia (Tchernjavski 1998), Tajikistan (Rahminov et al. 2000) and Armenia (Hovhannisyan et al. 2001). Georgia piloted with some success a voluntary drug reimbursement scheme in the region of Kutaisi in 1997, paying 50 per cent of the drug costs above a defined threshold for patients with high drug expenditures after a small fee was paid to join (World Health Organization 1999a). Humanitarian donations have been an important source of medicines for a number of these countries, particularly during the early stages of transition. Although private pharmacies are supposed to supply drugs free to the vulnerable, they often do not because of the delay in government reimbursement, as has occurred in Belarus (Karnitski 1997), Russia (Tchernjavski 1998) and Uzbekistan, unless the patient is willing to pay a fee (World Bank 2002b).

Given the limited funding available to meet health budgets in the public sector, the reliance on imports and the limited finances of households, drug prices are therefore decisive in determining access to pharmaceuticals. A study of retail drug prices in Kazakhstan found many to be significantly higher than the international median price (Hafner et al. 2002). Large drug price differences among countries, as discussed in Chapter 6, are due to a number of factors: import duties and tariffs, drug price regulation, high mark-ups along the distribution chain, and taxes.

There has been an attempt in some countries to institute price controls of both the manufacturer's price and the mark-ups along the distribution chain. Box 20.1 summarizes some of the strategies adopted in Russia. Belarus, Moldova and Uzbekistan fix the prices of some basic medicines (Goroshenko et al. 1996; Karnitski 1997; Skripachova 2002). Mark-ups along the distribution chain have also been fixed in some countries but remain high – accounting for 32 per cent of the final purchase cost in Armenia (Hovhannisyan et al. 2001) and 45 per cent in Uzbekistan (Skripachova 2002) – and may have introduced the perverse incentive for pharmacists to dispense a more expensive drug if the margin is higher (Karnitski 1997; see Chapter 11); this is of greater concern given the direct access pharmacists have to patients in many of these countries.

Drug prices and availability are to some extent dependent on procurement policies. In most countries, the centralized procurement of the Soviet Union has been replaced by direct purchasing from manufacturers and wholesalers by hospitals and pharmacies. Centralized procurement through collective, competitive and transparent tenders potentially adds leverage to reduce drug prices and corruption.[6] For example, in Turkmenistan, centralized procurement was

---

Box 20.1 Supply-side cost control strategies in Russia

- Drug manufacturers are required to register products and ex-factory prices at the federal level with the Ministry of Health; this was to counter high distributional mark-ups such that the manufacturer's price accounted on average for 25 per cent of the final price.
- Distribution margins are federally legislated: for drugs on the EDL, the maximum wholesaler's mark-up is 25 per cent and the retail mark-up is 30 per cent; the margins are higher for drugs not included on the EDL. The size of these distribution margins remain high compared with those in Western Europe (see Chapter 11). The ability to enforce these margins is questionable, given that distribution mark-ups of 120–200 per cent are not uncommon.
- Manufacturers are exempt from paying taxes on profits if they produce reasonably priced essential drugs; the effect of this policy was marginal
- In 2001, the Lower House of the Duma introduced a bill to limit the importation of drugs with analogues into Russia to improve the imbalance between domestically produced and imported products
- In 2002, a 10 per cent value-added tax was introduced on both domestic and imported pharmaceuticals; such a tax can increase the burden on the end-user.

Sources: Mossialos (1999), Tragakes and Lessof (2003).

---

based on an aggregated estimate of annual institutional demand for the whole country, where imported drugs were procured through barter in exchange for gas deliveries or credit loans (Mamedkuliev *et al.* 2000). The consequence of this approach was that choice of products, manufacturers and price negotiations was limited, and often there were shortages or surpluses of drugs. A similar problem was identified in Uzbekistan, where the government procurement of imports was hindered by exchange rate fluctuations and limited amounts of hard currency (World Bank 2002b). Problems also arose with the public procurement process in the Kyrgz Republic, where there was no competitive bidding until 1996, so that expensive branded generics were being purchased instead of less costly alternatives (Sargaldakova *et al.* 2000).

Prescription and distribution

High rates of drug prescription and patient expectations that a consultation should lead to a prescription were part of the legacy of the Soviet system (Karnitski 1997; Rahminov *et al.* 2000; Hovhannisyan *et al.* 2001). For example, in 56 per cent of encounters in Uzbekistan, patients were prescribed three or more drugs (the international average is 2.2) with 57 per cent of prescriptions for injectibles, compared with the international average of 17 per cent (Pavin *et al.* 2003).

Antibiotics were prescribed in 56.5 per cent of encounters, whereas the expected rate is 25–40 per cent internationally (Nurgozhin *et al.* 2001). Although these examples come from Uzbekistan, there is anecdotal evidence that similar figures are common throughout the CIS, raising concerns about appropriate prescription rates, antibiotic resistance, cost and safety (since oral formulations are safer and cheaper than injectibles).

While there has been some limited effort to promote rational prescription concepts to physicians, many confounding factors inhibit their adoption (Sargaldakova *et al.* 2000). Drug selection may be based on availability rather than usefulness (Mamedkuliev *et al.* 2000). The rapid influx of previously unavailable medicines has further impeded the development of rational prescription. A review of drug advertisements in Russian medical journals found that few provided information essential to making appropriate prescription decisions (Vlassov *et al.* 2001), and physicians, lacking other sources, have had to rely on manufacturers for information. There is a need to develop professional ethical standards that prevent marketing drugs by and through physicians. Alongside this there is a need to foster postgraduate medical education programmes for physicians and pharmacies on rational drug use.

Moreover, potent pharmaceuticals, including antibiotics, can often be purchased without a prescription (Nurgozhin *et al.* 2001). Drugs available on prescription elsewhere in Europe are often available over the counter in some of the countries. It is estimated that over-the-counter medicines account for over 60 per cent of dispensing in Russia (Mossialos 1999) and represent the fastest growing pharmaceutical segment in much of the CIS. Even where there is a requirement that a drug should be dispensed only if prescribed by a physician, this may not be strictly enforced, as in Georgia and Uzbekistan, where patients often go directly to the pharmacist or bazaar to avoid paying the physician's consultation fee (Gamkrelidze *et al.* 2002). The development of drug monitoring and evaluation systems for both prescription and dispensing are essential components of improving rational drug use.

There was much privatization of the pharmaceutical distribution system and of retail pharmacies after the dissolution of the Soviet Union. For example, in Kazakhstan approximately 90 per cent of the 10,000 licensed pharmacy retailers have been privatized (Tacis 1999a). The distribution system in many countries is fragmented with many small or medium-sized regional or local wholesalers. The number of pharmacists in the CIS is in general low compared with Western Europe (World Health Organization 2002b), but this is often offset by a number of kiosks (or other informal distribution networks) and prescribing physicians (Tchernjavski 1998). For example, in Russia there were 16,000 pharmacies and 25,000 kiosks in 1999 (Mossialos 1999). There is often a distinction between the stock of products available in state-owned versus private pharmacies. For example, in Ukraine in 1999, 44 per cent of pharmacies were private and in general stocked foreign products with higher margins, avoiding those products available to patients entitled to free medication. In contrast, state-run pharmacies stocked less expensive domestic and CEE products (Tacis 1999b). However, in other countries, public pharmacies do not necessarily supply medicines at lower prices than private pharmacies although the quality may be more reliable in the former. Also in the Ukraine, irrational prescription and supply shortages resulting from bottlenecks in the distribution network were associated with increasing rates of multidrug-resistant tuberculosis (World Bank 2000b). Given the high levels of OTC sales, and the pharmacist's often wide discretion in dispensing, concern has been raised about the adequacy of the pharmacy qualification in some CIS countries (Nurgozhin *et al.* 2001).

Discussion

Despite the fact that the EDL concept has been widely adopted across the CIS, non-transparent drug selection, poor management and monitoring of supplies, and few efforts directed at improving the rational use of medicines have undermined the basic initiatives to re-regulate the pharmaceutical sector. Developing an EDL is certainly important, but will have little impact in the absence of measures to ensure a cost-effective supply, efficient distribution and rational use of medicines. As most drugs included on the EDL are off-patent, a competitive tender arrangement should be part of a transparent procurement process. Components of good procurement practice include: restrictions to a limited list; determination of order quantities based on reliable needs estimation; competitive tendering from qualified suppliers; separation of key functions in the approval process; prompt payment, regular audits and a formal system of supplier qualification and monitoring (Quick *et al.* 1997). The EDL, like other reimbursement lists, should be based on cost- and clinical-effectiveness criteria and be revised regularly to ensure it is in line with national health needs and priorities. The development of reimbursement schemes around the EDL will be important to reduce the burden on individual households.

Securing an adequate supply of quality medicines remains an issue in most of the CIS. Improving domestic manufacturing capacity may help to improve access to essential medicines; however, the high costs of doing so may mean this is not an economically viable option for a number of countries. Prices of domestic or imported drugs need to reflect ability to pay. This means establishing competitive procurement, introducing price controls or expanding generic competition, but the latter will depend on the incentives along the distribution chain (see Chapter 11). Implementing price control strategies is likely to be more challenging in this region, given problems with governance, enforcement, transparency and corruption. Tools such as a corruption diagnostic (World Bank 2002c) can be useful for countries in assessing the extent of corruption in the pharmaceutical sector and in focusing policy development to improve transparency in drug registration, selection, procurement, distribution and service delivery. Countries that benefit from humanitarian donations of pharmaceuticals should begin to find ways of becoming self-sufficient to ensure longer-term sustainability of drug supplies.

Effective management of drug supply and distribution can result in wider savings to the health care system and the public, but there is a need for capacity building. Improving drug quality requires adequate quality control standards and equipment. Establishing GMP levels for WHO or the European Union is an important objective and international organizations can help to achieve these standards. Successful implementation of regulatory pharmaceutical policy requires appropriate clinical capacity, as well as enforcement capacity to ensure that drug safety and quality standards are met. Countering the corruption that undermines regulatory enforcement requires the development of appropriate incentives and higher pay for inspectors. Furthermore, the development of capacity in clinical epidemiology and evidence-based medicine is essential to ensure appropriate reimbursement criteria and prescription guidelines to improve pharmaceutical care.

As has been discussed so often in this book, expenditure control in pharmaceuticals must also consider volume. Rational drug prescription, dispensing and use are important. Continuing professional education of physicians and pharmacists is fundamental to improving rational drug use. Development of health promotion and patient education programmes about new drugs or new approaches to drug administration is necessary given the level of self-care, and there is certainly an important role for physicians, nurses and pharmacists in this. The issue of direct-to-consumer advertising should also be addressed, especially since, currently, there is little regulatory capacity in the CIS countries. Other measures aimed at rational prescription and dispensing – such as separating the functions where possible – and prescription monitoring are important to consider. Generic prescription or substitution may also be options, depending on the quality and price of the available generic equivalents and the incentives for pharmacists and physicians to use them. Finally, monitoring of indicators, including drug prices, supply levels, prescription and consumption, is crucial to measuring the impact of policies in the sector and is important for informing policy developments.

Notes

1   The authors would like to thank the following for their assistance in retrieving country information: Jan Bultman, Gizella Diaz, Yelena Fedeyeva, Tamar Gotsadze, Grace Hafner, Jack Langenbrunner, Tanya Loginova, Marat Mambetov, Nigor Mouzafarova, Katerina Rybalchenko, Vyacheslav Seppi, Mazim Zabigaylo and Baktybek Zhumadil.
2   US$2.15 per day is a threshold used by the World Bank to define absolute poverty in developing countries.
3   GMP is a term used to describe a set of principles and procedures for drug manufacturers to ensure that their products meet the required quality standards. The principles, procedures and standards vary depending on the body or country that defined them (Russia, European Union, WHO).
4   It is important to note that out-of-pocket payments are informal only if they are for services or items covered by the public system (Lewis 2001).
5   Given that the economic impact of pharmaceuticals can be substantial, particularly for a developing country, WHO published its first Model List of Essential Drugs in 1977 with the idea that the 208 individual drugs together could provide safe and effective treatment for the infectious and chronic diseases that affect the vast majority of the world's population. In 2002, WHO published its 12th Model List of Essential Drugs, which contained 325 individual drugs, including 12 antiretroviral medicines for the prevention and treatment of HIV/AIDS. For further information, see http:// www.who.int/medicines/.

6 Guides to procurement for pharmaceuticals have been produced by the World Health Organization (1999b) and the World Bank (2000a).

References

Association of International Pharmaceutical Manufacturers (AIPM) and Coalition for Intellectual Property Rights (CIPR) (2002) *Status Report: Action Plan to Fight Counterfeit Medicines in Russia* (available from www.cipr.org/activities/20020619/Status ReportEng.pdf) (accessed 2 December 2002).

Business Credit Co. (2001) *The Pharmaceutical Market – The 2000 Results* (available from www.ksk-market.com.ua/publications_en/009/pub1009.html) (accessed 2 December 2002).

Falkingham, J. (2002) Poverty, affordability and access to health care, in M. McKee, J. Healy and J. Falkingham (eds) *Health Care in Central Asia*. Buckingham: Open University Press.

Gamkrelidze, A., Atun, R., Gotsadze, G. and MacLehose, L. (2002) *Health Care Systems in Transition: Georgia*. Copenhagen: European Observatory on Health Care Systems.

Goroshenko, B., Volovei, V. and Mochniaga, A. (1996) *Health Care Systems in Transition: Republic of Moldova*. Copenhagen: European Observatory on Health Care Systems.

Hafner, G., Nurghozin, T., Gulyaev, A. and Laing, R. (2002) *Summary of Results: Prices and Availability of Pharmaceuticals in Kazakhstan's Pharmacies*. Almaty: ABT Associates.

Hovhannisyan, S.G., Tragakes, E., Lessof, S., Aslanian, H. and Mkrtchyan, A. (2001) *Health Care Systems in Transition: Armenia*. Copenhagen: European Observatory on Health Care Systems.

Ilkhamov, F.A. and Jakubowski, E. (2001) *Health Care Systems in Transition: Uzbekistan*. Copenhagen: European Observatory on Health Care Systems.

Jafarov, A. and Laing, R. (2002) *Drug Selection in the Former Soviet Central Asian Republics* (available from http://dcc2.bumc.bu.edu/richardl/DPI02/Eng_Read/sess11/DPI_Aziz_EN.doc) (accessed 23 July 2003).

Karnitski, G. (1997) *Health Care Systems in Transition: Belarus*. Copenhagen: European Observatory on Health Care Systems.

Lewis, M. (2001) Informal health payments in central and eastern Europe and the former Soviet Union: issues, trends and policy implications, in E. Mossialos, A. Dixon, J. Figueras and J. Kutzin (eds) *Funding Health Care: Options for Europe*. Buckingham: Open University Press.

Lotuashvili, A. (2001) *Overview of the Georgian Pharmaceutical Sector*. BISNIS Representative, US Embassy Tbilisi (available from www.bisnis.doc.gov/bisnis/isa/011217ggpharm.htm) (accessed 9 December 2002).

Mamedkuliev, C., Shevkun, E. and Hajioff, S. (2000) *Health Care Systems in Transition: Turkmenistan*. Copenhagen: European Observatory on Health Care Systems.

Mossialos, E. (1999) *The Pharmaceutical Sector in Russia*. Research paper prepared for USAID. Boston, MA: Boston University Legal Reform Project.

Nurgozhin, T., Pavin, M., Hafner, G. *et al.* (2001) *The Pharmaceutical Study in Ferghana Oblast, Uzbekistan*. Ferghana Oblast: ABT Associates.

Pavin, M., Nurgozhin, T., Hafner, G., Yusufy, F. and Laing, R. (2003) Prescribing practices of rural primary health care physicians in Uzbekistan, *Tropical Medicine and International Health*, 8(2): 182–90.

Quick, J.D., Rankin, J.R., Laing, R.O. *et al.* (eds) (1997) *Managing Drug Supply: The Selection, Procurement, Distribution and Use of Pharmaceuticals*, 2nd edn. West Hartford, CT: Kumarian Press.

Rahminov, R., Gedik, G. and Healy, J. (2000) *Health Care Systems in Transition: Tajikistan*. Copenhagen: European Observatory on Health Care Systems.

Sargaldakova, A., Healy, J., Kutzin, J. and Gedik, G. (2000) *Health Care Systems in Transition: Kyrgzstan*. Copenhagen: European Observatory on Health Care Systems.

Sari, N. and Langenbrunner, J.C. (2001) Consumer out-of-pocket spending for pharmaceuticals in Kazakhstan: implications for sectoral reform, *Health Policy and Planning*, 16(4): 428–34.

Savas, S., Gedik, G. and Craig, M. (2002) The reform process, in M. McKee, J. Healy and J. Falkingham (eds) *Health Care in Central Asia*. Buckingham: Open University Press.

Shkolnikov, V., McKee, M. and Leon, D.A. (2001) Changes in life expectancy in Russia in the mid-1990s, *Lancet*, 357: 917–21.

Skripachova, L. (2002) The pharmaceutical market of Uzbekistan: gradually about everything, *Kazakhstan Pharmaceutical Bulletin*, 2(150) (available from www.pharmnews.kz/Nomera150/ct0_eng.html) (accessed 9 December 2002).

Startseva, A. (2002) Fake drugs called a $250M business, *The Moscow Times*, 26 April.

Tacis (1999a) *The Country Profile of Kazakhstan*. Kiev: Ukraine-Tacis Enterprise Privatization and Restructuring Programme (available from www.delukr.cec.eu.int/data/vlib/020028/1/kazakhstan_profile.pdf) (accessed 9 December 2002).

Tacis (1999b) *The Country Profile of Ukraine*. Kiev: Ukraine-Tacis Enterprise Privatization and Restructuring Programme (available from www.delukr.cec.eu.int/data/vlib/020028/1/ukraine_profile.pdf) (accessed 9 December 2002).

Tchernjavski, V. (1998) *Health Care Systems in Transition: Russian Federation*. Copenhagen: European Observatory on Health Care Systems.

Tragakes, E. and Lessof, S. (2003) *Health Care Systems in Transition: Russian Federation*. Copenhagen: European Observatory on Health Care Systems.

US Commercial Service (2001) *Kazakhstan: Comparative Analysis of Pharmaceutical Imports*. Almaty: US & Foreign Commercial Services and US Department of State (available from www.bisnis.doc.gov/bisnis/isa/011126KZPharm.htm) (accessed 9 December 2002).

Vlassov, V., Mansfield, P., Lexchin, J. and Vlassova, A. (2001) Do drug advertisements in Russian medical journals provide essential information for safe prescribing?, *Western Journal of Medicine*, 174(6): 391–4.

World Bank (2000a) *Procurement of Health Sector Goods: Technical Note*. Washington, DC: World Bank.

World Bank (2000b) *Ukraine – TB & AIDS Control Project*. Project Implementation Document No. 9329. Washington, DC: World Bank.

World Bank (2002a) *Transition: The First Ten Years*. Washington, DC: World Bank.

World Bank (2002b) *Uzbekistan Living Standards Assessment: Health, Nutrition and Population*. Washington, DC: World Bank.

World Bank (2002c) *Improving Transparency in Pharmaceutical Systems: Strengthening Critical Decision Points Against Corruption*. Washington, DC: World Bank.

World Health Organization (1999a) *Drug Polis: Drug Reimbursement Pilot System, Kutaisi, Georgia: 1998 Annual Report*. Geneva: WHO.

World Health Organization (1999b) *Operational Principles for Good Pharmaceutical Procurement*. Geneva: WHO.

World Health Organization (2001) *Network for Monitoring the Impact of TRIPS and Globalization on Access to Medicines*. Geneva: WHO.

World Health Organization (2002a) *World Health Report*. Geneva: WHO.

World Health Organization (2002b) *Health for All Database*. http://hfadb.who.dk/hfa/) (accessed 4 December 2002).

twenty-one

A framework for containing costs fairly

Donald W. Light and Tom Walley

Introduction

This book describes how medicines are regulated across Europe, including government attempts to contain costs. To conclude, we feel it appropriate to consider an ethical framework within which governments can achieve their aims of ensuring access to medicines for their citizens at an affordable cost, while at the same time encouraging innovation and the development of new more effective and cost-effective medicines.

Most European countries have established universal health care systems that try to provide good medical services in cost-effective and equitable ways. From a global perspective, they are very successful in this, but many countries feel that these systems are under threat by rising costs, especially pharmaceutical costs. In response, governments have tried various ways to hold down costs. The term 'priority setting' perhaps describes the situation better than simple cost containment – one hopes that the responsible policy makers accept the need to choose between options for spending in some rational way to maintain or improve public health, and feel the need for fairness is a key concern (Tauber 2003). Some might equate 'priority setting' with 'rationing', but others consider rationing to include the complete denial of clinically needed services, which might not be necessary if priorities are clearly established. To avoid confusion, we have used the term priority setting throughout this chapter.

One could argue that any form of limitation on spending on health cannot have an ethical basis as long as we appear able to find funding for armies or projects to enhance national prestige, or that this whole question in a European context is trivial by comparison with questions of access to medicines in developing countries, or global price setting for HIV drugs. Nevertheless, the concern of this book is regulation of medicines in Europe, and cost containment in Europe: the reality is that this cost containment is happening now, so this chapter considers an ethical framework for how governments might achieve their varied and partly contradictory aims. On the way, we comment on the ethical concerns that arise from the different current approaches to this problem, analysed in detail in other chapters.

A whole book could be written on the ethics of pharmaceutical policy. Within the confines of a short chapter, it seems most useful to policy makers and professionals to offer a general ethical framework for how to prioritize resources for drug spending, and use that framework to assess current practices and issues raised in this book, and to identify policy priorities.

Accountable priority setting

Given the need to limit resources for drug therapy, how can it be done fairly? The moral dilemma here is that the needs of the individual are sometimes pitted against the needs of society as whole, and when these clash the prioritization that results is value-laden. Unfortunately, there is no consensus on which priorities should prevail. In the absence of such consensus, setting limits in an arbitrary or unilateral manner can undermine trust and the legitimacy of the health care system. Political parties and policy leaders are usually unwilling to take the heat for priority setting or rationing; so they try to disguise them. But the behind-closed doors paternalism of implicit prioritization, widely used in previous decades, no longer works so well in this era of patient advocacy groups, access to extensive information through the web and pro-active patients.

One solution, suggested by a philosopher and a doctor, concludes that the only way to set limits, contain costs or set priorities is by using open and fair procedures; so that whatever the decisions made, they are based on public, transparent deliberations and on full and relevant information, with fair procedures for revision and appeal (Daniels and Sabin 2002). While some implicit rationing will always take place, the argument here is that general and major priority setting should always be made explicitly in a publicly accountable way. Setting priorities therefore requires five conditions:

1 Decisions must be made publicly after sustained public debate based on as full and accurate information as possible.
2 Participants must endeavour to cooperate in finding mutually agreeable ways to hold costs down and work towards acceptable reasons for their choices.
3 Mechanisms must be provided for appealing, revising or improving the decisions made.
4 Past decisions, evidence and rationales should be used as a basis for deciding new cases to provide continuity, when relevant.
5 Processes must be put into action to ensure that conditions 1–4 are carried out.

Daniels and Sabin add that 'consumer participation' is not enough, unless attention is given to how representative the consumers are and how wide a spectrum of concerns are represented. The legitimacy of this approach is achieved by listening to and working through the concerns and objections of parties, which in health care can range dramatically.

For example, the UK National Institute for Clinical Excellence (NICE) considers clinical evidence but also has a process of formally consulting professional and patient groups and providing opportunity for the public to express views, before coming to a decision about whether a new technology should be funded in the UK National Health Service. There is also an appeals process, and NICE guidance is intended to be updated regularly. This process is far from perfect, and can even be undermined by government itself, as recent examples show (Walley 2004) but nevertheless it shows a willingness to set priorities within the type of framework proposed by Daniels and Sabin.

The National Institute for Clinical Excellence was set up to resolve problems of the previous system for rationing care, in which fragmented and often illogical and purely cost-driven decisions were made by local authorities ('post code prescribing'). These decisions often undermined the unity of a national health service, created uncertainty and dissatisfaction among patients, and led to many legal challenges. NICE illustrates well why such a fair and accountable procedure is better than many commonly used alternatives.

Two forms of irrational priority setting

An alternative is to allow priorities to be set by the market, as perhaps happens in the USA. Those who can and choose to pay can opt out of public priority setting. This is true in Europe also, where levels of private health insurance range from approximately 10 per cent of the population in the UK to over 50 per cent in Ireland. European nations, however, prize solidarity as well as public health and have created universal access to medical services and drug therapies as an alternative paradigm to the marketplace for serving the best interests of patients. Beneficial price competition in health care is difficult to achieve because health care markets do not meet most of the requirements envisioned by Adam Smith and his many intellectual descendents: full and free information about quality, performance and price; clear definitions of what one is buying beforehand; clear preferences that get exercised in the market; no externalities; many buyers; many sellers; easy entry; and easy exit. Health markets often have none of these (Light 1994; Rice 2003). Furthermore, uncertainties prevail and the distribution of risk is highly skewed towards the 2 per cent of any population that require about 40 per cent of all resources to be treated. Such markets lead not to beneficial but to *pernicious* competition, in which sellers exploit payers, patients and the market itself. As a rationing method, markets 'decide' that services and drugs are allocated to those who have better information, stronger networks and more money. Even when used within a system of universal access, markets favour powerful and wealthy individuals and institutions – in health care, the source of the inverse care law, whereby those who need health care least paradoxically have best access to it (Tudor Hart 2000). Setting priorities by market, therefore, meets none of the conditions defined by Daniels and Sabin, and it is perhaps a source of concern that in their rush to achieve efficiency, so many governments (e.g. UK, the Netherlands) seem to feel that some form of market approach to health care is the most appropriate.

Another alternative approach is implicit or paternalistic prioritization – Daddy (government ministers, chief executives, elite specialists or even your personal physician) knows what's best for you, or for a hospital, a community or a region. Some forms of paternalism are delegated, as when a budget is set and then clinicians must decide how to live within that budget. In this setting, individuals chosen for their technical expertise, or moral standing or by some other criteria act in what they perceive to be the best interests of the patient. This form of priority setting has always been around and will persist in the future, but in an era when authority is constantly challenged, when information is much more widely available, this is less and less acceptable to the public.

However, recent surveys suggest that, in the UK at least, some form of such implicit priority setting, implemented by doctors but not by politicians or bureaucrats, was seen as acceptable by three-quarters of those surveyed (King and Maynard 1999). Some argue that paternalism and implicit priority setting is superior to a more open approach, in part because an explicit approach will be controversial and difficult (Klein 1995; Mechanic 1997). An example in this book is the view that health technology assessment is ineffective because few politicians/decision makers are willing to say 'no' to a new technology in public. So implicit priority setting may be 'better' or easier for leaders of health care systems, or corporations, or patient care than explicit priority setting with its candid debate, controversy and possibility to lose votes. But ethically, it lacks principles, accountability or fairness, and Daniels and Sabin describe it as more troubling than explicit priority setting for these reasons.

Health economics or evidence-based medicine as a basis for priority setting

An increasingly common feature of explicit priority setting is the study of cost-effectiveness of drug therapies (Chapter 7). Economists develop outcome measures, calculate the cost–outcome ratios, and recommend resource allocation so as to provide the greatest benefit to the greatest number of people. But this, too, has its flaws (Freemantle and Maynard 1994). It is highly subject to technical manipulation by global corporations or governments of how 'benefits' and 'costs' are modelled and measured (almost all industry submissions to NICE cost £30,000 per quality adjusted life year, the unspoken limit that NICE is said to use – independent assessments are often wildly different (Raftery 2001)). The necessary information to conduct the evaluation may not be available. Cost-effectiveness studies may expose underfunding of the service and take no account of affordability within the health service. They cannot take account of all of the opportunity costs across all the services offered. It assumes that outcomes are the same for rather different kinds of patients with rather different life circumstances and values. Using trade-off studies to measure values has problems too. The results can impose the priorities and interests of those paying for the research, or those sampled to measure the priorities of everyone else. Daniels and Sabin (2002) review the morally troubling problems of this approach.

These problems are well known to policy makers, so although many reimbursement agencies ask for such studies, much of the time it is not clear how they are used, if at all. In Europe, the most advanced in using these studies is probably the UK's NICE: it examines the evidence of effectiveness and economic evaluations, but then undertakes an appraisal (i.e. the application of judgement) of these and other elements like public health need, social implications and public views before making its decision. This move away from apparent objectivity may seem unsatisfactory and almost a return to implicit priority setting by experts, but the methods of an explicit approach are also still underdeveloped. Although economic evaluation is technically weak, it provides useful information for stakeholders to debate, in an approach that Daniels and Sabin might approve.

Similar arguments could be made about priority setting by another approach, evidence-based medicine – that is, the view that only interventions of proven effectiveness should be provided by the health service and, conversely, that the health service should provide all interventions of proven effectiveness to everyone. This approach is rejected by Maynard (1999) on several grounds: the error of funding any intervention no matter how much it costs or how little added benefit it may bring; failure to consider affordability; inequity of distribution of resources that might result; and the undermining of patient autonomy. Evidence is necessary but not sufficient for ethical priority setting.

This briefly summarizes why an open, fair and accountable (but not rigidly defined by, for instance, economic evaluation or evidence-based medicine) set of procedures is superior to most forms of priority setting in most of Europe today. Some have looked at the UK model and proposed a Euro-NICE, but this is unlikely to develop. Nevertheless, these procedures need to be the focus of policy change in how prescription drugs are tested, approved, priced, reimbursed and listed. Authors in several of the chapters bemoan the lack of good information and open deliberation in each of these realms. Some, like McGuire *et al.* (Chapter 7), complain that public decisions become ossified and not evaluated or reviewed as circumstances change – flexibility is a key feature of the model recommended by Daniels and Sabin.

The best interests of patients

One basic starting point that might help guide deliberations on priorities is to place the best interests of patients above other goals, such as industrial growth. This title covers both the best interests of the individual patient and of the community as a whole – these are actually interdependent and complementary rather than in opposition, as the best interests of the individual are often best served by meeting the needs of the population (Tauber 2003). 'The best interests of patients' has the advantage of being embraced by major pharmaceutical firms, by politicians, by health plans, by clinicians and by patients themselves. 'The best interests of patients' is, however, a vague term that requires definition; perhaps its acceptability to so many stakeholders is precisely because of its vagueness. It can be interpreted to embody the four classic principles of medical ethics (National Commission for the Protection of Human Subjects of Biomedical and Behavioral Research 1978). One such principle is beneficence: persons are to be treated so as to maximize possible benefits both in the short and long term. A second is the just distribution among equals, not to impose a burden unduly or deny a benefit without good reason to the most disadvantaged. The key sticking point is the potential clash between giving priority to individual patients whose treatment is costly versus giving priority to the many who may benefit from an inexpensive medicine or vaccine. Good systems identify such dilemmas and try to negotiate a balance. In particular, the 1978 report noted that 'whenever research supported by public funds leads to the development of therapeutic devices and procedures, justice demands that these not provide advantages only to those who can afford them'. These principles require an assessment of risks and harms using 'a careful array of relevant data'.

Both of these principles must be applied while respecting the other two principles: the participants' autonomy must be promoted, and policy makers should also observe the principle of non-maleficence, which dictates that their policies should not harm those they affect. Setting priorities might be seen to offend against both of these – we are constraining the individual's right to access treatments as he or she wishes, and the individual may suffer harm as a result. Tauber (2003) argues that autonomy has less to do with individual freedom but more properly to do with respect for the rights of others and therefore places a premium on the cooperative nature of morality from which justice must be derived. This emphasis supports Daniels and Sabin's cooperative approach to setting limits so as to respect the autonomy of all.

Ethics and prescribing

The purpose of the regulation of prescribing is to allow the use of beneficial but often expensive and dangerous substances for the best interests of both individual patients and populations of patients. As Daniels and Sabin (2002) put it, 'public health is the final aim of medicinal products'. This has important implications. For example, it follows that in 'the widely-recognised clash between healthcare and industrial policy priorities' (Permanand and Altenstetter, Chapter 2), policies aimed at expanding the industry, the number of people it employs and its revenues, should be subordinate to the best interests of patients. It would seem perverse if the whole object of a pharmaceutical industry were industrial growth rather than improvement in health. On the other hand, one cannot totally ignore the benefits to the economies of many European countries such as the UK, Ireland or Germany, of large pharmaceutical industries in terms of generating wealth and employment – themselves factors that indirectly but powerfully promote health. Nevertheless, the best interests of patients (rather than shareholders) lead us to focus on prescribing affordable and effective drugs for disorders on which they have been tested, and on encouraging innovation aimed at finding better drugs than presently exist.

No more secrecy

Let us now turn to applying this ethical framework to European practices and policies discussed in this book. One pervasive obstacle to fair and informed efforts to compare the values of different drugs is the secrecy and the lack of data in the pubic domain about the safety, efficacy and costs of drugs. Both governments and companies contribute to high levels of secrecy, though recent efforts towards transparency have made some difference (see Chapter 4) and in general the European Medicines Evaluation Agency (EMEA) has done better than national agencies in Europe, though still far behind its US counterpart, the Food and Drug Administration (FDA). Garattini and Bertele' (Chapter 4), however, are critical of the secrecy that characterizes the EMEA, as are Abraham and Lewis (1998). The European Public Assessment Report provides some, but only limited, information, and access to the data submitted by companies to the EMEA or to national agencies would be desirable, and allow independent scrutiny of the process.

The principal justification for this secrecy is that information on safety and efficacy are 'proprietary'; but in the Daniels and Sabin model, this seems indefensible. Industries that serve vital needs of humankind cannot reasonably claim that results of clinical trials for safety and efficacy should not be universally available. There is a long, well-documented history of companies hiding or lying about damaging evidence, from the 1950s to 2003 (Stolberg 2002; Boseley 2003; Hilts 2003). Here we have a clear ethical choice about ending secrecy: do clinical and patient concerns take precedence over sales and profits or visa versa?

Thus, even in the event of extensive adverse reactions to a drug, patients 'may not be able to gain access to information they need about the product's safety'. An end to secrecy would probably reveal, as it has in the USA:

- trade-offs between safety and the rush to market as conflicting priorities, such as shortcuts in trial design, testing and safety (Office of Inspector General 2003);
- conflicts of interests embedded in pharmaceutical corporations paying the regulatory agencies and their reviewers (Stolberg 2002);
- low priority given to the principal concern of patients compared with the commercial needs of a manufacturer: how much better is this new drug than the best existing ones? Why have patients been put at risk by being exposed to a new chemical entity when, at the end of the day, there may be no therapeutic gain to patients, but only a commercial gain to a company?

There are also concerns about regulatory capture in the USA (i.e. the regulator coming to serve the industry rather than the public) (Moynihan 2002). Because of the lack of transparency, it is impossible to say whether this is a factor or to what extent it exists within the EMEA, but Garattini and Bertele' give enough cause for concern, even just by describing the composition of key EMEA committees; Daniels and Sabin rightly emphasize that the composition as well as the procedures of such bodies should reflect the goal of serving patients and the public.

If licensing decisions are opaque, decisions about drug pricing and around what to reimburse are even worse. These are in the hands of national agencies or social insurance companies on the one hand, and the companies themselves on the other. Governments are unwilling to allow market forces free rein in the drug market, and either control prices or profits or have some volume/price mix in their negotiations with suppliers. In the past, companies often demanded and received 'premium prices for premium products' (e.g. Glaxo's ranitidine was more expensive but had only very limited advantages over Smith Kline French's cimetidine). Indeed, achieving a premium price was seen as a marker of the new drug's superiority, as if prices were decided on the basis of the actual value of drug. One could also argue that capturing a large market share was also proof of the superiority of the drug, but as we have seen, health care is not a perfect market and there are too many examples of where neither market share nor price were justified by clinical superiority but only perhaps by marketing superiority.

In terms of pricing, things have improved in this regard, in at least some markets: companies with 'me-too' products can increasingly only secure a market share by charging a lower price or by offering some added value to the provider: this, and heavy marketing, has for instance secured the statin atorvastatin huge sales, second only to simvastatin – and despite the fact that until recently there was no evidence that atorvastatin could reduce mortality while the evidence for simvastatin was well established (Walley *et al*. 2004). Countries may encourage this either covertly or more openly: it allows them to secure access to the drug for their citizens at a more affordable price.

But these decisions, often in closed rooms, may undermine any attempts to manage local drug budgets (Walley *et al*. 2000) and there are discontinuities in public policies at a local and a national level. There is no easy or right way to decide reimbursement – but establishing transparent principles, such as rewarding useful innovation (using accurate data on net costs to corporations after allowing for public contributions or tax credits) and pricing so as to ensure public access to medicines (i.e. affordability), are important elements of this. Economic evaluation may have a role to play here.

Ethics of incentives

Turning to financial incentives, Walley and Mossialos (Chapter 10) emphasize how infrequently and incompletely the effects of incentives and disincentives to doctors and pharmacists on patient outcomes are measured. Furthermore, these incentives are often not disclosed to the patients who entrust their care to these providers. In their meticulous review of studies to measure the outcomes of various administrative measures to contain costs (all designed and applied behind closed doors and without patient consent), Kanavos *et al*. (Chapter 5) find most are poorly done, an issue analogous to questions about the methods and samples of clinical trials or cost-effectiveness studies. Most also reflect the USA, with its more fragmented and incomplete systems of provision of health care, more than Europe, with its more universalist approaches. This raises a related issue that is helped by having a fair process for deciding what and how to set priorities – that money should be put aside to specifically evaluate the effects of changing systems such as reimbursement or co-payments or physician incentives.

New drugs

Prescription drugs are vital tools in modern medicine, saving lives, relieving pain, curing illnesses and restoring patients to self-sufficiency. Thanks to several branches of biomedical research and to the pharmaceutical industry, major advances are made every few years. But we must not be blinded to the fact that many new drugs provide little added benefit over existing ones, even though they often cost much more (Mason and Freemantle 1998; see Chapter 8). New drugs are a particular challenge to ethical setting of priorities, and hence a particular focus for bodies like NICE.

A detailed study by a clinical team at Prescrire found that only 0.3 per cent of the 2693 new drugs approved and patented over the past 22 years provide a major therapeutic advance, and 2.7 per cent provide important therapeutic benefits with certain limitations (Prescrire International 2003). Another 7.9 per cent have some therapeutic value 'but do not fundamentally change the present therapeutic practice', and 16.0 per cent provide 'minimal additional value and should not change prescribing habits'. The rest (1584 of all new drugs) are therapeutically 'superfluous', and a few pose real disadvantages without evident benefit. These conclusions are similar to those of the US FDA in the past, although manufacturers would no doubt take issue with such descriptions of their products. To try to sell a drug with little or no clinical advantage over its competitors, the manufacturers resort to heavy marketing or low pricing to secure a share – the less the differentiation, the greater the marketing. This is often successful and as described in Chapter 1, one of the major drivers of drug costs in Europe is the change in product mix, as new drugs displace old, often for no valid medical reason. In theory, careful economic evaluation of new drugs should expose this as poor value. But what then? Will governments refuse to fund them? In practice, the efforts to contain costs described in this book, such as reimbursement lists, pricing schemes, user fees and incentives to doctors and pharmacists, are balanced against incentives for national industries which reward largely me-too 'innovation'. Governments are thus often reluctant to refuse access to a new therapy.

This is a larger view of the value of pharmaceuticals, to encompass not just the value of the individual drug but the value of the industry as a whole. This larger view will not be addressed here but needs to be noted, because it is the context in which efforts at cost containment or rationing of drug costs take place and suggests there are other, perhaps more ethical, ways to restrain costs. Again, this valuing of industry need not be of itself unethical, but it should be transparent.

Finally, some attempts have been made in the Netherlands to actively use ethics in drug resource allocation decisions, as discussed in Chapter 17. Walley argues for the appropriateness of such an approach but acknowledges that the advantages of involving ethics in this process may at first seem modest, and can even have adverse effects, such as misinterpretation of ethical analysis, for example concerning autonomy (Fijn *et al.* 2002a,b).

To summarize this section, regulating the cost and use of pharmaceuticals, especially in a system that rewards producing a large number of new drugs of limited value by allowing them high prices, involves difficult decisions. Getting these wrong may waste money, limit access to beneficial treatments, or may introduce perverse incentives. All parties involved need to become part of policy and evaluation boards that make such decisions, based on full information and the five features of a just system for making tough choices.

Penalizing the victim

Patient co-payments are a common way in which governments try to restrain the use and cost of drugs (Chapter 13), but just as clearly they penalize patients and undermine the basic ethics on which universal health care systems are based. Such systems have generally decided in the interests of public health and social solidarity that taxing the sick for seeking health care is wrong. Yet many national systems feel it necessary to have some means of curbing demand. Fine points of ethics can be made about the relative merits of flat fees versus percentage fees versus tiered co-payments; but except perhaps for an initial deductible to dampen pressure for every new drug featured in the press, these payments hit hardest those who are most sick and least well off. To maintain social solidarity, most European countries have extensive exemptions from co-payments, which may detract from their value as a means of containing demand. Most of the empirical evidence indicates that co-payments have adverse effects, such as inhibiting utilization of both essential and non-essential drugs – patients may not be able to distinguish between the two (Lexchin and Grootendorst 2003). They may therefore undermine public health.

Can we depend on doctors to control inappropriate demand? A critical part of clinical work is to learn how to handle a range of patients with uninformed expectations or demands in ways that make them more realistic self-clinicians about their problems. Developing this capacity is far better than the implicit model of giving patients whatever tests, procedures and drugs they demand but then charging them. Unfortunately, the view of the patient as a consumer as exemplified by the story of lifestyle drugs in Chapter 17 seems in the ascendant, and the ability of the doctor to curb this is limited. So it would appear that systems of co-payments or more restricted access to a narrower range of reimbursed medicines are likely to persist, but these too can be developed within the ethical framework outlined.

Ethics of off-patent and over-the-counter (OTC) drugs

In a fundamental way, Chapters 15 and 16 may be the most important for developing a just set of policies for drugs and so they deserve a concluding remark. The patent–generic–OTC continuum is undergoing dynamic change that started in the 1980s (Buono and Hartman 1985). Prescribed generics, by law, are as effective as the patented drugs on which they are based, but there are arguments against them that need to be acknowledged if only to be refuted. Governments are keen to promote generics, which, in turn, makes it more imperative for a company to maximize its profits as early in a product's life as possible, before it can be eroded. This will intensify arguments about pricing and marketing, but should also increase pressure on manufacturers to prove the added value of new drugs (or, conversely, to develop only drugs with added value).

Governments are pushing for more drugs gaining OTC status, in order to save money and to promote consumer choice as well as price competition (Rubin 2003). Companies push for OTC status as a product nears the end of its patent life and starts to face generic competitors, so as to enlarge the market and perhaps maintain brand loyalty. In practice, this does not save large amounts of money for governments, and if the policy in some countries is to stop reimbursing a drug once it goes over the counter, overall drug costs could rise as doctors and patients switch to a more expensive, still prescription-only drug.

The major pharmaceutical firms have worked with governments for decades to structure national markets around patented brand drugs that enable them to charge high prices and reap large profits. If the goal is to benefit the greatest number of patients within a limited budget in which spending more for drugs leaves less for other valued services, then governments need to re-think from the ground up the patented–generic–OTC continuum. Should pharmaceutical policies be centred on maximizing the number of patented drugs, as they are now, even though most are judged to offer little additional benefit? Or should the rewards for innovation be structured to reward real advances and should patents be regarded as a transient state on the road to price competition among generics as the central policy goal? The tactics used by pharmaceutical firms first to stall generic competitors and then to bump drugs over to OTC status indicate that the rules and incentives of the pharmaceutical system need to be re-examined and adjusted to be aligned with what is best for patients and the health care system.

Conclusions

We have tried to define a framework for setting priorities in an accountable and open way. Present systems often fall far below this standard, but there are signs of hope in some countries. Interventions to contain costs by setting priorities are inevitable, but require careful monitoring and evaluation in case there are perverse and unintended outcomes. Health economics can be a useful adjunct to evaluating drug therapies to allow ethical priority setting, but should not be allowed to become the sole arbiter. We have to be aware that the various kinds of efforts to contain the costs of prescription drugs are made in the context of an underlying set of regulations that have encouraged and produced a large proportion of new drugs with patent protection and high prices to replace older and cheaper drugs of similar benefit. So this is a complex and contentious area – and no doubt will be the subject of many more chapters and books!

References

Abraham, J. and Lewis, G. (1998) Secrecy and transparency of medicines licensing in the EU, *Lancet*, 352: 480–2.

Boseley, S. (2003) Drug review halted over company links, *The Guardian*, 26 March.

Buono, L. and Hartman, J.P. (1985) Hybrids: the new OTC option, *Pharmaceutical Executive*, 5: 46–8.

Daniels, N. and Sabin, J.E. (2002) *Setting Limits Fairly? Can We Learn to Share Medical Resources?* New York: Oxford University Press.

Fijn, R., van Epenhuysen, L.S., Peijnenburg, A.J., de Jong-van den Berg, L.T. and Brouwers, J.R. (2002a) Introducing ethics in hospital drug resource allocation decisions: keep expectations modest and beware of unintended effects. Part I: An explorative overview, *Pharmacoepidemiology and Drug Safety*, 11: 523–7.

Fijn, R., van Epenhuysen, L.S., Peijnenburg, A.J., de Jong-van den Berg, L.T. and Brouwers, J.R. (2002b) Introducing ethics in hospital drug resource allocation decisions: keep expectations modest and beware of unintended effects. Part II: The use of ethics. *Pharmacoepidemiology and Drug Safety*, 11: 617–20.

Freemantle, N. and Maynard, A. (1994) Something rotten in the state of clinical and economic evaluations?, *Health Economics*, 3(2): 63–7.

Hilts, P.J. (2003) *Protecting America's Health: The FDA, Business and One Hundred Years of Regulation*. New York: Alfred A. Knopf.

King, D. and Maynard, A. (1999) Public opinion and rationing in the United Kingdom, *Health Policy*, 50: 39–53.

Klein, R. (1995) Priorities and rationing: pragmatism or principles?, *British Medical Journal*, 311: 761–2.

Lexchin, J. and Grootendorst, P. (2003) The effects of prescription drug user fees on drug and health services use and health status in vulnerable populations: a systematic review of the evidence. Unpublished manuscript.

Light, D.W. (1994) Escaping the traps of postwar Western medicine, *European Journal of Public Health*, 3: 281–9.

Mason, J. and Freemantle, N. (1998) The dilemma of new drugs: are costs rising faster than effectiveness?, *Pharmacoeconomics*, 13: 653–7.

Maynard, A. (1999) Evidence-based medicine: an incomplete method for informing treatment choices, *Lancet*, 349: 126–8.

Mechanic, D. (1997) Muddling through elegantly: finding the proper balance in rationing, *Health Affairs*, 16: 83–92.

Moynihan, R. (2002) Alosetron: a case study in regulatory capture, or a victory for patients' rights?, *British Medical Journal*, 325: 592–5.

National Commission for the Protection of Human Subjects of Biomedical and Behavioral Research (1978) *The Belmont Report: Ethical Guidelines for the Protection of Human Subjects*. Washington, DC: US Government Printing Office.

Office of Inspector General (2003) *FDA's Review Process for New Drug Applications: A Management Review*. Washington, DC: Office of Inspector General.

Prescrire International (2003) A review of new drugs and indications in 2002: financial speculation or better patient care?, *Prescrire International*, 12: 74–7.

Raftery, J. (2001) NICE: faster access to modern treatments? Analysis of guidance on health technologies, *British Medical Journal*, 323: 1300–3.

Rice, T. (2003) *The Economics of Health Care Reconsidered*. Chicago, IL: Health Administration Press.

Rubin, R. (2003) FDA seeks to switch to over-counter, *USA Today*, 23 April, p. A1.

Stolberg, S.G. (2002) Study says clinical guides often hide ties of doctors, *New York Times*, 6 February.

Tauber A. (2003) A philosophical approach to rationing, *Medical Journal of Australia*, 178: 454–6.

Tudor Hart, J. (2000) Three decades of the inverse care law, *British Medical Journal*, 320: 18–19.

Walley, T. (2004) Prescribing of neuropsychotherapeutics in the UK: what has been the impact of NICE?, *CNS Drugs*, 18: 1–12.

Walley, T., Earl-Slater, A., Haycox, A. and Bagust, A. (2000) An integrated national pharmaceutical policy for the UK?, *British Medical Journal*, 321: 1523–6.

Walley, T., Folino-Gallo, P., Schwabe, U. and Van Ganse, E. (2004) Variation and increase in use of statins across Europe: data from administrative databases, *British Medical Journal*, 328: 385–6.

Index

Page numbers in *italics* refer to tables and boxes, those in **bold** denote main discussions. Chapter notes are indicated by *n/ns*.